HANDBOOK OF
CLINICAL
ANESTHESIA

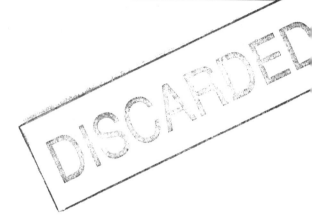

HANDBOOK OF
CLINICAL
ANESTHESIA

Second Edition

Paul G. Barash, M.D.
Professor and Chairman, Department of Anesthesiology
Associate Dean for Clinical Affairs
Yale University School of Medicine
Chief, Department of Anesthesiology
Yale–New Haven Hospital
New Haven, Connecticut

Bruce F. Cullen, M.D.
Professor
University of Washington School of Medicine
Anesthesiologist-in-Chief, Department of Anesthesiology
Harborview Medical Center
Seattle, Washington

Robert K. Stoelting, M.D.
Professor and Chairman, Department of Anesthesia
Indiana University School of Medicine
Indianapolis, Indiana

J. B. LIPPINCOTT COMPANY   Philadelphia

Acquisitions Editor: Mary K. Smith
Assistant Editor: Anne Geyer
Indexer: Maria Coughlin
Interior Designer: Susan Blaker
Senior Production Editor: Virginia Barishek
Production: P. M. Gordon Associates
Compositor: Compset, Inc.
Printer/Binder: R. R. Donnelley & Sons

Second Edition

6 5 4 3 2

Specific acknowledgments for reprinted material appear on
pages 617–618.

Library of Congress Cataloging-in-Publication Data
Handbook of clinical anesthesia / Paul G. Barash,
 Bruce F. Cullen, Robert K. Stoelting.—2nd ed.
   p.   cm.
   To accompany: Clinical anesthesia / edited by Paul G.
Barash, Bruce F. Cullen, Robert K. Stoelting. c1992.
   Includes index.
   ISBN 0–397–51297–X
   1. Anesthesiology—Handbooks, manuals, etc.
2. Anesthesia—Handbooks, manuals, etc.   I. Barash, Paul
G. II. Cullen, Bruce F.   III. Stoelting, Robert K.
IV. Clinical anesthesia.
   [DNLM: 1. Anesthesiology—handbooks.   WO 231 H236]
RD81.C58 1992 Suppl.
617.9′6—dc20
DNLM/DLC
for Library of Congress   92–49256
                                                          CIP

The authors and publisher have exerted every effort to ensure
that drug selection and dosage set forth in this text are in
accord with current recommendations and practice at the
time of publication. However, in view of ongoing research,
changes in government regulations, and the constant flow of
information relating to drug therapy and drug reactions, the
reader is urged to check the package insert for each drug for
any change in indications and dosage and for added warnings
and precautions. This is particularly important when the
recommended agent is a new or infrequently employed drug.

PREFACE

In the continuum of anesthesia education, the anesthesia practitioner or trainee may be overwhelmed by the volume of information that is required to manage patients. We designed the *Handbook of Clinical Anesthesia* to serve as a succinct guide for approaching both common and uncommon clinical problems and thus to help make this passage easier. It must be emphatically stated that the *Handbook* is not intended to replace a full-scale textbook; rather, the *Handbook* can serve as an extension of the textbook *Clinical Anesthesia,* as a "bridge" to the in-depth information that is needed for superb clinical care. We are proud of the enthusiastic reception that the first edition of both *Clinical Anesthesia* and the *Handbook of Clinical Anesthesia* received and feel that this indicates that we accomplished our goals.

Because we have extensively revised the textbook of *Clinical Anesthesia* (Second Edition), a new edition of the *Handbook* was mandated. Each chapter in the *Handbook* is referenced to the appropriate chapters in *Clinical Anesthesia* (Second Edition). Because the *Handbook* is desired for rapid acquisition of essential information, we have made extensive use of tables to facilitate rapid prioritization and understanding of crucial points pertaining to each clinical problem.

The *Handbook* comprises two major sections. The first section, the text, takes the reader in a systematic fashion through the perioperative period, including preoperative evaluation, intraoperative management, and anesthesia subspecialties, as well as postoperative care. In the Second Edition, a number of new chapters have been added, including cancer therapy and its anesthetic implications, anesthesia for organ transplantation, anesthesia for nonoperating room procedures, and management of acute postoperative pain. The second section, the appendixes, contains formulas, an ECG atlas, a drug list, and emergency protocols that will be useful for the practitioner as well as the trainee. With the kind permission of the American Heart Association, we have reproduced here the relevant Advanced Cardiac Life Support protocols pertinent to adult, pediatric, and neonatal resuscitation.

We would like to acknowledge the contributors of the textbook *Clinical Anesthesia*. Although the *Handbook of Clinical Anesthesia* is the product of the editors, its chapters were developed from the expert knowledge contained in the work of the original contributors, reorganized and rewritten in a style necessary for a text of this scope. We also would like to thank our secretaries, Gail Norup, Karen Frymoyer, and Deanna Walker, whose continued help has been a source of support. As always, a special word of thanks is due to our colleagues at the J.B. Lippincott Company—Mary K. Smith, Editor; Anne Geyer, Assistant Editor; and Virginia Barishek, Senior Production Editor; and thanks also to Mary McDonald, Production Editor. Their constructive comments during the process of writing and editing this book continue to demonstrate their commitment to medical education.

Paul G. Barash, M.D.
Bruce F. Cullen, M.D.
Robert K. Stoelting, M.D.

The editors would like to acknowledge gratefully the efforts of the contributors to the second edition of the textbook *Clinical Anesthesia:*

Stephen E. Abram, M.D.
J. Jeff Andrews, M.D.
Jeffrey Askanazi, M.D.
Michael J. Avram, Ph.D.
Max T. Baker, Ph.D.
Steven J. Barker, Ph.D., M.D.
Audrée A. Bendo, M.D.
Arnold J. Berry, M.D.
Frederic A. Berry, M.D.
David R. Bevan, M.B.,
  M.R.C.P., F.F.A.R.C.S.
Morris Brown, M.D.
F. Peter Buckley, M.B.,
  F.F.A.R.C.S.
Rod K. Calverley, M.D.,
  F.R.C.P.(C)
Frederick W. Campbell, III,
  M.D.
Randall L. Carpenter, M.D.
Frederick W. Cheney, M.D.
Edmond Cohen, M.D.
D. Ryan Cook, M.D.
James E. Cottrell, M.D.
Benjamin G. Covino, M.D.*
Stephen F. Dierdorf, M.D.
François Donati, Ph.D., M.D.,
  F.R.C.P.C.
Jan Ehrenwerth, M.D.
John H. Eichhorn, M.D.
James B. Eisenkraft, M.D.
John E. Ellis, M.D.
Norig Ellison, M.D.
Robert Feinstein, M.D., Ph.D.
Richard H. Fine, M.D.
Mieczyslaw Finster, M.D.
Leonard Firestone, M.D.
Susan Firestone, M.D.
Jeffrey E. Fletcher, Ph.D.
Arthur S. Foreman, M.D.
Robert J. Fragen, M.D.
Simon Gelman, M.D., Ph.D.
Hugh C. Gilbert, M.D.
Bruce S. A. Gillies, M.S.,
  M.D.
George J. Graf, M.D.

J. David Haddox, D.D.S.,
  M.D.
Ronald A. Harrison, M.D.
John Hartung, Ph.D.
Robert J. Hudson, M.D.,
  F.R.C.P.C.
Cindy W. Hughes, M.D.
Anthony D. Ivankovich, M.D.
Ira S. Kass, Ph.D.
Jonathan D. Katz, M.D.
Hoshang J. Khambatta, M.D.
Harry G. G. Kingston, M.B.,
  B.Ch., F.F.A.R.C.S.
Donald A. Kroll, M.D., Ph.D.
Carol L. Lake, M.D.
Donald H. Lambert, M.D.,
  Ph.D.
C. Philip Larson Jr., M.D.
Noel W. Lawson, M.D.
Jerrold H. Levy, M.D.
Wen-Shin Liu, M.D.
Timothy R. Lubenow, M.D.
Philip D. Lumb, M.B., B.S.
David C. Mackey, M.D.
Tuula Manner, M.D., Ph.D.
John T. Martin, M.D.
Robert J. McCarthy, Pharm.D.
Kathryn E. McGoldrick, M.D.
Charles H. McLeskey, M.D.
Roger S. Mecca, M.D.
John R. Moyers, M.D.
Michael F. Mulroy, M.D.
Michael R. Murphy, M.D.
Steven Neustein, M.D.
William D. Owens, M.D.
Nathan Leon Pace, M.D.
Hilda Pedersen, M.B., C.L.B.,
  F.F.A.R.C.S.
Lawrence L. Priano, M.D.,
  Ph.D.
Donald S. Prough, M.D.
James J. Richter, M.D., Ph.D.
Christine S. Rinder, M.D.
Michael F. Roizen, M.D.
Stanley H. Rosenbaum, M.D.
Henry Rosenberg, M.D.
Alan C. Santos, M.D.

*Deceased.

Mark S. Scheller, M.D.

Alan Jay Schwartz, M.D., M.S. Ed.

David T. Seitman, M.D.

Björn Skeie, M.D.

Howard S. Smith, M.D.

Theodore C. Smith, M.D.

Linda C. Stehling, M.D.

Wendell C. Stevens, M.D.

M. Christine Stock, M.D.

Stephen J. Thomas, M.D.

Kevin K. Tremper, Ph.D., M.D.

Russell A. Van Dyke, Ph.D.

Jeffrey S. Vender, M.D., F.C.C.M.

Bernard V. Wetchler, M.D.

K. C. Wong, M.D., Ph.D.

Doreen L. Wray, M.D.

James R. Zaidan, M.D.

Gary P. Zaloga, M.D.

CONTENTS

IV
MANAGEMENT OF ANESTHESIA

V
POSTANESTHESIA AND
CONSULTANT PRACTICE

VI
APPENDIXES

I

PREPARING FOR ANESTHESIA

1

Evaluation of the Patient and Preoperative Preparation

Implementation of an anesthetic always begins with preoperative evaluation of the patient and development of an anesthetic plan (Larson CP Jr: Evaluation of the patient and preoperative preparation. In: Barash PG, Cullen BF, Stoelting RK [eds]: Clinical Anesthesia, pp 545–562. Philadelphia, JB Lippincott, 1992.) The time expended and the level of detail of the evaluation vary with many factors, including the nature and severity of the patient's illness and the complexity, urgency, and expected duration of the proposed operation. Today, many patients have their preoperative evaluation and planning done in a presurgical screening clinic or ambulatory surgical facility one or more days before the scheduled operation. The use of a detailed or **automated health questionnaire** that is completed by the patient prior to seeing the anesthesiologist may be helpful.

I. CHART REVIEW

A. Preoperative evaluation of a patient begins with a review of the patient's chart.

B. The relevant history, physical examination findings, and laboratory studies should be recorded in the chart and available for review.

C. Previous hospital admissions are reviewed, with special emphasis on prior anesthetic experiences (e.g., difficult tracheal intubation, poor venous access, postoperative jaundice, allergic reactions to drugs).

II. HISTORY AND PHYSICAL EXAMINATION

A. The extent of the history taking and the physical examination that the anesthesiologist must perform depends in large measure on what is available from the chart review.

B. A useful approach to the preoperative patient interview incorporates a standard format so that nothing is forgotten but emphasis is placed on the circumstances of the individual patient (Table 1-1).

C. **Drug evaluation.** The anesthesiologist needs to know what treatments and/or drugs have been used, and in the case of drugs, their dose, duration, and effectiveness (Table 1-2). With rare exceptions (drugs with anticoagulant effects), preoperative drug therapy should be continued throughout the perioperative period.

D. **Review of organ systems** (Tables 1-1 and 1-3)

1. **Circulatory system.** Most anesthesiologists begin with the circulatory system because cardiovascular problems are so common in surgical patients. The two major determinations to be made are whether the patient has **hypertension and/or ischemic heart disease, with or without heart failure.**

   a. The most widely accepted definition of hypertension is a systolic blood pressure >160 mm Hg and/or a diastolic blood pressure >95 mm Hg (Table 1-4).

TABLE 1-1. General Outline of a Preoperative Patient Interview

1. Discuss planned surgery
2. Current medical problems
3. Current medications
4. Tobacco or alcohol use
5. Recreational drug use
6. Drug allergies
7. Prior anesthetic history
8. General health (organ system review)
   a. Circulatory system (hypertension, heart disease, angina pectoris, exercise tolerance)
   b. Respiratory system (cough, sputum, stridor, asthma, upper respiratory tract infection)
   c. Central nervous system (headache, dizziness, visual disturbances, stroke, seizures)
   d. Hepatic system (jaundice, hepatitis)
   e. Renal system
   f. Gastrointestinal system (nausea, vomiting, reflux, diarrhea, weight change)
   g. Endocrine system (diabetes mellitus, thyroid dysfunction, pheochromocytoma)
   h. Hematologic system (excessive bleeding, anemia)
   i. Musculoskeletal system (back or joint pain, arthritis)
   j. Dental system (loose teeth, caps)
   k. Reproductive system (menstrual history)
   l. Obesity

TABLE 1-2. Management of Drug Therapy in Relation to Anesthesia

Drug	Anesthetic Implication
Aspirin	Bleeding tendency; consider discontinuing several weeks before elective surgery
Aminoglycoside antibiotics	Can cause skeletal muscle weakness and potentiate the response to nondepolarizing muscle relaxants
Coumarin anticoagulants	Occult bleeding may result in anemia; obtain coagulation screen before surgery
Lithium	May cause sodium loss and skeletal muscle weakness
Monoamine oxidase inhibitors	Increased catecholamine stores may be reflected by hypertensive responses when sympathomimetics are administered; prolonged depressant effects of drugs may be due to decreased metabolism
Tricyclic antidepressants	Response to sympathomimetics may be exaggerated with acute treatment; chronic treatment may result in decreased response
Insulin	Hypoglycemia is the most significant consideration; adjust usual dose downward
Oral hypoglycemics	Hypoglycemia a risk; medication may be omitted preoperatively
Antihypertensives	Possible impairment of normal compensatory circulatory responses; continue therapy throughout perioperative period
Chemotherapeutic drugs	Anemia, thrombocytopenia; pulmonary, cardiac, renal, or hepatic toxicity
Benzodiazepines	Tolerance to anesthetic drugs
Beta antagonists	Bradycardia and myocardial depression; continue therapy throughout perioperative period
Calcium channel blockers	Hypotension
Cardiac glycosides	Risk of digitalis toxicity and cardiac dysrhythmias, especially if serum potassium level is low; continue therapy throughout perioperative period, especially if being administered for heart rate control

(*continued*)

TABLE 1-2. Management of Drug Therapy in Relation to Anesthesia (*continued*)

Drug	Anesthetic Implication
Potassium-losing diuretics	Hypokalemia and hypochloremic metabolic alkalosis; potassium supplementation may be considered preoperatively
Aldosterone antagonists	Hyperkalemia
Corticosteroids	Possible suppression of the pituitary-adrenal axis; consider perioperative supplementation

    b. The major organs at risk in the hypertensive patient are the heart, brain, and kidneys (Table 1-5).

    c. Despite numerous studies of hypertension, what should be done preoperatively for the patient with untreated or uncontrolled hypertension remains controversial. If the decision is to proceed with the anesthetic and operation, the anesthesiologist must anticipate greater absolute intraoperative blood pressure increases and decreases in such patients.

    d. Whether patients who evidence myocardial ischemia preoperatively are at increased risk for postoperative myocardial complications remains controversial.

    e. The patient should be asked specific questions about **exercise tolerance** and whether it is limited by angina pectoris or dyspnea. If a patient can climb **two or more flights of stairs without stopping** because of angina pectoris or dyspnea, cardiac reserve is probably good.

    f. **Stable angina pectoris** is not a contraindication to anesthesia and surgery.

    g. Any evidence of **congestive heart failure** (orthopnea) is a reason to delay elective surgery until heart disease has been fully evaluated.

    h. The history of a **prior myocardial infarction** is often cited as a reason for delaying elective surgery for up to 6 months after the event.

2. Respiratory system. Preoperative evaluation of the respiratory system is important because respiratory malfunction is a major cause of postopera-

TABLE 1-3. Preoperative Physical Examination

Circulatory System

Auscultation of the heart to determine heart rate, rhythm, and presence of cardiac murmurs (aortic stenosis may be asymptomatic)

Blood pressure (supine versus standing position)

Peripheral pulses (especially if arterial cannulation is planned)

Veins for access

Peripheral edema

Skin color

Respiratory System

Auscultation for evidence of pulmonary edema or bronchospasm

Pattern of breathing and anatomy of thorax (emphysema)

Central Nervous System

Level of consciousness

Evidence of peripheral sensory or motor dysfunction

Hepatic System

Jaundice

Ascites

Tremor

Diabetes Mellitus

Orthostatic hypotension (reflects autonomic nervous system dysfunction and possible associated gastroparesis)

Hematologic System

Bruising

Petechiae

Musculoskeletal System

Examine sites of planned regional anesthesia

Hoarseness (laryngeal involvement from rheumatoid arthritis)

Dental System

Neck flexion

Mouth opening

Temporomandibular joint mobility

Uvula visible

Dentition

Distance from the lower border of the mandible to the prominence of the thyroid cartilage with the neck fully extended (<6 cm may be a predictor of difficult visualization of the glottic opening during direct laryngoscopy)

TABLE 1-4. Etiology of Hypertension

Primary (Idiopathic, Essential Hypertension)

Secondary Hypertension
    Renal disease
    Endocrine disease
        Pheochromocytoma
        Cushing's syndrome
        Primary aldosteronism
    Pregnancy-induced hypertension
    Mechanical (coarctation of the aorta)
    Neurogenic (increased intracranial pressure)

TABLE 1-5. Consequences of Untreated Hypertension

Heart
    Myocardial hypertrophy
    Decreased intravascular fluid volume
    Ischemic heart disease

Brain
    Rightward shift of the autoregulation curve
    Stroke

Kidneys
    Decreased renal blood flow and glomerular filtration rate
    Impaired sodium-conserving ability

---

tive morbidity. Postoperative pulmonary complications are particularly common in the elderly, the obese, patients with a history of smoking, and patients undergoing operations in the upper abdomen or thorax.

  a. Dyspnea is a particularly revealing symptom. If dyspnea is absent on moderate exertion, the anesthesiologist can be confident that pre-existing lung disease is nonexistent or so minor that it will not present any problems during the anesthesia.

  b. Stridor suggests partial upper airway obstruction, which must be investigated before proceeding with general anesthesia.

    c. The patient with a **cough or coryza** suggestive of an upper respiratory tract infection may be at increased risk for postoperative pneumonia, although there is no general agreement as to whether elective surgery should be delayed for this reason.

    d. Patients with **asthma that is in remission** do not need any special preoperative therapy.

3. Central Nervous System

    a. Patients with symptomatic central nervous system diseases present with a variety of symptoms, including headache, nausea, and vomiting (which may reflect increased intracranial pressure), seizures, or a history of prior stroke.

    b. Peripheral neuropathy (caused by diabetes mellitus or drug-induced) may deter the anesthesiologist from recommending regional anesthesia.

4. Hepatic system. A history of jaundice or alcohol abuse suggests the possibility of underlying liver disease.

5. Renal system. Patients with renal dysfunction generally present with mild disorders (cystitis or incontinence in females, difficulty in voiding due to prostatism in males) that may require the use of a bladder catheter in the postoperative period. Those with a history of chronic renal failure often require dialysis (hyperkalemia is a risk).

6. Gastrointestinal system. Preoperative evaluation of the gastrointestinal system includes questioning about the occurrence of nausea and vomiting with prior use of anesthetics (consider prophylactic antiemetics), history of heartburn suggestive of a hiatal hernia (consider prophylactic antacids or H_2 antagonists), and any change in body weight. A detailed discussion of recent solid food and liquid intake is routine.

7. Endocrine system. The endocrine diseases of concern in the preoperative period include diabetes mellitus, thyroid or parathyroid diseases, pheochromocytoma, and adrenal cortical dysfunction (Tables 1-6, 1-7, and 1-8) (see Chapter 30).

8. Hematologic system. The two major issues related to the hematologic system that are of concern preoperatively are the presence of anemia (i.e., etiology, chronic or acute, will patient benefit from a delay in surgery to increase the hematocrit?) and

(Text continues on pg 12)

TABLE 1-6. Clinical Types of Diabetes Mellitus

| | Type I
Insulin-Dependent | Type II
Noninsulin-Dependent |
|---|---|---|
| Age at onset | Childhood | Middle age to elderly |
| Timing of onset | Abrupt | Gradual |
| Predisposing factors | Genetic | Obesity, pregnancy |
| Islet beta cell mass | 90% loss | Mild to moderate decrease |
| Plasma insulin level | Minimal to absent | Normal, increased, decreased |
| Control | Exogenous insulin required | Diet, exercise, exogenous insulin |
| Ketoacidosis | Common | Rare |

TABLE 1-7. Clinical Manifestations of Thyroid and Parathyroid Diseases

	Hyperthyroidism	Hypothyroidism	Hyperparathyroidism
General	Weight loss Heat intolerance Warm, moist skin	Cold intolerance	Weight loss Polydipsia
Cardiovascular	Tachycardia Atrial fibrillation Congestive heart failure	Bradycardia Pericardial or pleural effusions Cardiomegaly Congestive heart failure	Hypertension Heart block
Neurologic	Nervousness Tremor Hyperactive reflexes	Slow mental function Minimal reflexes	Weakness Lethargy Headache Insomnia Depression
Musculoskeletal	Skeletal muscle weakness Bone resorption	Large tongue Amyloidosis	Bone pain Arthritis Pathologic fractures
Gastrointestinal	Diarrhea	Delayed gastric emptying	Anorexia Nausea and vomiting Constipation Epigastric pain
Hematologic	Anemia Thrombocytopenia		
Renal		Impaired free water clearance	Polyuria Hematuria

TABLE 1-8. Clinical Manifestations (Usually Paroxysmal) of Pheochromocytoma	
Symptoms	**Signs**
Headache	Hypertension
Diaphoresis	Orthostatic hypotension
Weight loss	Tachycardia
Nervousness	Cardiac dysrhythmias
Irritability	Myocarditis
Palpitations	Hypovolemia
	Polycythemia
	Hyperglycemia

any disorder of hemostasis (delay elective surgery until bleeding disorder is characterized).

9. **Musculoskeletal system.** Determination of the most comfortable joint position is useful preoperative information in the patient with degenerative arthritis (osteoarthritis).

10. **Dental system.** The dental history includes questioning the patient about the presence of loose teeth, false teeth, or bridges that are removable and capped teeth that might be injured during intubation of the trachea. In selected patients, it is permissible to leave false teeth in place, especially if a brief mask anesthesia is planned. If the patient has had prior general anesthesia, it is vital to ask about any history of difficulty with intubation of the trachea.

11. **Reproductive system.** It is important to inquire about the menstrual history of all females of childbearing age (it is generally recommended that all elective surgery be postponed until the second trimester of pregnancy).

III. LABORATORY TESTS

A. **Laboratory tests should be ordered when evidence in the history or physical examination suggests that an abnormality exists** (Tables 1-1 and 1-3). Routine ordering of a battery of tests on all patients is medically unjustified and costly.

B. The reasons for ordering specific tests and how the results will influence the perioperative anesthetic plan should be clear when the tests are ordered.

C. Although there is no clear consensus of opinion, it is common practice to obtain an electrocardiogram, chest x-ray, and a blood chemistry panel (electrolytes, creatinine/blood urea nitrogen, glucose) in patients over the age of 50 years if they are asymptomatic except for their surgical condition.

1. It is recognized that the yield of these tests in terms of identification of unsuspected disease is very small, but they do serve as a useful baseline in the event that the patient develops unexpected complications in the perioperative period.

2. Whether or not to proceed with anesthesia and surgery in the presence of an abnormal laboratory finding depends on the severity of the abnormality, whether it is likely to influence perioperative morbidity if uncorrected, and whether there is a reasonable chance that it can be corrected or improved preoperatively.

IV. CHOICE OF ANESTHETIC TECHNIQUE

A. The choice of anesthetic technique (general, regional, monitored anesthetic care) is based on the patient's physiologic status and planned operation as well as

---

TABLE 1-9. Risks of Anesthesia

Less Serious Risks
> Nausea and vomiting
> Bruising or superficial thrombophlebitis at the intravenous access site
> Sore throat
> Dental injury
> Corneal abrasion
> Headache

More Serious Risks
> Peripheral neuropathy (ulnar neuropathy most common)
> Cardiac dysrhythmias
> Myocardial infarction
> Atelectasis/pneumonia
> Renal or hepatic insufficiency
> Stroke
> Allergic drug reactions
> Malignant hyperthermia
> Blood reactions

Mortality

TABLE 1-10. American Society of Anesthesiologists' Physical Status Classification*

ASA 1	A normal healthy patient
ASA 2	A patient with mild systemic disease (mild diabetes mellitus, controlled hypertension, anemia, chronic bronchitis, morbid obesity)
ASA 3	A patient with severe systemic disease that limits activity (angina pectoris, obstructive pulmonary disease, prior myocardial infarction)
ASA 4	A patient with an incapacitating disease that is a constant threat to life (congestive heart failure, renal failure)
ASA 5	A moribund patient not expected to survive longer than 24 hours (ruptured aortic aneurysm, head trauma with increased intracranial pressure)

*For emergency operations, add the letter E before classification.

TABLE 1-11. Preinduction Anesthesia Checklist

1. Check functional state of anesthesia machine, monitors, and suction.
2. Prepare appropriate fluid infusion system.
3. Prepare appropriate intravenous drugs (anesthetics, muscle relaxants, anticholinergic, vasopressor).
4. Assemble equipment for general anesthesia or regional anesthesia.
5. Check room temperature, operating table function, special needs (warming/cooling blanket on table).
6. Identify and position patient on the operating table.
7. Examine chart to determine any recent information or changes and to verify administration and timing of premedication.
8. Start intravenous infusion.
9. Apply monitors and chart baseline values.
10. Discuss any changes in surgical plans or patient's condition with the surgeon.

---

the skills of the anesthesiologist and the wishes of the patient.

B. Outcome does not seem to be influenced by the choice of anesthetic technique, with the possible exception of patients undergoing peripheral vascular surgery, who may benefit from continuous epidural analgesia into the postoperative period.

V. THE RISKS OF ANESTHESIA

    A. A final portion of the preoperative visit includes a discussion of the risks of anesthesia that is guided by the patient's wishes to pursue this area (Table 1-9).

    B. Anesthetic-related mortality is estimated to be 1 in 10,000 anesthetics, and this may be even lower with the introduction of pulse oximetry and capnography.

VI. AMERICAN SOCIETY OF ANESTHESIOLOGISTS' PHYSICAL STATUS

    A. The purpose of this classification is to standardize physical status categories (not anesthetic risk) to allow comparison of outcome based on one standard criterion (physical status).

    B. Despite its shortcomings (it lacks preciseness), the physical status classification is sufficiently important that at the conclusion of the preoperative evaluation the anesthesiologist should assign each patient to one of the categories (Table 1-10).

VII. IMMEDIATE PREINDUCTION CHECKLIST

Prior to and after arrival of the patient in the operating room, the anesthesiologist must do several things to make delivery of the anesthetic as safe as possible (Table 1-11).

2

Pharmacogenetics

Certain inherited disorders are enhanced or instigated by drugs administered by anesthesiologists (Rosenberg H, Seitman D, Fletcher J: Pharmacogenetics. In Barash PG, Cullen BF, Stoelting RK [eds]: Clinical Anesthesia, pp 589–613. Philadelphia, JB Lippincott, 1992).

I. MALIGNANT HYPERTHERMIA (MH)

A. Clinical manifestations. MH is a hypermetabolic disorder of skeletal muscle that may or may not have a heritable component. When triggered, typically by succinylcholine (SCh) or a volatile anesthetic, intracellular hypercalcemia activates pathways that deplete adenosine triphosphate (ATP).

B. Classic MH most often manifests in the operating room but can also occur within the first few hours of recovery from anesthesia (Table 2-1).

1. SCh may accelerate the onset of MH (entire course over 5–10 minutes) in some patients, whereas in others a volatile anesthetic plus SCh is necessary to trigger the response. Some susceptible patients may develop MH despite multiple prior uneventful exposures to triggering drugs.

2. Even with successful treatment, patients with MH are at risk for myoglobinuric renal failure and disseminated intravascular coagulation. Creatine phosphokinase levels may exceed 20,000 units in the first 12–24 hours. Recrudescence of the syndrome may occur in the first 24–36 hours.

C. Masseter muscle rigidity may occur after administration of SCh, especially in children undergoing strabismus surgery. This response is considered **premonitory of MH.**

1. Recovery is usually uneventful following masseter muscle rigidity if the anesthetic is immediately discontinued. Nevertheless, creatine phosphokinase elevation (>20,000 units virtually confirms the diag-

    nosis of MH) and myoglobinuria are usually present for 4–12 hours. Patients should be observed for 12–24 hours, and some recommend administration of dantrolene, 1–2 mg·kg^{-1} iv.

  2. An alternative to canceling elective surgery when masseter muscle rigidity occurs is continuing the anesthetic with nontriggering drugs and monitoring with capnography.

  3. Several events may mimic masseter muscle rigidity (Table 2-2).

D. Drugs that trigger MH (Table 2-3)

E. Incidence and epidemiology. MH is estimated to occur in 1 in every 15,000 anesthetics in children and 1 in every 50,000 anesthetics in adults, with a mortality rate of about 10%.

F. Inheritance of MH is autosomal dominant with variable penetrance such that 50% of children of MH-susceptible parents are potentially at risk. Molecular biologic techniques are being applied to identify the genes for MH (possibly a defect in the ryanodine receptor).

TABLE 2-1. Manifestations of Malignant Hyperthermia

Hypercarbia (reflects hypermetabolism and is responsible for many of the signs of sympathetic nervous system stimulation)

Tachycardia

Tachypnea

Temperature elevation (1–2°C increase every 5 minutes)

Hypertension

Cardiac dysrhythmias

Acidosis

Hypoxemia

Hyperkalemia

Skeletal muscle rigidity

Myoglobinuria

TABLE 2-2. Events That Mimic Masseter Spasm

Inadequate dose of SCh

Inadequate time for onset of SCh

Temporomandibular joint dysfunction

Myotonic syndrome

TABLE 2-3. Drugs That May or May Not Trigger Malignant Hyperthermia

Unsafe Drugs
   SCh
   Volatile anesthetics

Insufficient Data/Controversial
   d-Tubocurarine
   Phenothiazines

Safe Drugs
   Antibiotics
   Antihistamines
   Antipyretics
   Atracurium
   Barbiturates
   Benzodiazepines
   Droperidol
   Ketamine (inherent circulatory effects may mimic MH)
   Local anesthetics
   Nitrous oxide
   Opioids
   Pancuronium
   Propofol
   Propranolol
   Vasoactive drugs
   Vecuronium

G. **Diagnostic tests for MH.** Although several tests have been described, the halothane-caffeine contracture test remains the standard. Skeletal muscle biopsy specimens (usually of the vastus lateralis) are bathed in a solution containing 1–3% halothane and caffeine or, alternatively, either drug alone.

H. **MH treatment.** When MH is diagnosed early and treated promptly, the mortality rate should be near zero. **Whenever anesthesia is administered, dantrolene should be readily available as well as a protocol for management** (see inside back cover for Malignant Hyperthermia Protocol).

   1. **The initial episode** (Table 2-4)
   2. **Management after the initial episode** (Table 2-5)

I. **Dantrolene** acts in the skeletal muscle cell to reduce intracellular levels of Ca^{2+}, most likely by reduction of sarcoplasmic reticulum Ca^{2+} release or inhibition of ex-

---

TABLE 2-4. Management of the Initial Manifestations of Malignant Hyperthermia

Discontinue inhaled anesthetics and SCh

Hyperventilate the lungs with oxygen

Administer dantrolene, 2.5 mg·kg^{-1} iv with repeated doses (up to a maximum of 10 mg·kg^{-1}) based on PaCO$_2$, heart rate, and body temperature (each ampule of 20 mg is mixed with 50 ml of distilled water)

Treat persistent acidosis with sodium bicarbonate (1–2 mEq·kg^{-1})

Control body temperature (gastric lavage, external ice packs until 38°C)

Replace anesthetic circuit and canister

Monitor with capnography and arterial blood gas determinations

Be prepared to treat hyperkalemia and cardiac dysrhythmias

TABLE 2-5. Management of Malignant Hyperthermia After the Initial Episode

Continue dantrolene, 1–2 mg·kg^{-1} iv every 4 hours, for at least 24 hours

Anticipate complications
    Recrudescence
    Disseminated intravascular coagulation
    Myoglobinuric renal failure
    Skeletal muscle weakness
    Electrolyte abnormalities

---

citation-contracture coupling at the transverse tubular level. The therapeutic level of dantrolene (2.5 μg·ml^{-1}) usually persists for 4–6 hours after an intravenous dose of 2.5 mg·kg^{-1}, which is the reason to supplement every 4 hours. Prophylaxis for MH should be carried out with intravenous or oral dantrolene (5 mg·kg^{-1}·d^{-1}).

J. Management of MH-susceptible patients (Table 2-6)

    1. There have been no deaths from MH in previously diagnosed MH-susceptible patients when the anesthesiologist was prospectively aware of the problem. This information is useful to allay patients' preoperative anxiety.

    2. Dantrolene need not be repeated after the anesthetic is terminated if there were no signs of MH during surgery.

TABLE 2-6. **Management of Malignant Hyperthermia—
Susceptible Patients**

Standard preoperative medication
Dantrolene, 2.5 mg·kg^{-1} iv 15–30 minutes before induction of anesthesia
Clean anesthesia machine (disposable circuit, new soda lime, drain vaporizers, oxygen flow of 3–5 l·min^{-1} for several hours to flush system)
Capnography (increased end-tidal carbon dioxide pressure is the earliest sign of malignant hyperthermia)
Monitor body temperature
Use nontriggering drugs and techniques (regional if possible)
Observe closely postoperatively

3. In a MH-susceptible parturient, an acceptable approach to management of routine labor is epidural anesthesia without dantrolene pretreatment and close monitoring of vital signs. If general anesthesia is necessary for delivery, an acceptable approach is to administer dantrolene intravenously and use nontriggering drugs. No adverse fetal effects of dantrolene have been observed.

II. DISORDERS OF PLASMA CHOLINESTERASE

A. **SCh-related apnea.** Hydrolysis of SCh by plasma cholinesterase is slowed to absent in patients with inherited alterations on the gene locus responsible for production of this enzyme (Table 2-7).
   1. When there is a question about the rate of hydrolysis of SCh, the plasma cholinesterase activity as well as dibucaine and fluoride numbers should be measured.
   2. Patients who are homozygous for atypical cholinesterase enzyme should wear **Medic-Alert** bracelets indicating that SCh administration will lead to prolonged apnea (often >120 minutes).
   3. Depression of plasma cholinesterase activity in the absence of atypical genotypes can be seen following administration of anticholinesterases or plasmapheresis and in the presence of advanced liver disease. This usually results in only moderate prolongation of SCh-induced paralysis (rarely >30 minutes).

TABLE 2-7. Genotypes for Plasma Cholinesterase Enzyme

Genotype	Dibucaine Number	Fluoride Number	Cholinesterase Activity	Response to SCh	Incidence
EuEu	78–86	55–65	Normal	Normal	96%
EaEa	18–26	16–32	Decreased	Greatly prolonged	1 in 2000
EuEa	51–70	38–55	Intermediate	Slightly prolonged	1 in 25
EuEf	74–80	47–48	Intermediate	Slightly prolonged	1 in 200
EfEa	49–59	25–33	Intermediate	Greatly prolonged	1 in 20,000
EfEs	63	26	Decreased	Moderately prolonged	1 in 150,000

Eu, normal enzyme gene; Ea, atypical enzyme gene; Ef, fluoride-sensitive gene; Es, silent gene.

21

TABLE 2-8. Manifestations of Porphyria	
Abdominal pain	Fever
Vomiting	Confusion
Tachycardia	Seizures
Hypertension	Somnolence
Neuropathy	

B. **C5 variant** is a disorder with an isoenzyme of plasma cholinesterase that is associated with accelerated hydrolysis of SCh.

C. **Plasma cholinesterase abnormalities and the metabolism of local anesthetics.** Ester local anesthetics are metabolized by plasma cholinesterase. Despite the theoretical argument that the action of these drugs might be prolonged, there is evidence that the response of homozygous atypical patients is usually normal.

III. PORPHYRIAS

Porphyrias are inherited defects of heme synthesis with manifestations that can mimic surgical diseases and that can be provoked by administration of certain drugs (Table 2-8).

A. **Management of patients with porphyria** is designed to avoid triggering drugs such as the barbiturates and perhaps benzodiazepines and ketamine. Nontriggering drugs include nitrous oxide, volatile anesthetics, opioids, and muscle relaxants. Regional anesthesia may be avoided to prevent confusion in case neurologic changes occur.

B. Glucose infusions are important in prevention (starvation can induce an attack) and treatment of porphyria.

3

Preoperative Medication

Preoperative medication consists of **psychological preparation** and **pharmacologic preparation** of patients before surgery (Moyers JR: Preoperative medication. In Barash PG, Cullen BF, Stoelting RK [eds]: Clinical Anesthesia, pp 615–635. Philadelphia, JB Lippincott, 1992). Ideally, all patients should enter the preoperative period free from apprehension, sedated but easily arousable, and fully cooperative.

I. PSYCHOLOGICAL PREPARATION

The preoperative visit and interview with patients and family members serves as a nonpharmacologic antidote to apprehension (Table 3-1).

II. PHARMACOLOGIC PREPARATION

A. Drugs selected for preoperative medication are typically administered orally or intramuscularly in a patient's room 1–2 hours before the anticipated induction of anesthesia. For outpatient surgery, drugs may be administered intravenously in the immediate preoperative period. Alternatively, a physician may prescribe drugs for a patient to take orally before arriving at the outpatient center.

B. **Various goals for pharmacologic premedication** (Table 3-2)

C. **Determinants of drug choice and dose** (Table 3-3)

D. Several classes of drugs are available to facilitate achievement of the desired goals for pharmacologic premedication in each patient (Table 3-4).

1. There is no best drug or drug combination for preoperative medication. The choice may be influenced by tradition and an anesthesiologist's previous experience. **Timing of drug selection is as important as drug selection.**

2. Ideally, the specific drugs selected are based on the goals of premedication balanced against potential

TABLE 3-1. Areas to Be Discussed During a Preoperative Interview

Review medical history with patient
    Coexisting diseases
    Chronic drug therapy
    Prior anesthesia experiences
Describe anesthetic techniques available and associated risks
Review planned preoperative medication and time scheduled for surgery
Describe what to expect on arrival in operating room
Describe anticipated duration of surgery and expected time to return to room
Describe methods available to manage postoperative pain
    Patient-controlled analgesia
    Neuraxial opioids

TABLE 3-2. Goals for Pharmacologic Premedication

Anxiety relief
Sedation
Amnesia
Analgesia
Drying of airway secretions (antisialagogue effect)
Prevention of autonomic nervous system reflex responses
Reduction of gastric fluid volume and increase in pH
Antiemetic effects
Reduction of anesthetic requirements
Facilitate induction of anesthesia
Prophylaxis against allergic reactions

TABLE 3-3. Determinants of Drug Choice and Dose

Patient age and weight
American Society of Anesthesiologists' physical status
Level of anxiety
Tolerance for depressant drugs
Prior adverse experiences with premedication
Drug allergies
Elective vs. emergency surgery
Inpatient vs. outpatient surgery

TABLE 3-4. Drugs Used for Pharmacologic Premedication

Drug	Route of Administration	Adult Dose (mg)
Diazepam	oral	5–20
Lorazepam	oral, im	1–4
Midazolam	im	3–5
	iv	1–2.5
Secobarbital	oral, im	50–200
Pentobarbital	oral, im	50–200
Morphine	im	5–15
Meperidine	im	50–150
Cimetidine	oral, im, iv	150–300
Ranitidine	oral	50–200
Famotidine	oral	20–40
Metoclopramide	oral, im, iv	5–20
Atropine	im, iv	0.3–0.6
Glycopyrrolate	im, iv	0.1–0.3
Scopolamine	im, iv	0.3–0.6
Antacids	oral	10–30 ml

undesirable effects these drugs may produce. It must be recognized that some patients may not need (elderly) or should not receive (decreased level of consciousness, intracranial pathology, severe pulmonary disease, hypovolemia) depressant drugs for preoperative medication.

E. **Benzodiazepines** act on specific brain (gamma aminobutyric acid [GABA]) receptors to produce selective antianxiety effects at doses that do not produce excessive sedation, depression of ventilation, or adverse cardiac effects.

1. **Diazepam** produces a peak effect in 30–60 minutes after oral administration. Because diazepam is insoluble in water and must be dissolved in organic solvents, pain may occur with intramuscular or intravenous injection.

2. **Lorazepam** produces intense amnesia, but sedation and prolonged duration of action detract from its use for short surgical procedures or in outpatients. Peak effects after oral administration may not occur for 2–4 hours.

3. **Midazolam.** After intramuscular injection, the onset of effect is 5–10 minutes, a peak effect occurs

---

TABLE 3-5. Side Effects of Opioids As Used for Pharmacologic Premedication

Depression of ventilation
Nausea and vomiting
Orthostatic hypotension
Delayed gastric emptying
Pruritus
Choledochoduodenal sphincter spasm

---

in 30–60 minutes, and the duration is usually brief. Unlike with diazepam, intramuscular or intravenous injection is not unusually painful.

F. **Barbiturates,** which are long acting and provide little amnesia, have been largely replaced by benzodiazepines for preoperative medication.

G. **Butyrophenones,** such as droperidol, provide good antiemetic effects but can evoke dysphoria in patients who are scheduled for surgery and who otherwise appear sedated and comfortable.

H. **Opioids** are used for preoperative medication when there is a need to provide analgesia, as before institution of a regional anesthetic or when patients have pain owing to their surgical disease. Anesthesiologists often use a combination of opioid, benzodiazepine, and scopolamine for preoperative medication of patients who are likely to be unusually apprehensive, as before cardiac surgery or cancer surgery. Administration of opioids has the potential to produce multiple side effects (Table 3-5).

1. **Morphine** produces peak effects within 45–90 minutes after intramuscular injection. Inclusion of morphine in the preoperative medication reduces the likelihood that undesirable increases in heart rate will accompany surgical stimulation.

2. **Meperidine** is often used in combination with promethazine. Peak effects after intramuscular injection of meperidine may be unpredictable.

III. GASTRIC FLUID pH AND VOLUME

A. It is estimated that 40–80% of patients scheduled for elective surgery may be at risk for aspiration pneumonitis based on the presence of a gastric fluid pH

<2.5 and a gastric fluid volume ≥25 ml. Anticholinergics, H_2 receptor antagonists, antacids, and gastrokinetic drugs all have been used to raise gastric pH or lower gastric fluid volume in hopes of reducing the likelihood of acid pneumonitis should aspiration occur. Nevertheless, **clinically significant pulmonary aspiration of gastric contents is very rare in healthy patients** having elective surgical procedures, and routine prophylaxis is questionable.

1. **Anticholinergics** do not reliably increase gastric fluid pH in the doses used for preoperative medication and may relax the lower esophageal sphincter, making gastroesophageal reflux more likely.

2. **H_2 receptor antagonists** increase gastric fluid pH by blocking histamine-induced secretion of gastric fluid with a high H^+ content. Gastric fluid volume is not influenced.

    a. **Cimetidine.** Oral administration 1–1.5 hours before surgery increases gastric fluid pH above 2.5 in about 80% of patients. Cimetidine crosses the placenta, but adverse fetal effects have not been proved. Cimetidine inhibits mixed-function oxidase enzyme systems and reduces hepatic blood flow; as a result, the elimination half-time of some drugs may be prolonged.

    b. **Ranitidine** is more potent and longer lasting than cimetidine.

3. **Antacids,** when administered 15–30 minutes before induction of anesthesia, raise gastric fluid pH above 2.5 in nearly all patients. Unlike H_2 receptor antagonists, there is no lag time for the effect of antacids on gastric fluid pH, with fluid present before the administration of antacid being neutralized. Efficacy of antacids may depend to some extent on patient movement so as to facilitate complete mixing with gastric fluid. Nonparticulate antacids are recommended because they do not produce pulmonary damage if fluid containing these antacids is inhaled.

4. **Gastrokinetic drugs** reduce gastric fluid volume by relaxing the pyloric sphincter and promoting gastric motility. Lower esophageal sphincter tone is increased. Gastric fluid pH is not altered. Gastrokinetic drugs are particularly useful for those patients likely to have large gastric fluid volumes as a result of slow gastric emptying (Table 3-6).

    a. **Metoclopramide,** when administered orally, has an onset of 30–60 minutes compared with 3–5 minutes when injected intravenously. Metoclo-

TABLE 3-6. Factors That May Delay Gastric Emptying	
Opioids	Trauma
Pregnancy	Pain
Obesity	Anxiety
Diabetes	

pramide does not guarantee gastric emptying, and its beneficial effects may be offset by concomitant or prior administration of anticholinergics, opioids, or antacids.

  b. **Metoclopramide and an H$_2$ antagonist** in combination may be the most reliable approach for reducing gastric fluid volume and elevating gastric fluid pH.

B. **Oral fluids.** The necessity of **prolonged fasting** (nothing by mouth after midnight) prior to induction of anesthesia for elective surgery has been challenged. Up to 150 ml of water administered with oral premedication drugs 2–3 hours before induction of anesthesia does not increase gastric fluid volume. In fact, fluid may stimulate the stomach to empty. For this reason, it does not seem logical to forbid ingestion of small volumes of clear fluids before elective surgery. This recommendation does not apply to solid foods or to patients at known risk for slow gastric emptying.

IV. ANTIEMETICS

Certain types of patients and operations may benefit from antiemetics administered near the conclusion of surgery (Table 3-7).

A. **Droperidol** in low doses (10–15 μg·kg^{-1}) administered intravenously 5 minutes before the conclusion of surgery may reduce the incidence of postoperative nausea and vomiting. Sedation may accompany this dose of droperidol.

B. **Metoclopramide.** Administer intravenously near the end of surgery.

C. **Transdermal scopolamine patch** may be applied before induction of anesthesia.

V. ANTICHOLINERGICS

A. Routine inclusion of anticholinergics as part of the pharmacologic premedication is not mandatory but

rather should be individualized based on a patient's
needs and the pharmacology of the anticholinergics
(Table 3-8).

B. Indications for anticholinergics
  1. **Antisialagogue effect.** This is useful to reduce air-
     way secretions associated with endotracheal intu-
     bation, intraoral operations, and bronchoscopy.
     Patients scheduled for regional anesthesia do not
     benefit from an antisialagogue effect.
  2. **Sedation and amnesia.** Scopolamine, especially in
     combination with morphine, is useful. The dose
     should be reduced in elderly patients.
  3. **Vagolytic action.** Prevention of reflex bradycardia
     with intramuscular doses of anticholinergics is un-
     reliable, given the drug dosage and timing usually

**TABLE 3-7. Patients Who May Benefit from
Prophylactic Antiemetics**

Patients undergoing ophthalmologic surgery
Patients undergoing gynecologic surgery
Obese patients
Patients with a prior history of vomiting

TABLE 3-8. Comparative Effects of Anticholinergics*

	Atropine	Scopolamine	Glycopyrrolate
Antisialagogue effect	+	+ + +	+ +
Sedative and amnesic effects	+	+ + +	0
Central nervous system toxicity	+	+ +	0
Relaxation of gastro-esophageal sphincter	+ +	+ +	+ +
Mydriasis and cycloplegia	+	+ +	0
Increased heart rate	+ + +	+	+ +

0 none; + mild; + + moderate; + + + marked
  *Intravenous administration

involved with preoperative medication administered on the ward. Many anesthesiologists prefer
to administer atropine or glycopyrrolate intravenously just before induction of anesthesia.

C. **Side effects of anticholinergic drugs**
1. **Central nervous system toxicity** is characterized
   by confusion and restlessness manifested postoperatively, especially in elderly patients receiving
   scopolamine and to a lesser degree atropine. Glycopyrrolate does not easily cross the blood-brain
   barrier and is therefore not associated with this
   side effect. Some anesthesiologists have successfully treated this toxic effect with 15–60 $\mu g \cdot kg^{-1}$ of
   physostigmine administered intravenously.
2. **Relaxation of the lower esophageal sphincter.**
   Although it has not been proved to be clinically
   significant, this effect of anticholinergics could
   theoretically increase the incidence of gastroesophageal reflux and the likelihood of acid pneumonitis.
3. **Mydriasis and cycloplegia.** Anticholinergics could
   increase intraocular pressure in patients with glaucoma, but this seems unlikely with doses used for
   premedication. Miotic eyedrops should be continued in patients with glaucoma.
4. **Increased physiologic dead space** reflects relaxation of bronchial smooth muscle by reduction in
   vagal tone to airways. This response could be
   viewed as therapeutic in patients with asthma.
5. **Drying of airway secretions.**
6. **Interferes with sweating.** Sweat glands are innervated by cholinergic nerves through the sympathetic nervous system. Prevention of sweating by
   this mechanism is an important consideration in
   administering anticholinergic premedication to febrile patients, especially children.
7. **Increased heart rate.** This response is unlikely after intramuscular administration. In fact, heart rate
   may transiently decrease after administration as a
   result of a peripheral agonist effect of the anticholinergic.

VI. ATTENUATED SYMPATHETIC NERVOUS SYSTEM REFLEX RESPONSES AND REDUCTION OF ANESTHETIC REQUIREMENTS

Clonidine is a centrally acting alpha$_2$ agonist that attenuates blood pressure and heart rate responses to noxious
stimulation and reduces by about 40% requirements for

inhaled or injected anesthetics when it is administered as an oral preoperative medication (5 $\mu g \cdot kg^{-1}$). Experience is too limited to recommend use of clonidine or other alpha$_2$ agonists (e.g., dexmedetomidine) as part of routine preoperative medication.

VII. PROPHYLAXIS AGAINST ALLERGIC REACTIONS

For patients considered at high risk for allergic reactions (from radiographic dye studies, chemonucleolysis), anesthesiologists may include H$_1$ and H$_2$ receptor antagonists plus corticosteroids in the preoperative medication. The efficacy of this approach is not proved.

VIII. DIFFERENCES IN PREOPERATIVE MEDICATION BETWEEN PEDIATRIC AND ADULT PATIENTS (see Chapter 33)

A. Children differ from adults with regard to preoperative medication in terms of (1) psychological preparation, (2) greater use of oral medications, and (3) more frequent use of anticholinergics for their vagolytic activity. The need to assess the requirements of each child and to tailor the preoperative medication accordingly is equally important in children and adults.

B. **Psychological factors in pediatric patients**
1. Age is probably the most important factor in the success of a preoperative visit and interview. Patients younger than 6 months of age are not upset by separation from their parents, whereas those older than 5 years are amenable to explanation and reassurance. Preschool-age children are likely to be upset by separation from parents.
2. Children who do not ask questions or appear nonchalant during the preoperative interview may be masking a high level of apprehension.
3. Some children wish to take an active part in the induction of anesthesia. In this regard, it may be helpful to have the parents accompany these children to the operating room.

C. **Differences in pharmacologic preparation**
1. Use of pharmacologic premedication in children after 6 months of age is controversial and has not been proved to reduce unwanted psychological outcome. More important in avoiding long-lasting psychological problems is a pleasant induction of anesthesia.

2. Oral administration is preferred to intramuscular injections in children. An oral "cocktail" consisting of an opioid, sedative-hypnotic, and anticholinergic may be useful.
3. Rectal methohexital (20–30 mg·kg^{-1}) may be useful in selected patients and can be administered while the child is still in a parent's arms.
4. **Easily induced vagal reflexes** in response to airway manipulation, halothane, and succinylcholine are the reasons many anesthesiologists administer atropine intravenously or intramuscularly just before induction of anesthesia.

IX. PREOPERATIVE MEDICATION FOR OUTPATIENTS (see Chapter 35)

Pharmacologic premedication for outpatients is controversial, with the greatest concern being delayed awakening owing to lingering drug effects. The use of intravenous meperidine, oral diazepam, or intravenous fentanyl does not appear to adversely delay awakening in outpatients. Droperidol or metoclopramide may reduce the incidence of postoperative nausea and vomiting, which is a common reason for delaying discharge after outpatient surgery. Routine administration of antacids and gastrokinetic drugs to outpatients is of questionable value.

X. EXAMPLE OF PREOPERATIVE MEDICATION SEQUENCE FOR AN ADULT INPATIENT

A. Preoperative visit and interview.
B. Oral benzodiazepine to treat insomnia the night before surgery.
C. Oral benzodiazepine 1–2 hours before surgery. Water, up to 150 ml, may stimulate gastric emptying. Substitute or add an intramuscular opioid if analgesia is desired.
D. Intramuscular scopolamine 1–2 hours before surgery if reliable sedation and amnesia are desired.
E. If antisialagogue effect only is desired, administer glycopyrrolate (or atropine) intramuscularly before a patient leaves the room for transport to surgery or administer intravenously before induction of anesthesia.
F. Consider the possible value of an oral H$_2$ antagonist and/or metoclopramide. For emergency surgery, these drugs may be administered intravenously.

4

Anesthesia Systems

An understanding of the components of the anesthesia system (machine, vaporizers, ventilators, circuit) is essential to the safe practice of anesthesia (Andrews JJ: Anesthesia systems. In Barash PG, Cullen BF, Stoelting RK [eds]: Clinical Anesthesia, pp 637–683. Philadelphia, JB Lippincott, 1992).

I. THE ANESTHESIA MACHINE (Fig. 4-1)

A. **Gases** such as oxygen (O_2), nitrous oxide (N_2O), and air are usually supplied from a central pipeline, with cylinders on the machine as a back-up. The pipeline source is usually at 50 psig (pounds per square inch gauge). A full O_2 cylinder contains only gas, and the tank pressure decreases linearly from a maximum of approximately 2000 psig as it is consumed. N_2O is compressed to a liquid in tanks and maintains a pressure of 750 psig until all the liquid is dissipated. **Regulators** downstream from the O_2 supply source adjust the pressure to approximately 15–25 psig before entering the flow meter assembly. **Flow meters** route the gases through a common manifold and then to a calibrated, agent-specific, variable bypass **vaporizer** containing a volatile halogenated anesthetic. The mixture then flows to a **common gas outlet.** A **check valve** is located proximal to the common gas outlet to prevent back pressure from increasing anesthetic delivery during positive pressure ventilation. An **O_2 flush valve** is also present. It diverts O_2 past the flow meter assembly directly to the common gas outlet. An O_2 supply **failsafe** device is located downstream from the non-O_2 supply source. It shuts off the supply of those gases if the O_2 supply pressure falls below a certain minimum. Newer anesthetic machines are also equipped with

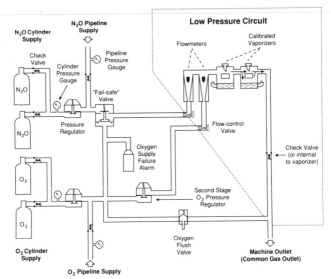

Figure 4-1. Schematic diagram of a generic two-gas anesthesia machine.

pressure **alarms** warning of low O_2 supply and mechanical or pneumatic **proportioning devices,** which lower the delivery of gases other than O_2 if the ratio of O_2 flow to the flow of other gases decreases below some arbitrary minimum of about 25%.

B. **Flow meters** precisely measure gas flow to the common gas outlet. Depending on the setting of the flow control valve, gases flow through **variable orifice,** tapered tubes at a rate indicated by the position of a **float indicator** in relation to a calibrated scale. At low flow rates, the **viscosity** of the gas is dominant in determining flow, whereas **density** is dominant at high flow rates. **Safety features** include use of standardized colors for each gas, an O_2 flow meter valve that is distinct from the others, and positioning of the O_2 flow meter immediately proximal to the common gas outlet to minimize the chance of delivery of hypoxic mixtures in the event of leaks in the flow meter assembly.

C. **Vaporizers** on contemporary anesthesia machines are calibrated, variable bypass, agent-specific, and temperature compensated and have a flow-over design. They contain volatile anesthetics that are liquid at room temperature (isoflurane, enflurane, and halothane). As the valve is turned, a portion of the inflowing gas is diverted into a vaporizing chamber, where it "picks up" anesthetic vapor before rejoining the bypassed gas at the vaporizer outlet. The amount of gas diverted into the vaporizing chamber is primarily a function of the anesthetic **vapor pressure.** Most vaporizers are accurate if inflow rates exceed 250 ml·min^{-1}. Addition of N_2O to the inflow gas mixture reduces the concentration of volatile anesthetic delivered from the vaporizer to slightly less than that shown on the dial.

   1. Hazards of vaporizers (Table 4-1).
   2. **Desflurane vaporizers** are electrically heated (23–25° C) and pressurized (1550 mm Hg) to create conditions in which this anesthetic (vapor pressure 664 mm Hg) has a relatively lower volatility.

II. ANESTHETIC CIRCUITS

A. An anesthetic circuit is interposed between the anesthesia machine, common gas outlet, and the patient. The function of the circuit is to deliver anesthetic gases and O_2 to a patient and to remove exhaled CO_2.

B. **Mapleson** described several different **non–rebreathing** anesthesia arrangements, which are highly dependent on the fresh gas flow rate (Fig. 4-2).

   1. System F is the **Jackson-Rees** modification, which is popular for use with pediatric patients. With this latter system, it is usually necessary to administer

---

TABLE 4-1. Possible Hazards of Vaporizers

Filled with incorrect anesthetic

Contamination of the bypass chamber with liquid anesthetic if the vaporizer is tipped

Simultaneous administration of two anesthetics if the interlock mechanism is not operative

Development of leaks, as when filter cap is off or loose

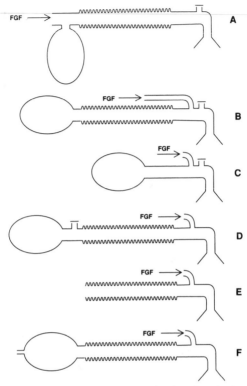

Figure 4-2. Mapleson breathing systems showing sites of entry of fresh gas flow (FGF).

a fresh gas flow rate that is at least twice the patient's minute ventilation.

2. The **Bain circuit** is a modification of the Mapleson D circuit, in which fresh gas flow is delivered at the end nearest the patient through a small inner tube located within the larger corrugated tubing (Fig. 4-3).

3. The **advantages** of all these systems are that they are lightweight and convenient. The main **disadvantage** is that high fresh gas flows are required.

C. The **circle system** consists of a fresh gas inflow, inspiratory and expiratory unidirectional valves, inspiratory and expiratory corrugated tubing, a Y-piece connector,

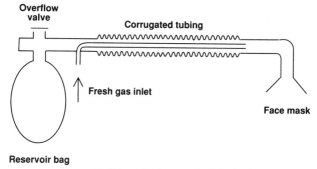

Figure 4-3. Schematic diagram of a Bain circuit.

an overflow or pop-off valve, a reservoir bag, and a canister containing CO_2 absorbent (Table 4-2). The unidirectional valves are placed so that gases flow in only one direction and through the CO_2 absorber (Fig. 4-4).

1. If the valves are functioning properly, the only dead space in the system is between the Y-piece and the patient.
2. A **closed system** exists when the fresh gas flow equals that being consumed by the patient (about $300\ ml \cdot min^{-1}$ of O_2 plus uptake of anesthetic gases) and the overflow (pop-off) valve is closed. If high fresh gas flows are used, the system is called **semiclosed** or **semiopen**.

D. CO_2 **absorption** is accomplished in a circle system by a chemical reaction that has water and heat as by-products (Tables 4-3 and 4-4).

TABLE 4-2. Characteristics of a Circle System	
Advantages	**Disadvantages**
Conservation of gases	Tubing disconnection
Conservation of heat	Leaks
Conservation of moisture	Carbon dioxide absorbent exhaustion
Minimal operating room pollution	Failure of unidirectional valves
	Poor portability

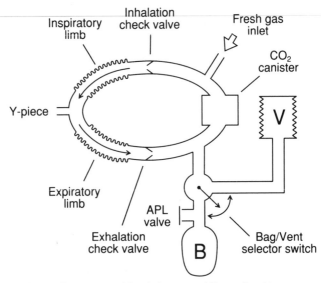

Figure 4-4. Components of the circle system. APL = adjustable pressure-limiting valve.

TABLE 4-3. Chemical Reaction of CO_2 with Soda Lime

$CO_2 + H_2O \rightarrow H_2CO_3$
$H_2CO_3 + 2NaOH(KOH) \rightarrow Na_2CO_3(K_2CO_3) + 2H_2O + heat$
$Na_2CO_3(K_2CO_3) + Ca(OH)_2 \rightarrow CaCO_3 + 2NaOH(KOH)$

TABLE 4-4. Chemical Reaction of CO_2 with Baralyme

$Ba(OH)_2 + 8H_2O + CO_2 \rightarrow BaCO_3 + 9H_2O + heat$
$9H_2O + 9CO_2 \rightarrow 9H_2CO_3$
Then, by direct reactions and by KOH and NaOH
$9H_2CO_3 + 9Ca(OH)_2 \rightarrow CaCO_3 + 18H_2O + heat$

---

1. **Indicators** are placed in the CO_2 absorbent; they change color when the absorbent is exhausted.
2. Other indications of absorbent exhaustion include an elevated inspired CO_2 concentration and physiologic changes in a patient suggestive of CO_2 re-

breathing (tachypnea, tachycardia, and hypertension).

III. VENTILATORS

A. Anesthesia ventilators may be **powered** by electricity, compressed gas, or both. Typically, a **bellows** containing anesthetic gases and attached to the anesthetic circuit is housed in a clear plastic chamber. During inspiration, a **driving gas** is delivered into the chamber, which causes the bellows to be compressed. It is safest to have O_2 as the driving gas because the fraction of inspired O_2 (FIO_2) will be enriched if there is a leak in the bellows. During exhalation, the driving gas is vented into the room, and the bellows refill as the patient exhales.

B. Ventilators with bellows that **rise** during expiration are safest because an accidental disconnection of the circuit from a patient is more readily detected. A low-pressure **disconnect alarm** may also sound. This alarm is activated when pressure in the anesthetic circuit, as sensed by a tube connected to the ventilator, does not increase within a set period of time. Some ventilators are also equipped with a **high-pressure alarm,** which sounds when airway pressure exceeds an arbitrary maximum. Most newer ventilators are **time cycled. Hazards** associated with anesthesia ventilators include those listed in Table 4-5.

IV. SCAVENGING SYSTEMS

Scavenging is the collection and subsequent removal of vented gases from the operating room. Scavenging systems minimize operating room pollution but increase the complexity of the anesthesia system (Table 4-6).

TABLE 4-5. Hazards Associated with Ventilators

Accidental disconnection
Delivery of excessive pressure
Leaks in the bellows
Erroneous connection of tubing to anesthetic circuit
Failure of the ventilator relief valve
Failure of the driving mechanism

TABLE 4-6. Hazards Introduced by Scavenging Systems

Transmission of excessive positive pressure to the breathing system (obstruction of scavenging pathways)
Application of excessive negative pressure to the breathing system (relief valve or port becomes obstructed)
Loss of means of monitoring (conceals odor of excessive anesthetic concentration)

TABLE 4-7. Effects of Dry Gas Inhalation

Impairs ciliary function
Desiccates the mucus blanket of the trachea
Induces an inflammatory reaction
Predisposes patients to atelectasis and/or pneumonia
Decreases body temperature

V. CHECKING ANESTHESIA MACHINES

A complete test of the anesthesia apparatus is recommended before starting the first case of the day (see Appendix D).

VI. HUMIDIFICATION

A. Persistent inhalation of dry gases can result in undesirable changes (Table 4-7).
B. To minimize postoperative pulmonary problems, warmth and humidity must be added to the inspired gases by using a circle system with **low fresh gas flows** or by bypassing the gases through an **external humidifier.**
C. There are two basic types of humidifying devices.
   1. Heated **nebulizers** deliver water in droplet form as an aerosol. Although effective, they have significant drawbacks (Table 4-8).
   2. **Humidifiers** can be of the **blow-over, bubble,** or **heated cascade** variety. They are designed to provide only enough humidity to make inhalation of the gas comfortable. Cascade humidifiers break the

TABLE 4-8. Disadvantages of Heated Nebulizers

Overheating
Overhydration
Infection
Increased airway resistance

inspired gas into tiny bubbles and pass them through heated water to produce 100% humidity. The main **disadvantage** of bubble or cascade humidifiers is that they may provide added airway resistance, which can be significant if a patient is breathing spontaneously.

VII. CLOSED CIRCUIT ANESTHESIA (Table 4-9)

TABLE 4-9. Closed Circuit Anesthesia

Advantages	Disadvantages
Decreased cost	More complex (frequent adjustments necessary to match dynamic aspects of uptake and distribution)
Decreased pollution	
Improved humidification	
Accurate measurement of volume	
	Dosage errors
Direct monitoring of oxygen consumption (early detection of malignant hyperthermia)	Hypoxic mixture possible (prior denitrogenation; avoid nitrous oxide?)
	Inability to rapidly change inspired gas concentrations
Gradual change in delivered anesthetic concentrations	Accumulation of waste products or metabolites

5

Management of the Airway

Maintenance of a patent upper airway and intubation of the trachea (translaryngeal intubation) depend on a knowledge of the anatomy of the upper airway and appropriate use of equipment and drugs, especially muscle relaxants (Stehling LC: Management of the airway. In Barash PG, Cullen BF, Stoelting RK [eds]: Clinical Anesthesia, pp 685–708. Philadelphia, JB Lippincott, 1992). It is important to prospectively recognize patients in whom airway management may be difficult and to be able to formulate and implement alternative plans in various clinical situations.

I. LARYNX

A. **Adults.** Located at the level of C4–6, the larynx is bounded anteriorly by the epiglottis, posteriorly by the mucous membrane that extends between the arytenoid cartilages, and laterally by the aryepiglottic folds. The glottic opening is the triangular space between the vocal cords, representing the narrowest part of the airway (Fig. 5-1).

B. **Infants.** Compared with an adult, an infant's larynx is located more cephalad, the epiglottis is longer and narrower, and the glottic opening is more anterior. The cricoid cartilage is the narrowest point in the larynx; thus, a tube that passes through the glottic opening may subsequently resist advancement at this site.

C. **Innervation** of the larynx is provided by the vagus nerves. Sensation above the vocal cords is provided by the internal branch of the superior laryngeal nerves, whereas sensation below the vocal cords is from the recurrent laryngeal nerves.

D. **Function.** The principal function of the larynx is to protect the lungs by preventing foreign material from entering.

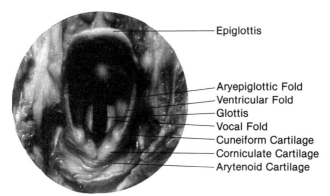

Epiglottis

Aryepiglottic Fold
Ventricular Fold
Glottis
Vocal Fold
Cuneiform Cartilage
Corniculate Cartilage
Arytenoid Cartilage

Figure 5-1. Anatomy of an adult larynx.

II. AIRWAY ASSESSMENT

A. **History.** Was airway management difficult during previous anesthetics? Verify with the patient and previous anesthesia records.

B. **Physical examination**

1. **Anatomic characteristics** that impair alignment of the oral, laryngeal, and pharyngeal axes and make visualization of the glottic opening by direct laryngoscopy difficult must be evaluated (Table 5-1).

2. Any type of head movement that produces paresthesias must be noted so that similar positioning is avoided during direct laryngoscopy.

3. The probable ease of tracheal intubation can be assessed by measurement of the distance between the lower border of the mandible and the thyroid notch with the patient's neck fully extended. If the

---

TABLE 5-1. Anatomic Characteristics Associated with Difficult Exposure of the Glottic Opening

Short, muscular neck
Receding mandible
Protruding maxillary incisors
Inability to visualize uvula
Limited temporomandibular joint mobility (<40 mm)
Limited cervical spine mobility

measurement in an adult is less than 6 cm (about three finger breadths), it will probably not be possible to visualize the glottic opening by direct laryngoscopic examination (Fig. 5-2).

4. **Dental examination.** Loose, capped, and prosthetic teeth must be noted, as they are vulnerable to dislodgment or damage during direct laryngoscopy. Nonfixed dental prostheses usually should be removed before induction of anesthesia, although some anesthesiologists recommend leaving dentures in place so as to facilitate fitting a mask to the patient's face.

III. AIRWAY EQUIPMENT

Airway equipment must be available for every anesthetic regardless of the anesthetic technique employed (local, regional, or general).

A. **Masks.** The availability of clear plastic face masks in various sizes allows selection of the size that best fits an individual patient and permits an anesthesiologist to visualize evidence of exhalation (condensation or "fogging" on the mask), regurgitation, and pressure injury on the lips.

B. **Airways.** Oropharyngeal and nasopharyngeal airways are available in various sizes. These devices help to keep the airway patent by providing a passageway between the tongue and posterior pharynx.

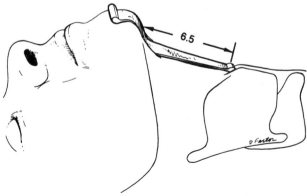

Figure 5-2. An intubation gauge can be used to estimate the degree of difficulty with endotracheal intubation.

C. **Laryngoscopes** consist of a battery-containing handle
   that powers the light source on interchangeable blades
   of various sizes. Curved (MacIntosh) and straight
   (Miller) blades are the most commonly used. The personal preference of the anesthesiologist primarily
   determines the type of blade used for intubating the
   trachea of adults. The straight blade is usually chosen
   for children.
D. **Endotracheal tubes** are numbered according to the internal diameter (ID), which is marked on each tube.
   The tracheal tube also has lengthwise centimeter
   markings starting at the distal tracheal end to permit
   accurate determination of the tube length inserted
   past the lips or incisors. Selection of the approximate
   size and length of the orotracheal tube should be determined by the patient's age and size (Table 5-2).
   1. After about 14 years of age, the trachea is adult
      size. In general, a 7.0–8.5-mm ID tube is appropri-
      ate for women and an 8.0–10.0-mm ID tube for
      men. In women, the length from the alveolar ridge
      to the tip of the tube should be approximately 21
      cm, and in men, 23 cm. A radiographic marker at
      the end of the tube facilitates radiographic verifi-
      cation of the tube position above the carina.
   2. Most endotracheal tubes are made of clear non-
      toxic plastic (IT for implant tested or Z-79 for the
      committee that signifies the tube material is non-
      toxic to tissue) and are disposable. Anode or ar-

TABLE 5-2. Tracheal Tube Size and Length

Age	Internal Diameter (mm)	Length (cm)*
Premature	2.5	10
Neonate	3.0–3.5	10–11
6–12 months	3.5–4.0	11–12
2 years	4.5	13
4 years	5.0	14
6 years	5.5	15
8 years	6.0	16
10 years	6.5	17
12 years	7.0	18

*Distance inserted from lips to place distal end in the midtrachea. Naso-
tracheal tubes should be about 3 cm longer.

mored tubes, designed to minimize kinking, have a wire coil embedded in the wall.

3. **Double-lumen tubes** permit isolation and selective ventilation of the lungs, as during thoracic surgery (see Chapter 20).

4. **Tracheal tube cuff.** Cuffs, built into the distal end of tracheal tubes, are inflated with air to create a seal against the underlying tracheal mucosa. This seal facilitates positive-pressure ventilation of the lungs and reduces the likelihood of pulmonary aspiration. When a cuffed tube is used, the size of the tube must be smaller in order to compensate for the added bulk of the cuff. Uncuffed tracheal tubes may be selected for use in children in an attempt to reduce the risk of subglottic edema.

   a. Transmission of cuff pressure to the underlying tracheal mucosa may produce mucosal ischemia whenever the pressure on the tracheal wall exceeds capillary arteriolar pressure (about 32 mm Hg). Persistent ischemia of the tracheal mucosa has been implicated as a cause of tracheal stenosis.

   b. There is probably no period of tracheal intubation that does not produce some laryngotracheal damage. For example, ciliary denudation has been found to occur predominantly over the tracheal rings and underlying cuff site after only 2 hours of tracheal intubation and tracheal wall pressures of less than 25 mm Hg.

E. **Ancillary equipment**

   1. **Suction** must always be immediately available.

   2. **A stylet** to help maintain the desired curve of the endotracheal tube.

   3. **A tooth protector** to reduce damage to teeth during direct laryngoscopy.

IV. AIRWAY OBSTRUCTION

A. The anesthesiologist is responsible for maintaining a patent upper airway and promptly recognizing any signs of airway obstruction (Table 5-3).

   1. **Upper airway obstruction** is likely to occur with the induction of anesthesia when there is relaxation of the mandible and tongue so that the base of the tongue falls back against the posterior pharynx. To relieve upper airway obstruction, an anesthesiologist often extends the patient's head and elevates the mandible (head-tilt–jaw-thrust) so as to

TABLE 5-3. Signs of Airway Obstruction

Stridor (snoring)
Flaring of the nostrils
Tracheal retraction
Thoracic retraction–abdominal flaring (rocking-boat respirations)
Failure to detect exhaled air against palm of hand used to extend head
Decreased or absent breath sounds
Absence of carbon dioxide in exhaled gases

tense the muscles attached to the tongue and thus displace it away from the posterior pharynx. Other methods to relieve upper airway obstruction include positive airway pressure to "distend the soft tissue" and insertion of an oropharyngeal or nasopharyngeal (better tolerated than an oropharyngeal airway in lightly anesthetized patients) airway.

2. **Laryngospasm** is reflex closure of the vocal cords that may occur in anesthetized patients when the vocal cords are irritated by secretions or when a patient experiences a painful stimulus. Partial laryngospasm is characterized by high-pitched phonation ("crowing"). Total occlusion due to laryngospasm is characterized by absence of sound because there is no air movement.

   a. **Treatment of laryngospasm** is by application of the head-tilt–jaw-thrust maneuver while applying positive airway pressure by means of a face mask connected to a delivery system containing 100% oxygen.

   b. If laryngospasm persists despite this treatment and signs of arterial oxygen desaturation develop, it is **imperative to administer a short-acting muscle relaxant** intravenously, such as succinylcholine (SCh) 0.2–0.5 mg·kg^{-1}. Intramuscular (deltoid) or sublingual injection of SCh (2–4 mg·kg^{-1}) is an alternative when an intravenous site is not available.

B. **Transtracheal oxygenation (cricothyrotomy) (see inside front cover).** A temporary method to provide oxygen until more definitive steps are taken to reverse total upper airway obstruction is placement of a 12–14-gauge catheter over the needle (extracath) through the **cricothyroid membrane.** The needle is removed and the catheter connected either to a jet injection device or to a 3-ml syringe with the plunger removed. A 15-mm endotracheal tube adapter fits into the barrel of the syringe and permits connection of an anesthesia breathing circuit. If the upper airway is totally obstructed, passive exhalation must be allowed to occur through the catheter to avoid development of excessive airway pressures.

V. ENDOTRACHEAL INTUBATION

A. **Indications for tracheal intubation are multiple** (Table 5-4).
B. **General anesthesia** does not mandate intubation of the trachea. Nevertheless, most general anesthetics are conducted with a tracheal tube in place.
C. Once it is determined that endotracheal intubation is necessary, an anesthesiologist must consider the following questions:
  1. **Type of laryngoscope blade.**
  2. **Type and size of tracheal tube.**
  3. **Nasotracheal versus orotracheal intubation.**
    a. Orotracheal intubation is selected unless the site of surgery is intraoral (an orotracheal tube could be easily displaced or interfere with a surgeon's access) or the patient's mouth cannot be opened.
    b. Nasotracheal intubation can be performed "blind" or under direct vision during direct laryngoscopy.
  4. **Intubate the trachea while a patient is awake or after induction of anesthesia?**
    a. Tracheal intubation after induction of anesthesia is selected unless the anesthesiologist de-

---

TABLE 5-4. Indications for Tracheal Intubation

Provide patent airway
Prevent aspiration
Facilitate positive-pressure ventilation
Operative position other than supine
Operative site near or involving the upper airway
Airway maintenance by mask difficult
Disease involving the upper airway

cides that the presence of certain factors (e.g., congenital or acquired upper airway abnormalities, cervical spine abnormalities, facial trauma, intestinal obstruction, recent food ingestion) dictate against rendering a patient unconscious before a tube (usually cuffed) is placed in the trachea.

  b. When intubation of the trachea while the patient is awake is selected, local anesthetics may be applied topically (aerosol lidocaine to the tongue, cocaine or phenylephrine to the nasal mucosa if appropriate), infiltrated (superior laryngeal nerve block), or instilled (translaryngeal injection of lidocaine through the cricothyroid membrane) to improve a patient's comfort (see Chapter 18). When aspiration of gastric contents is a consideration, a superior laryngeal nerve block and translaryngeal injection of local anesthetic should probably not be employed because this would anesthetize the vocal cords and remove the protective effect of reflex laryngeal closure.

D. Induction of anesthesia before orotracheal (or nasotracheal) intubation.

  1. Rapid-sequence induction. Intravenous injection of an induction drug (barbiturate, benzodiazepine, etomidate, propofol) followed in rapid sequence by a muscle relaxant (SCh or a short-acting nondepolarizing muscle relaxant) is a common method for induction of anesthesia. A defasciculating dose of a nondepolarizing muscle relaxant is commonly administered before SCh.

   a. The lungs are denitrogenated **(preoxygenation)** before the injection of drugs. In this regard, four maximal breaths of oxygen over 30 seconds are as effective as breathing oxygen spontaneously for 2–5 minutes.

   b. When a patient is considered to be at increased risk for regurgitation, an assistant applies **cricoid pressure** (Sellick's maneuver) to compress the esophagus against the cervical vertebrae until the cuffed tracheal tube is in place (Fig. 5-3).

  2. Inhalation induction. Volatile anesthetics (with or without N_2O) are administered in gradually increasing concentrations until a concentration of anesthetic adequate for surgery is established. Skeletal muscle relaxation to facilitate tracheal in-

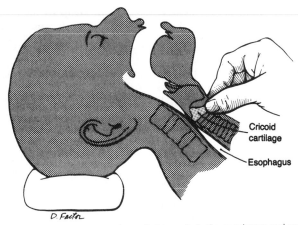

D. Factor

Figure 5-3. Cricoid pressure is applied to occlude the esophagus and prevent aspiration.

tubation is provided by the volatile anesthetic or by injection of a muscle relaxant.

  a. Initial intravenous injection of a reduced dose of an induction drug may be used to improve the patient's acceptance of the inhaled drug.

  b. An inhalation induction is not a likely selection when a patient is considered to be at risk for regurgitation.

VI. OROTRACHEAL INTUBATION

  A. Position of the patient. The height of the operating table is adjusted so that the patient's face is at the level of the standing anesthesiologist's xiphoid cartilage.

  1. Elevating the patient's head about 10 cm with pads under the occiput and extension of the head at the atlanto-occipital joint (**sniffing position**) serve to align the oral, pharyngeal, and laryngeal axes so that the passage from the lips to the glottic opening is almost a straight line.

  2. If it is not opened by extension of the head, the patient's mouth may be manually opened by depressing the mandible with the right thumb. The patient's lower lip can simultaneously be rolled away with the anesthesiologist's right index finger to prevent bruising it with the laryngoscope blade.

3. Routine use of gloves during all airway manipulations is recommended, as contact with saliva and blood may be the mechanism for exposure to infectious diseases (hepatitis, acquired immunodeficiency syndrome).

B. **Direct laryngoscopy.** The laryngoscope is held in the anesthesiologist's left hand (near the junction between the handle and blade) and inserted on the right side of the patient's mouth so as to avoid the incisor teeth and deflect the tongue to the left.

C. **Visualize the epiglottis.** The laryngoscope blade is advanced in the midline until the epiglottis is visualized. Depending on the type of blade selected, the tip of the blade is advanced into the vallecula (curved blade) or beneath the epiglottis (straight blade).

   1. When the blade is properly positioned, forward and upward movement exerted along the long axis of the laryngoscope handle (**"lift toward the feet— never lever"**) serves to elevate the epiglottis and expose the glottic opening.

   2. Depression or lateral movement of a patient's thyroid cartilage externally on the neck with the anesthesiologist's right hand may facilitate exposure of the glottic opening.

D. **Placement of the tracheal tube.** A previously selected tracheal tube is held in the anesthesiologist's right hand (like a pencil) and introduced on the right side of the patient's mouth (midline insertion obscures vision of the glottic opening), with the built-in curve directed anteriorly. The tube is advanced through the glottic opening until the cuff just passes the vocal cords. The amount of tube inserted should correspond to the distance predicted to place the distal end of the tube midway between the vocal cords and carina (21–23 cm from the lips in an adult). At this point, the laryngoscope blade is removed from the patient's mouth, the tube is secured to the patient's face with tape, and the tracheal tube cuff is inflated with air to form a seal with the tracheal mucosa. An adequate seal is confirmed by the absence of an audible air leak around the tube when positive airway pressure to 20–30 cm H_2O is applied.

E. **Confirmation of tracheal placement of the tube** (Table 5-5)

   1. Placement of the tube in the trachea rather than the esophagus is most reliably verified by the **presence of carbon dioxide (CO_2)** in the exhaled gases exiting through the tube. Documentation of exhaled CO_2 in three consecutive breaths (**PETCO_2 > 30 mm**

TABLE 5-5.   Evidence of Successful Tracheal Intubation

Carbon dioxide in exhaled gases
Bilateral breath sounds
Absence of air movement during epigastric auscultation
Condensation (fogging) of water vapor in tube during
  exhalation
Refilling of reservoir bag during exhalation
Maintenance of arterial oxygenation

Hg and recorded on a patient's anesthesia record)
should reduce the incidence of unrecognized
esophageal intubation to near zero. Esophageal intubation is indicated by a PET_{CO_2} reading near
zero.

   a. Recent ingestion of carbonated beverages may
result in an initial appearance of exhaled CO_2
from the esophagus.

   b. A single use device interposed between the endotracheal tube and anesthetic circuit that indicates the presence of CO_2 by a colorimetric
change is an alternative to capnography in areas
of the hospital other than the operating room
and during out-of-hospital resuscitation.

  2. Tracheal placement is further confirmed by the
presence of bilateral and equal breath sounds and
the absence of sounds over the epigastrium. Listen-
ing for breath sounds in each axilla minimizes the
chances of being misled by breath sounds transmitted from the opposite lung.

  3. After confirmation that the tube is in the trachea,
it is **mandatory to confirm that the distal end of
the tube is positioned in the midtrachea.** Detection
by external palpation of cuff distention in the suprasternal notch during rapid inflation of the cuff
is evidence that the distal end of the tracheal tube
is positioned midway between the vocal cords and
the carina. If the distance from the teeth to the distal end of the tube is 21–23 cm, endobronchial intubation is unlikely. It is important to recognize
that PET_{CO_2} is unlikely to be altered by endobronchial intubation.

   a. The presence of unequal breath sounds or
breath sounds only on one side of the thorax is
evidence that the tube may have been inserted
into a mainstem bronchus.

    b. Unexplained low oxygen saturation or decreases in pulmonary compliance should suggest an unrecognized endobronchial intubation.

VII. EXTUBATION OF THE TRACHEA

  A. When reintubation would be difficult or pulmonary aspiration is a risk, it is often recommended that extubation of the trachea be delayed until the patient is fully awake (reacting to the presence of the tube in the trachea). The trachea of a child is often extubated when the child is awake to minimize the likelihood of laryngospasm, which seems to occur more often in lightly anesthetized patients.

  B. Removal of the tube from the patient's trachea before awakening from anesthesia is acceptable in selected patients, especially if their reacting to the presence of the tube would elicit undesirable increases in blood pressure, intraocular pressure, or intracranial pressure.

  C. Suctioning of the pharynx is important before proceeding with tracheal extubation, because secretions could be aspirated or predispose to laryngospasm.

VIII. COMPLICATIONS OF ENDOTRACHEAL INTUBATION (Table 5-6)

  A. A patient's age influences the significance of certain complications. For example, 1 mm of edema decreases

---

TABLE 5-6. Complications of Endotracheal Intubation

During Intubation
Aspiration
Dental damage
Laceration of the lips or gums
Laryngeal injury
Esophageal intubation
Endobronchial intubation
Activation of the sympathetic nervous system
Bronchospasm

After Extubation
Aspiration
Laryngospasm
Transient vocal cord incompetence
Glottic or subglottic edema
Pharyngitis or tracheitis

the cross-sectional area of the glottic opening about 70% in an infant.

B. Some complications vary with a patient's gender. For example, sore throat is more common in females.

C. Duration of tracheal intubation influences the likelihood of certain complications such as vocal cord dysfunction and tracheal stenosis. For periods of a week or less, translaryngeal intubation of the trachea is generally preferred to tracheostomy.

IX. THE DIFFICULT AIRWAY (see Appendix G)

A. Difficulty in exposure of the glottic opening occurs in 1–3% of patients (may be more frequent in the parturient) and is usually predictable (see Table 5-1).

B. The degree of difficulty with intubation of the trachea may be classified on the basis of the view obtained at laryngoscopy (Fig. 5-4).

C. An organized approach to alternative methods of securing the airway is important when glottic exposure

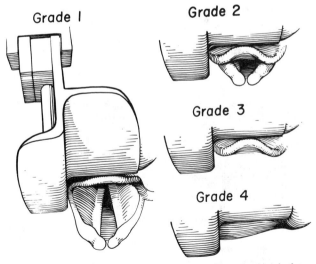

Figure 5-4. The degree of difficulty associated with tracheal intubation can be classified on the basis of the view obtained at laryngoscopy. A grade 4 view mandates the utilization of methods alternative to conventional direct laryngoscopy (e.g. fiberoptic laryngoscopy).

by direct laryngoscopy is difficult or impossible (see Appendix G).

X. FIBEROPTIC ENDOSCOPY

A. Intubation of the trachea using a flexible fiberoptic laryngoscope is useful for patients in whom the glottic opening cannot be visualized because of anatomic abnormalities. Provision of topical anesthesia greatly facilitates the procedure if a patient is awake. A fiberoptic laryngoscope can be passed through the nose or mouth.

B. When induction of anesthesia before fiberoptic laryngoscopy is appropriate, it may be helpful to use an endoscopic airway and endoscopic mask with a separate port for insertion of a fiberoptic laryngoscope, thus allowing continued delivery of anesthesia and uninterrupted ventilation of the lungs during the procedure (Fig. 5-5).

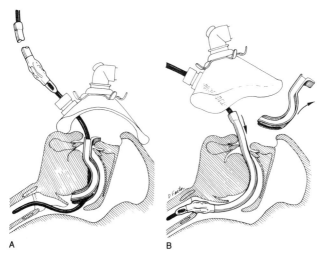

A   B

Figure 5-5. Fiberoptic laryngoscopy during general anesthesia is facilitated by use of an endoscopic mask with an introductory port plus an endoscopic airway that maintains the midline position of the fiberscope.

**TABLE 5-7. Steps in Performing Fiberoptic
Laryngoscopy and Tracheal Intubation**

Administer an antisialagogue

Use largest fiberscope that will fit easily into the tracheal tube

Lubricate sheath of fiberscope (avoid lens)

Focus lens and apply antifogging agent

Thread fiberscope into tube and confirm that tip moves up and down (not sideways)

Insert tracheal tube orally, keeping orientation in midline (endoscopic airway) and advance fiberscope until vocal cords are visible.

Advance fiberscope until tracheal rings or carina is visible

Hold fiberscope firmly in a neutral position and thread tube into the trachea (retraction of the tongue and anterior displacement of the mandible may be necessary to change the angle between the oropharynx and trachea)

    C. A step-by-step procedure should be followed when fiberoptic endoscopic examination is performed (Table 5-7).

6

Patient Positioning

Positioning is important for surgical exposure but, at the same time, may introduce physiologic compromises and the potential for nerve damage (Martin JT: Patient positioning. In Barash PG, Cullen BF, Stoelting RK [eds]: Clinical Anesthesia, pp 709–736. Philadelphia, JB Lippincott, 1992). **Decubitus** indicates that part of the patient that is in contact with the operating table.

I. DORSAL DECUBITUS POSITIONS
A. Physiology
1. **Circulation.** In patients in the supine position, the influence of gravity on the vascular system is minimal. Intravascular pressures change by **2 mm Hg for every 2.5 cm** that a given site varies in vertical height above or below the reference point at the heart. **This is the reason to place transducers at the level of vital organs to be perfused (heart or brain).** Head-down tilt (Trendelenburg position) increases cerebral venous pressure and intracranial pressure. An accompanying increase in central blood volume activates baroreceptors to produce peripheral vasodilation and an unchanged to decreased cardiac output.
2. **Respiration.** Movement of abdominal viscera toward or away from the diaphragm in association with the head-up or head-down position influences the effectiveness of spontaneous ventilation.
B. Variations of the dorsal decubitus position (Table 6-1)
C. Complications of the dorsal decubitus positions (Table 6-2)
1. **Ulnar nerve injury** is a frequent cause of postsurgical litigation, emphasizing the importance of protecting this nerve during anesthesia.
   a. Supination of the hand shifts the weight of the

TABLE 6-1. Dorsal Decubitus Positions

Supine

Horizontal (does not place hips and knees in a neutral
position, poorly tolerated in awake patients)

Contoured (slightly flex hips and knees, good for routine
use)

Frog leg (knees bent and soles of feet together; permits
access to the perineum and vagina for the surgeon
standing at the side of the patient's abdomen).

Lithotomy (worsens pain of a herniated disk)

Standard (legs flexed at hips and knees and simultaneously
elevated to expose perineum; at the end of surgery, both
legs should be lowered together to minimize torsion stress
on the lumbar spine)

Exaggerated (stresses the lumbar spine and restricts
ventilation because of abdominal compression by the
thighs)

Trendelenburg (shoulder braces are placed over the
acromioclavicular joint to avoid compression of the brachial
plexus)

TABLE 6-2. Complications of Dorsal Decubitus Position

Postural hypotension (most common complication of head-up
position; lower legs simultaneously from lithotomy position
if patient is hypovolemic)

Pressure alopecia (use padded head supports)

Pressure-point reactions (heels, elbows, sacrum)

Brachial plexus injuries (most likely if the head is turned away
from an excessively abducted arm; may be associated with
first rib fracture during median sternotomy)

Radial nerve compression (vertical bar of screen forces nerve
against the humerus; wristdrop)

Ulnar nerve compression (trauma occurs as the nerve passes
behind the medial epicondyle of the humerus; sensory loss
over the fifth finger)

Lumbar backache (ligamentous relaxation during anesthesia)

elbow onto the olecranon process and protects
the ulnar nerve (Fig. 6-1).

   b. Soft padding is added routinely to the pressure
point of each elbow.

  2. A preoperative history of ulnar neuropathies is associated with the possibility of a postoperative re-

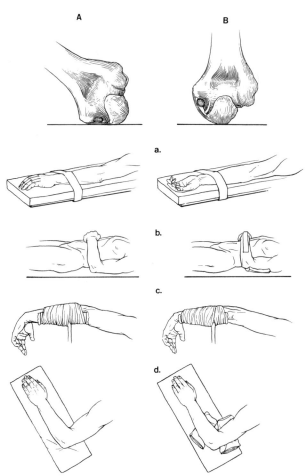

Figure 6-1. The ulnar nerve at the cubital tunnel. Column A shows positions (pronation) that may increase the likelihood of nerve compression at the cubital tunnel. Column B shows positions and techniques (supination and padding) that may decrease the likelihood of nerve compression at the cubital tunnel.

currence despite special precautions of padding and positioning.

3. Prompt recognition of ulnar hypesthesia after the conclusion of anesthesia (opioids cannot mask loss of sensation due to nerve dysfunction) suggests an intraoperative etiology.

II. LATERAL DECUBITUS POSITIONS

A. Physiology
1. **Circulation.** In the low-pressure pulmonary circuit, there is overperfusion of the dependent lung and relative hypoperfusion of the lung that is positioned superiorly. A small support should be placed just caudad to the down-side axilla so as to lift the thorax enough to relieve pressure on the axillary neurovascular bundle and prevent reduced blood flow to the hand. Dependent venous pooling is minimized by compressive wrappings applied to the legs and thighs.
2. **Respiration.** Ventilation tends to be directed to the more compliant superiorly positioned lung, resulting in hyperventilation of this underperfused lung and hypoventilation of the overperfused dependent lung.

B. Variations of the lateral decubitus positions (Table 6-3)

C. Complications of the lateral decubitus position (Table 6-4)

III. VENTRAL DECUBITUS POSITIONS

A. Physiology
1. **Circulation.** Pressure on compressed viscera is transmitted to mesenteric and paravertebral vessels, resulting in increased venous bleeding.
2. **Respiration.** Compressed abdominal viscera force the diaphragm cephalad. Support provided by pads under the shoulder girdle and pelvis allow the abdomen to hang free, thus minimizing loss of func-

---

TABLE 6-3. Lateral Decubitus Positions

Standard lateral position
   Flex the down-side thigh and knee, pillows placed between the legs and under the head to maintain alignment of the cervical and thoracic spines

Flexed lateral positions
   Lateral jackknife (down-side iliac crest is over the table hinge to allow stretch of the up-side flank; venous pooling occurs in the legs)
   Kidney (elevated table rest under the iliac crest further increases lateral flexion to expose kidney; venous pooling and ventilation/perfusion mismatch may occur)

TABLE 6-4. Complications of Lateral Decubitus Position

Damage to the eyes and/or ears (avoid pressure)

Neck injury (lateral flexion is a risk, especially in arthritic patients)

Suprascapular nerve injury (a pad caudad to the dependent axilla prevents circumduction of the nerve; injury manifests as diffuse shoulder pain)

Atelectasis

Aseptic necrosis of up-side femoral head (restraining tape forces the head of the femur into the acetabulum and obstructs the nutrient artery; place restraining tape across the soft tissue in the space between the head of the femur and the crest of the ileum)

Peroneal nerve injury (compressed against the mattress as it passes laterally around the neck of fibula; loss of sensation over the dorsum of the foot)

TABLE 6-5. Ventral Decubitus Positions

Full prone (use supportive pads under the abdomen)

Prone jackknife

Kneeling

TABLE 6-6. Complications of Ventral Decubitus Positions

Eyes and ears (avoid pressure)

Neck injury (an arthritic neck may be best managed in the sagittal plane; head rotation may reduce carotid and vertebral blood flows)

Brachial plexus injuries

Thoracic outlet syndrome

Breast injuries

Impaired venous return (use supportive pads under the abdomen)

tional residual capacity and obstruction to venous return.

B. Variations of the ventral decubitus positions (Table 6-5)

C. Complications of the ventral decubitus position (Table 6-6)

IV. HEAD-ELEVATED POSITIONS

A. **The sitting position** permits improved surgical exposure for operations involving the posterior fossa and cervical spine. Mean arterial pressure should be measured at the level of the circle of Willis (transducer placed at level of external ear canal), as this site is the best to indicate perfusion pressure at the brain. Compressive wraps about the legs reduce pooling of blood in the lower extremities.

B. **Complications** (Table 6-7)

TABLE 6-7. Complications of the Sitting Position

Postural hypotension (normal compensatory reflexes are inhibited by anesthesia)

Air embolus (air can pass through a probe patent foramen ovale if right atrial pressure exceeds left atrial pressure)

Pneumocephalus

Ocular compression

Edema of the face and tongue

Midcervical tetraplegia

Sciatic nerve injury

7

Monitoring the Anesthetized Patient

Monitoring represents the process by which anesthesiologists recognize and evaluate potential physiologic problems by identifying prognostic trends in patients in a timely manner (Gilbert HC, Vender JS: Monitoring the anesthetized patient. In: Barash PG, Cullen BF, Stoelting RK [eds]: Clinical Anesthesia, pp 737–770. Philadelphia, JB Lippincott, 1992). Effective monitoring of both the patient and the equipment used for administering anesthesia should, in theory, diminish preventable mishaps as well as reduce poor outcomes that may follow surgical procedures, disease processes, or adverse effects related to administration of anesthesia. The question of choice of monitors and their usefulness is a matter of convention, technology, politics, litigation, and personal taste. Standards for intraoperative monitoring have been adopted by The American Society of Anesthesiologists (Appendix F).

I. INSPIRATORY AND EXPIRED GAS MONITORING

A. Inspired Oxygen Monitoring

1. The concentration of oxygen in the anesthetic circuit is measured with a sensor placed in the expiratory limb or more commonly in the inspiratory limb.

   a. When the sensor is placed in the inspiratory limb, the use of oxygen analyzers is helpful in detecting a disconnection of the fresh gas flow.

   b. If the sensor is placed in the expiratory limb, endotracheal tube disconnects may also be identified.

2. Use of an **oxygen analyzer** ensures that a hypoxic oxygen concentration is not delivered to the patient but does not guarantee the adequacy of arterial oxygenation.

  3. Three types of oxygen analyzers have been intro-
     duced for clinical use: paramagnetic, polarographic,
     and galvanic cell monitors.
B. **Monitoring of Expired Gases**
  1. **Infrared Capnography**
     a. Expiratory CO_2 monitoring has evolved as an im-
        portant physiologic and safety monitor for **iden-
        tifying appropriate placement of endotracheal
        tubes** and assessing variables such as ventilation
        (i.e., indirect measurement of Pa_{CO_2}, rebreath-
        ing), cardiac output, distribution of blood flow,
        and metabolic activity.
     b. **Capnometry** is the measurement and numeric
        representation of the CO_2 concentration (mm
        Hg).
     c. A **capnogram** is a continuous concentration-
        time display of the CO_2 concentration (divided
        into four distinct phrases) sampled at the pa-
        tient's airway during ventilation (Fig. 7-1).
     d. **Capnography** is the continuous monitoring of
        the patient's capnogram.
     e. **End-tidal CO_2** provides a clinical estimate of the
        Pa_{CO_2}, assuming ventilation and perfusion in the
        lungs are appropriately matched (normal gra-
        dient, 5–10 mm Hg) and no sampling errors oc-
        cur during measurement (sidestream analyzers
        can dilute a patient's tidal breath with fresh gas,

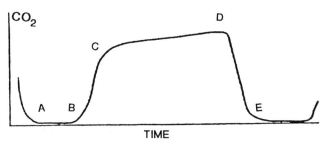

Figure 7-1. The capnogram is divided into four distinct phases. The first
phase (A-B) represents the initial stage of expiration (gas from anatomic
dead space) and is usually devoid of CO_2. At point B, CO_2-containing gas
is present at the sampling site, and a sharp upstroke (BC) is seen in the
capnogram. Phase C-D represents the ventilation-weighted average concentration of CO_2 in alveolar gas. Point D is the highest value and is desig-
nated the end-tidal CO_2 concentration. At point D, the patient begins to
inspire CO_2-free gas, and there is a steep downstroke (D-E) back to baseline. Normally, unless rebreathing of CO_2 occurs, the baseline approaches
zero.

especially when tidal volume is small, as in the young patient; loose connections and system leaks also dilute end-tidal CO_2).

f. **Dead space** (ventilation without perfusion) and a resulting increase in the $Paco_2$-end-tidal CO_2 gradient (the greater the dead space, the lower the end-tidal CO_2) may reflect hypoperfusion states, chronic obstructive pulmonary disease, and embolic phenomena (thrombus, air).

g. **Shunt** (perfusion without ventilation) causes minimal changes in the $Paco_2$-end-tidal CO_2 gradient.

h. Capnography has **decreased the potential for unrecognized accidental esophageal intubation.** Since the esophageal or gastric gas concentration is primarily composed of inspired gas, it should contain exceedingly small amounts of CO_2. Following an esophageal intubation, the first one or two "breaths" may contain some CO_2, but the concentration should approach zero after four or five "breaths." **A continuous stable CO_2 waveform** ensures the presence of alveolar ventilation (tube in the trachea) but does not necessarily indicate that the endotracheal tube is properly positioned above the carina in the trachea.

i. Common etiologies of **gradual increases or decreases in end-tidal CO_2** reflect **changes in CO_2 production** or **changes in CO_2 elimination** (Table 7-1).

j. A **sudden decrease in end-tidal CO_2 to near zero or zero** requires a rapid assessment of possible causes (Table 7-2).

TABLE 7-1. Changing End-Tidal CO_2 Concentrations

Increases in End-Tidal CO_2	Decreases in End-Tidal CO_2
Hyperthermia	Hypothermia
Sepsis	Hypometabolism
Malignant hyperthermia	Hyperventilation
Skeletal muscle activity	Hypoperfusion
Hypoventilation	Embolism
Rebreathing	

TABLE 7-2. Causes of Sudden Decrease in End-Tidal CO$_2$

Malposition of tracheal tube in pharynx or esophagus
Disruption of airway integrity (disconnection or obstruction)
Disruption of sampling line
Pulmonary embolism
Low cardiac output
Cardiac arrest

---

    k. The adequacy of cardiopulmonary resuscitation can be assessed by capnography, as reflected by a reappearance or an increase in end-tidal CO$_2$ with restoration of pulmonary blood flow (see Chapter 44).

    l. The size and shape of the capnogram waveform can be informative (Table 7-3).

  2. Multiple Expired Gas Analysis

    a. Intraoperative breath-by-breath analysis of respiratory (O$_2$, CO$_2$, N$_2$) and anesthetic gases is achieved by mass spectrometry or Raman spectroscopy (RASCAL is an instrument using this technology).

    b. Many critical events can be detected by analysis of respiratory and anesthetic gases (Table 7-4).

    c. Nitrogen monitoring provides quantification of washout during **preoxygenation.** A sudden rise in the nitrogen concentration in the exhaled gas indicates either introduction of air from **leaks in the anesthesia delivery system** or **venous air embolism.**

C. Oxygen Monitoring

  1. Pulse Oximetry

    a. This monitor is the **standard of care for monitoring oxygenation** during anesthesia.

    b. Pulse oximetry combines the use of plethysmography and spectrophotometric analysis (light-emitting diodes are sources of two wavelengths of light that are passed through an arterial bed; absorption of specific wavelengths of light relative to the ratio of oxyhemoglobin to reduced hemoglobin is transmitted to a photodetector) to calculate oxygen saturation of hemoglobin (SpO$_2$) on a noninvasive, continuous basis.

TABLE 7-3. Information Derived from the Capnogram Waveform

Slow Rate of Rise of Upstroke
  Chronic obstructive pulmonary disease
  Acute airway obstruction

Normally Shaped but Increased End-Tidal CO_2
  Alveolar hypoventilation
  Increased CO_2 production

Transient Increases in End-Tidal CO_2
  Tourniquet release/aortic unclamping
  Administration of bicarbonate
  CO_2 insufflation during laparoscopy

Failure of the Baseline to Return to Zero
  Rebreathing

TABLE 7-4. Gas Analysis and the Detection of Critical Events

Event	Monitored Gas
Error in gas delivery system	Oxygen
Anesthesia machine malfunction	Carbon dioxide
	Nitrogen
	Inhaled anesthetic
Vaporizer malfunction or contamination	Volatile anesthetic
Anesthesia circuit leaks	Nitrogen
Endotracheal tube cuff leaks	Carbon dioxide
Poor mask fit	
Air embolism	
Hypoventilation	Carbon dioxide
Airway obstruction	
Disconnection	
Malignant hyperthermia	
Circuit hypoxia	Oxygen

    c. A relationship exists between hemoglobin saturation and oxygen tension as depicted by the **oxyhemoglobin dissociation curve** (Fig. 7-2).
    d. Pulse oximetry measures functional saturation of hemoglobin (but does not distinguish between hemoglobin saturated with oxygen or other molecules), which may be higher than the SaO_2 measured by a laboratory co-oximeter.

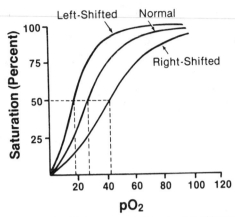

Figure 7-2. The relationship between arterial saturation of hemoglobin with oxygen (%) and P_{O_2} is represented by the sigmoid-shaped oxyhemoglobin dissociation curve.

    e. Many factors may influence the accuracy or ability of the pulse oximeter to calculate SpO_2 (Table 7-5).

    f. Fetal hemoglobin has limited influence on the accuracy of SpO_2.

    g. Pulse oximetry does not ensure adequacy of oxygen delivery to or utilization by the tissues, nor is this monitor a replacement for blood gas measurements.

  2. Transcutaneous Gas Monitoring

    a. Transcutaneous oxygen tension ($PtcO_2$) is not identical to PaO_2, although similar trends may be reflected.

    b. Heating the cutaneous electrode to 43° C improves the accuracy of the sensor but introduces the risk of skin burns.

    c. Transconjunctival oxygen monitoring does not require heating, but the measured value is always less than the measured PaO_2.

II. BLOOD PRESSURE MONITORING

  A. Intraoperative measurement and recording of arterial blood pressure (lateral pressure exerted on arteries as

TABLE 7-5. Factors That Influence Accuracy of Pulse Oximetry

Absence of a Pulsatile Waveform
 Hypothermia
 Hypotension
 Altered vascular resistance (vasoactive drugs)

Factitiously High Sp_{O_2}
 Increased carboxyhemoglobin concentration
 Increased methemoglobin concentration (Sp_{O_2} tends to be
  85% regardless of actual Sa_{O_2} or Pa_{O_2})

Motion
 Awake patient
 Shivering

Extraneous Light Sources

Factitiously Low Sp_{O_2}
 Methylene blue
 Nail polish

it flows) is an essential aspect of anesthesia care and is
mandated as an important indicator of the adequacy of
circulation during anesthesia.

1. Traditionally, anesthesiologists routinely measure
   and record **systolic blood pressure** (SBP) and **diastolic blood pressure** (DBP) at 5-minute intervals.
2. Changes in SBP correlate with changes in myocardial oxygen requirements.
3. Changes in DBP reflect coronary perfusion pressure.
4. **Mean arterial pressure** (MAP) is the hydrostatic
   force that provides for diffusion and filtration functions.
5. MAP is utilized in calculating resistance to blood
   flow (R), using the equation R = MAP divided by
   blood flow (Q). Rearranged, this equation is Q =
   MAP/R.

B. Arterial Pressure Wave
1. As blood pressure is examined from the aorta to the
   distal arteries, it appears to increase.

2. The tapering of peripheral arteries confines the pressure trace energy, producing an increase in SBP.

3. Intra-arterial measurements in peripheral arteries demonstrate that SBP is higher and MAP is lower than in the aorta, reflecting the effects of forward wave propagation and wave reflection.

C. **Indirect Measurement of Arterial Blood Pressure**

1. The simplest method of blood pressure determination estimates SBP by palpating the return of the arterial pulse or Doppler sounds while an occluding cuff is deflated.

2. **Auscultation** of the Korotkoff sounds (which result from turbulent flow within an artery in response to the mechanical deformation from the blood pressure cuff) is a common method of blood pressure measurement.

   a. SBP is signaled by the appearance of the first Korotkoff sound, whereas disappearance of the sounds or a muffled tone signals the DBP.

   b. The detection of sound changes is subjective, requires pulsatile flow (unreliable during low flow), and is prone to mechanical errors (Table 7-6).

   c. Comparison of direct intra-arterial pressure recordings with blood pressure determined by auscultation can show considerable divergence, whereas correlation of direct arterial measurement of SBP with the value determined by Doppler sphygmomanometry is good.

TABLE 7-6. **Mechanical Errors Associated with Auscultatory Measurement of Blood Pressure**

Falsely High Estimates of Blood Pressure
Cuff too small (bladder width should approximate 40% of the circumference of the extremity)
Cuff applied too loosely
Uneven compression of the underlying artery
Extremity is below heart level

Falsely Low Estimates of Blood Pressure
Cuff too large
Cuff deflation >3 mm Hg·s^{-1}
Extremity is above heart level

3. **Automated oscillometry** (*Dinamap*) has replaced auscultatory and palpatory techniques for routine intraoperative blood pressure monitoring.
   a. Oscillometry accurately measures SBP, DBP, and MAP (error less than 5 mm Hg when compared with a centrally placed arterial line).
   b. A variety of cuff sizes makes it possible to utilize oscillometry in all age groups.
4. **Indirect Continuous Noninvasive Techniques**
   a. *Finapres* uses infrared light and detects oscillations within a finger cuff.
   b. *Artrac* estimates SBP and DBP by measuring the pulse wave velocity and changes in blood volume using two photometric sensors placed on the forehead and a digit.
5. **Problems Associated with Noninvasive Monitoring** (Table 7-7)

D. **Invasive Measurement of Arterial Blood Pressure**
   1. Indwelling arterial cannulation not only offers anesthesiologists the opportunity to monitor beat-to-beat changes in arterial blood pressure but also provides vascular access for arterial blood sampling.
   2. Although they are thought of as the gold standard, intra-arterial techniques are subject to many sources of error based on the physical properties of fluid motion and the performance of the catheter-transducer-amplification system used to sense, process, and display the pressure pulse wave.
      a. Ideally, the catheters and tubings are very stiff, the mass of the fluid is small, the number of

---

TABLE 7-7. Problems Associated with Noninvasive Automatic Cycled Cuff-Based Pressure Monitoring Systems

Edema of the extremity

Petechiae formation

Ulnar neuropathy (apply encircling cuff proximal to the ulnar groove)

Interference with timing of intravenous drug administration when access site is located in the same extremity as monitoring system

Hydrostatic effect (correct by adding or subtracting 0.7 mm Hg for every centimeter the cuff is above or below the heart)

stopcocks is limited, and the connecting tubing length is not excessive.

b. In clinical practice, underdamped catheter-transducer systems tend to overestimate SBP by 15–30 mm Hg and to amplify artifact (catheter whip).

c. Air bubbles cause overdamping and underestimation of the SBP.

d. MAP is accurately measured even in the presence of overdamping or underdamping.

e. In clinical practice, it is sufficient to calibrate the transducer to atmospheric pressure, usually with the transducer located at the level of the right atrium.

f. **Since many therapeutic decisions are based on changes in arterial blood pressure, it is imperative that anesthesiologists understand the physical limitations imposed by fluid-filled pressure transducer systems.**

2. The **radial artery** remains the most popular site for cannulation because of its accessibility and the presence of a collateral blood supply (Figure 7-3 and Table 7-8).

a. The prognostic value of the **Allen test** in assessing the adequacy of the ulnar collateral circulation may have been overestimated.

b. Abnormal radial artery blood flow following the removal of an arterial catheter (nontapered 20–22 gauge Teflon catheter recommended) occurs

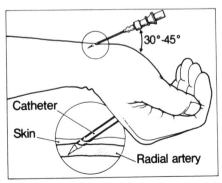

Figure 7-3. Technique for radial artery cannulation.

TABLE 7-8. Cannulation Sites for Direct Arterial Blood Pressure Monitoring

Site	Clinical Points
Radial artery	Ischemia most likely reflects arterial thrombosis Aneurysm formation Arteriovenous fistula formation Infection Fluid overload in neonates from continuous flush techniques (3–6 ml·h^{-1})
Ulnar artery	Complications similar to those for radial artery Primary source of hand blood flow
Brachial artery	Insertion site medial to biceps tendon Median nerve damage
Axillary artery	Insertion site at junction of pectoralis major and deltoid muscles
Femoral artery	Easy access in low-flow states Potential for local and retroperitoneal hemorrhage Longer catheters preferred
Dorsalis pedis artery	Higher systolic blood pressure

frequently (presumably a reflection of radial artery thrombosis), with normalization of blood flow usually occurring in 3–70 days.

3. Direct arterial pressure monitoring requires constant vigilance and correlation of the measured blood pressure with other clinical parameters before therapeutic interventions are initiated.

   a. Sudden increases or decreases in blood pressure may represent a hydrostatic error because the position of the transducer was not adjusted following changes in the position of the operating room table.

   b. A sudden decrease in blood pressure may be caused by a damped tracing because the arterial catheter is partially occluded or kinked.

   c. **Before initiating therapy,** the transducer systems should be calibrated and the patency of the arterial cannula verified.

III. CENTRAL VENOUS AND PULMONARY ARTERY MONITORING

A. The **right internal jugular vein** is preferred as an access site (Figures 7-4, 7-5, and 7-6 and Table 7-9).

B. **Central Venous Pressure Monitoring**

   1. Central venous pressure (CVP) is essentially equivalent to right atrial pressure, and the normal waveform consists of three peaks (a, c, and v waves) and two descents (x, y) (Fig. 7-7 and Table 7-10).

      a. The possibility of venous air embolism is decreased by positioning the patient in a head-down position during central venous catheter placement or removal.

      b. Central venous catheter placement is an important source of nosocomial infection and sepsis;

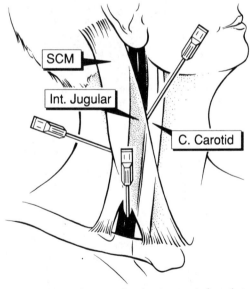

Figure 7-4. Three anatomic approaches for placement of a catheter in the internal jugular vein. The patient is placed head down with the head turned away from the intended venipuncture site. A 22-gauge **locator needle** may be inserted initially to identify the vein and thus minimize the likelihood of accidental carotid artery puncture when placing the larger needle. Return of desaturated blood or transduction of the catheter (venous pressure) confirms entry into the internal jugular vein.

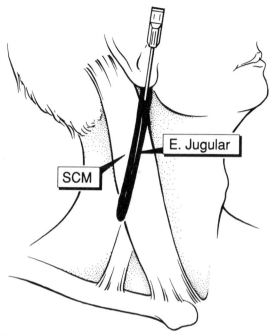

Figure 7-5. Placement of a catheter in the external jugular vein.

this underscores the importance of sterile technique during catheter placement and of the application of appropriate dressings (Table 7-11).

C. Pulmonary Artery Monitoring

    1. **Indications** for placement of a pulmonary artery catheter are broadly defined (the need to measure intracardiac pressures, thermodilution cardiac output, and mixed venous oxygen saturation; calculation of derived hemodynamic indices). The derived information is utilized to help define the clinical problem, monitor the progression of hemodynamic dysfunction, and guide the response to therapy.

    2. Correct placement of the pulmonary artery catheter is most often guided by using changes in vascular waveforms (Fig. 7-8).

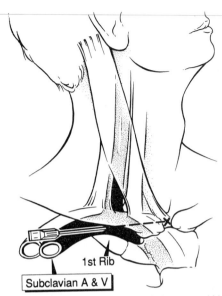

Figure 7-6. Placement of a catheter (infraclavicular approach) in the subclavian vein. The patient is placed head down with the head turned away from the intended venipuncture site. Placing a roll between the scapulas opens the space between the clavicle and first rib. The needle is inserted 1 cm below the midpoint of the clavicle and advanced toward the anesthesiologist's finger in the suprasternal notch keeping close to the posterior surface of the clavicle. Return of desaturated blood or transduction of the catheter (venous pressure) confirms entry into the subclavian vein.

3. Pulmonary capillary wedge pressure (PCWP) is used to indirectly assess left ventricular end-diastolic volume by reflecting changes in left ventricular end-diastolic pressure.
   a. Right-sided pressures often are poor indicators of left ventricular filling, either as absolute numbers or in terms of direction of change in response to therapy.
   b. **Increased pulmonary vascular resistance** distorts the usual correlation between PCWP and pulmonary artery end-diastolic pressure (PAEDP).
   c. PCWP and PAEDP measurements are affected by the position of the catheter tip in the pulmonary artery (confirm by a lateral chest x-ray) and changes in intrathoracic pressure (positive pres-

TABLE 7-9. Central Venous Cannulation Sites

Site	Advantages	Disadvantages
Right internal jugular vein	Accessible from head of operating room table Predictable anatomy High success rate in both adults and children Good landmarks	Carotid artery puncture Trauma to brachial plexus Pneumothorax
Left internal jugular vein	Same as for right internal jugular vein	Thoracic duct damage Difficulty in maneuvering catheter through the jugular-subclavian junction Carotid artery puncture and embolization of the left dominant cerebral hemisphere
External jugular vein	Superficial location Safety	Lower success rate Kinks at subclavian vein
Subclavian vein	Accessible Good landmarks	Pneumothorax Hemothorax Chylothorax Pleural effusion
Antecubital vein	Few complications	Lowest success rate Thrombosis Thrombophlebitis
Femoral vein	High success rate	Catheter sepsis Thrombophlebitis

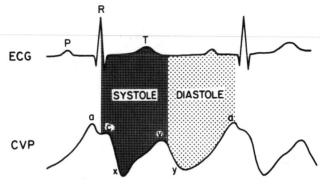

Figure 7-7. Central venous pressure (CVP) waveforms in relation to electrical events on the electrocardiogram (ECG).

TABLE 7-10. Diagnostic Value of Central Venous Pressure Waveform	
Waveform	**Associated Conditions**
Large a Waves	Tricuspid stenosis
	Pulmonic stenosis
	Pulmonary hypertension
	Decreased right ventricular compliance
Large v Waves	Tricuspid regurgitation
	Right ventricular papillary muscle ischemia and/or right ventricular failure
	Constrictive pericarditis
	Cardiac tamponade

TABLE 7-11. Complications Common to All Central Venous Pressure Catheter Placement Techniques

Accidental arterial puncture (hematoma, false aneurysm, arteriovenous fistula)

Poor positioning of catheter during placement (vascular or cardiac chamber perforation, cardiac dysrhythmias)

Injury to surrounding structures

Clot and fibrinous sleeve formation

Thrombosis of the vein (embolus)

Catheter-related sepsis

Bleeding

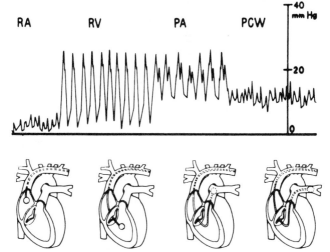

Figure 7-8. Pressure tracing observed during flotation of a pulmonary artery catheter through the right atrium (RA), right ventricle (RV), pulmonary artery (PA), and into a pulmonary capillary wedge (PCW) position.

sure ventilation, positive end-expiratory pressure; measure PCWP at end expiration).

4. **Cardiac dysrhythmias** are the most common complication associated with pulmonary artery catheter passage. Pulmonary artery perforation and hemorrhage represent the most life-threatening complication (Tables 7-12 and 7-13).

5. Advances in fiberoptic technology have led to the development of pulmonary artery catheters that can continuously measure **mixed venous oxygen saturation** (Sv_{O_2}). Mixed venous oximetry is a powerful tool for both diagnostic and therapeutic assessments in critically ill patients.

   a. Sv_{O_2} varies directly with cardiac output, hemoglobin concentration, and Sa_{O_2} and inversely with minute oxygen consumption.

   b. When all other variables are constant, Sv_{O_2} reflects changes in cardiac output.

   c. The normal Sv_{O_2} is 75%, and anaerobic metabolism occurs when Sv_{O_2} is <30%.

**TABLE 7-12. Complications of Pulmonary Artery
Catheter Passage**

Cardiac dysrhythmias
Catheter knotting, kinking, or coiling
Cardiac valve damage
Heart block
Perforation of pulmonary artery, right atrium, or right ventricle

---

**TABLE 7-13. Complications of Pulmonary Artery
Catheter Presence**

Thrombosis	Pulmonary infarction
Pulmonary artery rupture	Thrombocytopenia
Sepsis	Cardiac valve damage
Endocarditis	Thromboembolism
Balloon rupture	Cardiac dysrhythmias

IV. MONITORING CARDIAC FUNCTION

   A. Cardiac output and hemodynamic variables derived
      from estimates of blood pressure and blood flow are
      important indices of myocardial performance and the
      status of the circulatory system.
   B. **Thermodilution cardiac output determination** is the
      most widely utilized adaptation of the indicator dilu-
      tion principle (cooled 5% dextrose or 0.9% saline is
      injected into the CVP port of a thermodilution pulmo-
      nary artery catheter and a thermistor in the pulmonary
      artery records the decrease in temperature between the
      two points, which is proportional to blood flow or car-
      diac output).
      1. Comparison studies suggest that either room tem-
         perature or an iced injectate can be used, but the
         iced injectate produces a more exacting curve with
         a better signal-to-noise ratio.
      2. When properly performed (maintaining consis-
         tency of injection volume and injection rate), ther-
         modilution cardiac output measurements correlate
         well with direct Fick's and dye dilution determi-
         nations.
         a. False high thermodilution cardiac output deter-
            minations occur when the injectate volume is
            too small (incomplete filling of syringe, leaks) or
            there is a thrombus insulating the pulmonary ar-
            tery catheter thermistor.

      b. Alterations in right-sided cardiac output vary during inhalation and exhalation, such that thermodilution cardiac measurements at peak inspiration and end-expiration have less variability.

      c. Repetition of injections should be delayed for at least 90 seconds to allow for a steady thermal environment.

      d. In clinical practice, triplicate determinations are averaged to increase precision (differences <15% are not of clinical significance).

      e. It is important to consider sources of inaccuracies in measurement of thermodilution cardiac output before initiating changes in clinical treatment based on this measurement.

  C. Intraoperative cardiac imaging utilizing **two-dimensional transesophageal echocardiography** has added a new dimension to monitoring cardiac function during anesthesia and surgery (Table 7-14).

V. MONITORING NEUROLOGIC FUNCTION

  A. **Intracranial pressure (ICP) monitoring** was initially utilized in the management of trauma where the relationship between uncontrolled ICP elevation and fatality has been firmly established.

    1. ICP can be monitored by insertion of a subarachnoid bolt (Richmond bolt), insertion of a ventricular catheter, insertion of an epidural transducer, or placement of a fiberoptic sensor in the epidural space.

      a. Each of these techniques is invasive and requires a burr hole.

TABLE 7-14. Clinical Application of Intraoperative Transesophageal Echocardiography

Global Cardiac Function
  Ejection fraction
  Cardiac output
  Effects of anesthesia and surgery

Regional Wall Motion
  Segmental wall ischemia versus changes in afterload

Anatomic Assessment
  Mitral valve function
  Aortic valve function
  Aortic aneurysms and dissections
  Congenital heart disease
  Intracardiac air

        b. Normal ICP is <15 mm Hg.

        c. An acute increase in cerebral blood volume may result in a sustained increase of 50–100 mm Hg in the ICP (plateau wave).

    2. ICP monitoring does not measure neural function or neural recovery.

B. The electroencephalogram (EEG) represents the spontaneous electrical activity of pyramidal cells located in the outer cerebral cortex.

    1. The EEG signal is difficult to measure and evaluate accurately in the operating room because of low voltages (10–100 μV; 1000 times lower than electrocardiogram signals) and the variation in frequencies (1–30 Hz) as recorded from scalp electrodes.

        a. During periods of ischemia or while the patient is under general anesthesia, EEG activity generally decreases in both amplitude and frequency (see Tables 19-4 and 19-5).

        b. Generation of EEG activity is responsible for approximately 50% of the total oxygen consumption of the cerebral cortex.

    2. EEG monitoring has been advocated for the intraoperative detection of cerebral ischemia during deliberate hypotension or during carotid endarterectomy; for the intraoperative or perioperative assessment of pharmacologic interventions; for the identification of epileptic foci; or for the assessment of coma or brain death.

    3. Several signal processing techniques (compressed spectral array) have been utilized to produce displays of EEG information so as to improve the ability to interpret changes or evaluate trends.

C. Evoked potentials are useful because they monitor the functional integrity of specific brain stem, visual, or peripheral neural pathways.

    1. Evoked potentials represent a small electrical signal generated in neural pathways following periodic neural stimulation.

        a. In the cortex and subcortex, the evoked potential signals are much smaller than the background EEG, such that computer signal averaging and filtering are used to remove the random background electrical activity.

        b. The averaged evoked response is then displayed as a plot of voltage over time.

    2. Three sensory pathways are commonly utilized intraoperatively to monitor neural function (Table 7-15).

3. Anesthetic drugs, blood pressure changes, and temperature changes may interfere with interpretation and assessment of evoked potentials in the intraoperative period (see Table 19-6).

VI. NEUROMUSCULAR MONITORING

A. It is desirable to monitor the status of the neuromuscular junction with a **nerve stimulator** when using neuromuscular blocking agents during anesthesia (Table 7-16). Nerve stimulators permit precise, individualized dosing of neuromuscular blocking agents.

TABLE 7-15. Commonly Monitored Evoked Potentials

Brain Stem Auditory Evoked Responses

Produced by stimulation of the cochlea using pulsed sound
Assess auditory pathway (ear and brain stem)
Useful for monitoring comatose patients or those undergoing surgical procedures on the cerebellopontine angle, floor of fourth ventricle, or cranial nerves V, VII, or VIII
May remain normal despite severe cortical dysfunction and deep anesthesia

Visual Evoked Potentials

Produced by flashing light to stimulate the retina
Assess integrity of the visual pathways
Useful for monitoring procedures on the visual system, during resection of pituitary tumors, and during procedures in the vicinity of the optic tracts (e.g., anterior cerebral artery aneurysms)
Very sensitive to depressant effects of anesthetics

Somatosensory Evoked Potentials

Produced by stimulation of a peripheral nerve (median, ulnar, common peroneal, posterior tibial) using small electrical impulses
Useful for monitoring cerebral function and ischemia associated with cerebral procedures and hemorrhage, spinal cord function during instrumentation of the spine or during thoracoabdominal vascular surgery
Injury or ischemia to the spinal cord manifests as decreased amplitude and increased latency of the evoked potential tracing
Does not monitor function of motor pathways

TABLE 7-16. Information Derived from Nerve Stimulator

Onset time

Guide to titration of neuromuscular blockade (match clinical needs in presence of individual differences in sensitivity to neuromuscular blocking drugs)

Assess optimal time to initiate drug-enhanced reversal

Determine adequacy of drug-enhanced reversal

    B. Various stimulus patterns have been described for the clinical assessment of neuromuscular function (Table 7-17).

        1. In clinical practice, the ulnar nerve at the wrist or elbow or the facial nerve at the stylomastoid process or at the lateral canthal fold is the most frequently selected stimulation site.

        2. Clinical judgments based on responses of the adductor pollicis or facial muscles overestimate the degree of blockade of the diaphragm, which is particularly resistant to neuromuscular blockade.

VII. MONITORING TEMPERATURE

    A. The potential for accidental heat loss or the risk of triggering malignant hyperthermia requires the continued observation of temperature changes.

    B. **Perioperative hypothermia** commonly results from anesthetic-induced inhibition of thermoregulation as well as a cold ambient environment in the operating room and heat loss owing to surgical exposure.

        1. Anesthetized patients often behave like poikilotherms until core temperature approaches a new set-point for thermoregulation.

        2. Those at greatest risk for perioperative hypothermia include the elderly, burn patients, neonates, and patients with spinal cord injuries.

    C. **Perioperative hyperthermia** occurs rarely; potential explanations other than malignant hyperthermia include exposure to endogenous pyrogens, increases in metabolic rate secondary to thyrotoxicosis or pheochromocytoma, and anticholinergic blockade of sweating.

    D. Central temperature is customarily measured using temperature probes placed in the nasopharynx, esoph-

---

TABLE 7-17. Stimulus Patterns Delivered by a Nerve Stimulator

Single Twitch Stimulation

Depicts onset, depth, and recovery (spontaneous and drug-enhanced)
Identifies ideal conditions for tracheal intubation
Response is dependent on stimulus frequency

Train-of-Four (four supramaximal stimuli separated by 0.5 second)

Degree of nondepolarizing blockade is determined by estimating the ratio of the fourth response to the first response (fade)
Ratio does not change with depolarizing blockade, since all four twitch responses are similarly decreased
Fade occurring in the presence of depolarizing blockade reflects phase II blockade
Reflects magnitude of maintenance relaxation and extent of recovery (spontaneous and drug-enhanced)

Tetanic Stimulation (5 seconds at 50 Hz)

Assess neuromuscular transmission following intense neuromuscular blockade
Perform only in anesthetized patients because it is very painful

Double-Burst Stimulation (three 0.2 msec volleys of tetanic stimulation, 750 μsec pause, repeat volley)

Designed to enhance the ability to detect residual neuromuscular blockade
If fade occurs, the train-of-four ratio is < 0.7
Detects residual neuromuscular blockade in postanesthesia care unit without producing pain

---

agus, blood (pulmonary artery catheter), bladder, or rectum.

1. During routine noncardiac surgery, temperature differences among these sites are small.
2. During and following cardiopulmonary bypass or deliberate hypothermia, gradients among these sites are to be anticipated.
   a. During cooling in anesthetized patients, changes in rectal temperature often lag behind changes in central (core) temperature.
   b. During rewarming, probe locations residing in regions of high blood flow often reflect blood temperature rather than central temperature, emphasizing that the adequacy of rewarming is best judged by measuring temperature at more than one location.

BASIC PRINCIPLES IN ANESTHESIA PRACTICE

8

Fluids and Electrolytes

Trauma and surgery acutely alter the volume and composition of the intracellular fluid (ICF) and extracellular fluid (ECF) spaces (Zaloga GP, Prough DS: Fluids and electrolytes. In: Barash PG, Cullen BF, Stoelting RK, [eds]: Clinical Anesthesia, pp 203–236. Philadelphia, JB Lippincott, 1992). Subsequent therapeutic infusion of fluids, primarily intended to replenish blood volume and maintain cardiac output, further alters compartmental volumes and composition. Hypovolemia, which increases the risk of organ hypoperfusion, and hypervolemia, which increases the risk of pulmonary edema, are potential hazards of perioperative fluid therapy. Surgical patients may also develop potentially harmful disorders of the plasma concentrations and total body content of important electrolytes.

I. PHYSIOLOGY

A. **Body fluid compartments.** Accurate replacement of fluid deficits necessitates an understanding of the distribution spaces of water, sodium, and colloid.

1. **Total body water** approximates 60% of total body weight, or 42 l in a 70-kg adult. Total body water consists of ICF (28 l) and ECF (14 l) (Fig. 8-1). Plasma volume is about 3 l, whereas red blood cell volume is about 2 l.

2. **Sodium** is present principally in the ECF (140 $mEq \cdot l^{-1}$), whereas **potassium** is principally present in the ICF (150 $mEq \cdot l^{-1}$).

3. **Albumin** is the most important oncotically active constituent of ECF (4 $g \cdot dl^{-1}$).

B. **Regulation of extracellular fluid volume** is influenced by aldosterone (enhances sodium reabsorption), antidiuretic hormone (enhances water reabsorption), and atrial natriuretic peptide (enhances sodium and water excretion).

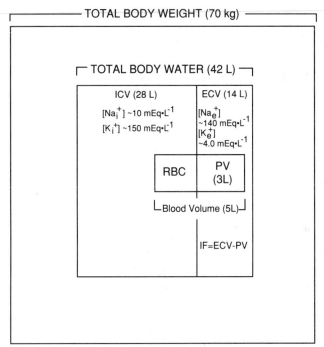

Figure 8-1. The distribution volume of water, approximately 60% of total body weight, includes both the extracellular volume (ECV) and intracellular volume (ICV). Sodium is distributed primarily in the ECV. If capillary integrity is preserved, the concentration of colloid is higher in the plasma volume (PV) than in interstitial fluid (IF).

II. FLUID REPLACEMENT THERAPY

A. Maintenance Fluid Requirements

1. **Water maintenance requirements** are often calculated on the basis of body weight. For a 70-kg adult water maintenance requirements are about 2500 $ml \cdot day^{-1}$ (Table 8-1).

2. **Renal sodium conservation** is highly efficient, such that the **average daily maintenance requirement** in an adult is about 75 mEq.

3. **The average daily maintenance requirement of potassium** in an adult is about 40 mEq. Physiologic di-

TABLE 8-1. Maintenance Water Requirements		
	ml·kg^{-1}·h^{-1}	ml·kg^{-1}·day^{-1}
1–10 kg	4	100
11–20 kg	2	50
>20 kg	1	20

uresis induces an obligate potassium loss of at least 10 mEq for every 1000 ml of urine.

4. Electrolytes such as chloride, calcium, and magnesium require no short-term replacement, although they must be supplied during chronic intravenous fluid maintenance.

5. **Addition of glucose** to maintenance fluid solutions is indicated only in those patients considered to be at risk for the development of hypoglycemia (infants, patients on insulin therapy). The influence, if any, of hyperglycemia on the extent of neurologic injury following a global or focal neurologic insult in humans is not clearly defined.

B. **Surgical Fluid Requirements**

1. Surgical patients require replacement of plasma volume and ECF secondary to hemorrhage and tissue manipulation **(third-space loss).**

   a. **Lactated Ringer's solution** is often selected for replacement of third-space losses as well as of gastrointestinal secretions.

   b. In addition to maintenance fluids and replacement of estimated blood loss, a **guideline for third-space loss** is 4 ml·kg^{-1}·h^{-1} for operations involving minimal tissue trauma, 6 ml·kg^{-1}·h^{-1} for those involving moderate trauma, and 8 ml·kg^{-1}·h for those involving extreme tissue trauma.

2. **Chronic gastric fluid losses** may produce hypochloremic metabolic alkalosis (treat with 0.9% saline), whereas **chronic diarrhea** may produce hyperchloremic metabolic acidosis (treat with a lactate-containing solution).

3. The reverse of third-space translocation of fluid (mobilization and return of accumulated fluid to the ECF volume and plasma; "deresuscitation") occurs about 72 hours postoperatively. Hypervolemia and/or pulmonary edema may occur at this time in a patient with compromised renal and/or cardiac function.

III. COLLOIDS, CRYSTALLOIDS, AND HYPERTONIC SOLUTIONS

  A. Intravenous fluids vary in oncotic pressure, osmolarity, and tonicity. When the capillary membrane is intact, fluids containing colloid, such as albumin or hydroxyethyl starch, preferentially expand plasma volume rather than ICF volume. Despite relative advantages and disadvantages, there is **no evidence to support the superiority** of either colloid-containing or crystalloid-containing solutions (Table 8-2).

  B. Despite a commonly believed clinical notion, the **risk of pulmonary edema seems to be independent** of the selection of a crystalloid- or colloid-containing solution.

   1. Colloid-induced expansion of the plasma volume redistributes slowly, such that diuretic therapy is often required if pulmonary edema develops.

   2. There appears to be no important clinical difference in pulmonary function after administration of crystalloid or colloid solutions in the absence of hypervolemia.

  C. Despite a commonly believed clinical notion, the **risk of increased intracranial pressure** seems to be inde-

TABLE 8-2. Advantages and Disadvantages of Colloid Versus Crystalloid Solutions for Intravenous Infusion

	Advantages	Disadvantages
Colloid	Smaller infused volume Prolonged increase in plasma volume Minimal peripheral edema Lower intracranial pressure*	Expensive Coagulopathy (dextran>hetastarch) Pulmonary edema (capillary leak states)
Crystalloid	Inexpensive Greater urine output Replaces interstitial fluid	Short-lived hemodynamic improvement Peripheral edema Pulmonary edema*

*Conflicting data.

pendent of the selection of a crystalloid- or colloid-containing solution.

D. **Hypertonic saline** may be a preferable fluid selection for correction of hypovolemia caused by acute, severe hemorrhage. The transient effects of hypertonic saline administration on plasma volume may be prolonged by its combination with dextran.

IV. FLUID STATUS: ASSESSMENT AND MONITORING

A. **The preoperative clinical assessment of blood volume and ECF volume** begins with the recognition of conditions in which deficits are likely to occur (Table 8-3).

B. **Physical signs of hypovolemia** are insensitive and nonspecific (Table 8-4).

1. A normal blood pressure reading may represent relative hypotension in an elderly or chronically hypertensive patient. Conversely, substantial hypovolemia may occur despite an apparently normal blood pressure and heart rate.

2. Elderly patients may demonstrate orthostatic hypotension despite a normal blood volume.

3. Young healthy subjects can tolerate an acute blood

TABLE 8-3. Conditions Associated with Deficits in Blood Volume and Extracellular Fluid Volume

Trauma	Pancreatitis
Burns	Bowel obstruction
Sepsis	Chronic systemic hypertension
Prolonged gastrointestinal losses	Chronic diuretic use

TABLE 8-4. Physical Signs of Hypovolemia

Oliguria (rule out renal failure, stress-induced endocrine responses)

Supine hypotension (implies blood volume deficit >30%)

Positive tilt test (increase in heart rate >20 beats·min^{-1} and decrease in systolic blood pressure >20 mm Hg when the patient assumes the standing position)

loss equivalent to 20% of their blood volume while exhibiting only postural tachycardia and variable postural hypotension.

4. Orthostatic changes in central venous pressure (CVP), coupled with assessment of the response to fluid infusion, may represent a useful test of the adequacy of blood volume.

C. **Laboratory Evidence of Hypovolemia** (Table 8-5)

1. **Hematocrit (Hct)** is a poor indicator of blood volume because it is influenced by the time elapsed since hemorrhage and the volume of asanguineous fluid replacement.

   a. Hct is virtually unchanged by acute hemorrhage; later, hemodilution occurs as fluids are administered or as fluid shifts from the interstitial to the intravascular space.

   b. If the intravascular fluid volume has been restored, Hct measurement will reflect red blood cell mass more accurately and can be used to guide transfusion.

2. **Blood urea nitrogen and serum creatinine** levels may be increased if hypovolemia is sufficiently prolonged (both measurements may be influenced by events unrelated to blood volume). Although hypovolemia does not cause metabolic alkalosis, ECF volume depletion is a potent stimulus for the maintenance of metabolic alkalosis.

D. **Visual estimation** is the simplest technique for quantifying intraoperative blood loss, as seen on sponges.

E. **Adequacy of intraoperative blood volume replacement** cannot be ascertained by any single modality (Table 8-6).

TABLE 8-5. Laboratory Evidence of Hypovolemia

Hemoconcentration (hematocrit is a poor indicator of blood volume)

Azotemia (may be influenced by events unrelated to blood volume)

Low urine sodium concentration (<20 mEq for every 1000 ml of urine)

Metabolic alkalosis

Metabolic acidosis (reflects organ hypoperfusion)

**TABLE 8-6. Clinical Indicators of the Adequacy of
Intraoperative Blood Volume Replacement**

Heart rate (tachycardia is insensitive and nonspecific)
Blood pressure
Central venous pressure
Urinary output
Arterial oxygenation and pH

---

1. Preservation of the blood pressure, accompanied by
   a CVP of 6–12 mm Hg in the presence of a volatile
   anesthetic, suggests an adequate blood volume. During profound hypovolemia, indirect measurement of
   blood pressure may significantly underestimate true
   blood pressure, emphasizing the potential value of
   direct blood pressure measurements in selected patients.
2. **Urinary output** usually declines precipitously (<0.5
   $ml\cdot kg^{-1}\cdot h^{-1}$) in the presence of moderate to severe
   hypovolemia.

V. ELECTROLYTES

A. **Physiologic role of electrolytes** (Table 8-7).
B. Regulation of the quantity and concentration of electrolytes is accomplished primarily by the endocrine and
   renal systems.
C. **Hyponatremia (<120 mEq$\cdot$l^{-1})** is usually the result of
   excess total body water.
   1. **The signs and symptoms of hyponatremia** depend
      on the rate at which the plasma sodium concentra-
      tion decreases and the severity of the decrease (Table
      8-8).
   2. Many patients develop hyponatremia as a result of
      the **syndrome of inappropriate antidiuretic hor-
      mone secretion** (SIADH).
      a. The cornerstone of SIADH management is free
         water restriction and elimination of precipitating
         causes (Table 8-9).
      b. Demeclocycline and lithium have been used ef-
         fectively to reverse SIADH in patients in whom
         the primary disease process is irreversible.
   3. Inappropriately rapid correction of hyponatremia
      (>12 mEq$\cdot$l^{-1} in 24 hours or 25 mEq$\cdot$l^{-1} in 48 hours)
      may result in neurologic sequelae (central pontine

TABLE 8-7. Physiologic Role of Electrolytes

Sodium	Osmolarity
	Extracellular fluid volume
	Action potential
Potassium	Transmembrane potential
	Action potential
Calcium	Excitation-contraction
	Neurotransmission
	Enzyme function
	Cardiac pacemaker activity
	Cardiac action potential
	Bone structure
Phosphorus	Stores energy (adenosine triphosphate)
	Component of second messengers (cyclic adenosine monophosphate)
	Component of cell membranes (phospholipids)
Magnesium	Enzyme cofactor (sodium-potassium pump)
	Controls potassium movement into cells
	Membrane excitability
	Bone structure

TABLE 8-8. Hyponatremia: Clinical Manifestations

Neurologic
Altered consciousness (sedation to coma)
Seizures
Cerebral edema

Gastrointestinal
Loss of appetite
Nausea and vomiting

Muscular
Cramps
Weakness

---

myelinolysis or the osmotic demyelination syndrome).

a. Hypertonic saline (1–2 ml·kg^{-1}·h^{-1}) is indicated in patients with severe hyponatremia (<120 mEq·l^{-1}) who have developed seizures. Intravenous administration of furosemide may be useful by increasing free water clearance.

b. Once the plasma sodium concentration exceeds 120–125 mEq·l^{-1}, water restriction alone is usually sufficient to normalize it.

TABLE 8-9. Precipitating Causes of Inappropriate Antidiuretic Hormone Secretion

Hypovolemia
Pulmonary disease
Central nervous system trauma
Endocrine dysfunction
Drugs that mimic antidiuretic hormone

D. **Hypernatremia (>150 mEq·l⁻¹)** is usually the result of decreased total body water.
   1. **The signs and symptoms of hypernatremia** most likely reflect the effect of dehydration on neurons and the presence of hypoperfusion caused by hypovolemia (Table 8-10). When hypernatremia develops abruptly, the associated sudden brain shrinkage may stretch and disrupt cerebral vessels, leading to subdural hematoma, subarachnoid hemorrhage, and venous thrombosis.
   2. Postoperative neurosurgical patients who have undergone pituitary surgery are at particular risk of developing transient or prolonged **diabetes insipidus,** leading to hypernatremia.
   3. **Treatment of hypernatremia** is influenced by the clinical assessment of ECF volume (Table 8-11).
E. **Hypokalemia (<3.0 mEq·l⁻¹)** may result from acute redistribution of potassium from the ECF to the ICF (total body potassium concentration is normal) or from chronic depletion of body potassium. With chronic potassium loss the ratio of intracellular to extracellular

TABLE 8-10. Hypernatremia: Clinical Manifestations

Neurologic
  Thirst
  Weakness
  Hyper-reflexia
  Seizures
  Intracranial hemorrhage

Cardiovascular
  Hypovolemia

Renal
  Polyuria or oliguria
  Renal insufficiency

TABLE 8-11. Hypernatremia: Treatment

Sodium Depletion (Hypovolemia)
  Hypovolemia correction (0.9% saline)
  Hypernatremia correction (hypotonic fluids)

Sodium Overload (Hypervolemia)
  Enhance sodium removal (loop diuretics, dialysis)
  Replace water deficit (hypotonic fluids)

Normal Total Body Sodium (Euvolemia)
  Replace water deficit (hypotonic fluids)
  Control diabetes insipidus (DDAVP, vasopressin,
    chlorpropamide)
  Control nephrogenic diabetes insipidus (restrict sodium and
    water intake, thiazide diuretics)

---

potassium remains relatively constant, whereas acute redistribution of potassium substantially changes the resting potential difference across cell membranes.
1. **The signs and symptoms of hypokalemia** reflect the diffuse effects of potassium on cell membranes and excitable tissue (Table 8-12).
   a. **Cardiac rhythm disturbances** are among the most dangerous complications of hypokalemia. De-

---

TABLE 8-12. Hypokalemia: Clinical Manifestations

Cardiovascular
  Cardiac dysrhythmias (premature ventricular contractions)
  Electrocardiogram changes (widened QRS segment, ST
    segment depression, first-degree atrioventricular heart
    block)
  Potentiates digitalis toxicity
  Postural hypotension

Neuromuscular
  Skeletal muscle weakness (hypoventilation)
  Hyporeflexia
  Confusion

Renal
  Polyuria
  Concentrating defect

Metabolic
  Glucose intolerance
  Potentiation of hypercalcemia and hypomagnesemia

spite the commonly believed notion that chronic hypokalemia increases the incidence of intraoperative cardiac dysrhythmias, prospective studies fail to support this concept.

   b. Potassium depletion induces defects in renal concentrating ability, resulting in polyuria.

   c. Hypokalemia causes skeletal muscle weakness and when severe, may even cause paralysis.

2. The plasma potassium concentration (98% of potassium is intracellular) correlates poorly with total body potassium stores.

   a. Total body potassium approximates 50–55 $mEq \cdot kg^{-1}$.

   b. As a guideline, a chronic decrease in serum potassium of 1 $mEq \cdot l^{-1}$ corresponds to a total body deficit of about 200–300 mEq.

3. **The treatment of hypokalemia** consists of potassium repletion, correction of alkalemia, and discontinuation of offending drugs (diuretics, aminoglycosides) (Table 8-13).

   a. Hypokalemia secondary only to acute redistribution may not require treatment.

   b. Oral potassium chloride (chloride deficiency may limit the ability of the kidneys to conserve potassium) is preferable to intravenous replacement if total body potassium stores are decreased.

   c. Intravenous potassium replacement at a rate of >20 $mEq \cdot h^{-1}$ should be continuously monitored with an electrocardiogram.

F. **Hyperkalemia** (>5 $mEq \cdot l^{-1}$) is most often due to renal insufficiency or drugs that limit potassium excretion (nonsteroidal anti-inflammatory drugs, angiotensin-

---

TABLE 8-13. Hypokalemia: Treatment

Correct Precipitating Factors
Alkalemia
Hypomagnesemia
Drugs

Mild Hypokalemia (>2 $mEq \cdot l^{-1}$)
Infuse potassium chloride up to 10 $mEq \cdot h^{-1}$

Severe Hypokalemia (<2 $mEq \cdot l^{-1}$, electrocardiogram changes, intense skeletal muscle weakness)
Infuse potassium chloride up to 40 $mEq \cdot h^{-1}$
Continuously monitor the electrocardiogram

TABLE 8-14. Hyperkalemia: Clinical Manifestations

Cardiovascular
  Cardiac dysrhythmias (heart block)
  Electrocardiogram changes (widened QRS segment, tall
    peaked T waves, atrial asystole, prolongation of P-R
    interval)

Neuromuscular
  Skeletal muscle weakness
  Paresthesias
  Confusion

---

converting enzyme inhibitors, cyclosporine, potassium-sparing drugs such as triamterine).
1. **The signs and symptoms of hyperkalemia** primarily involve the central nervous and cardiovascular systems (Table 8-14).
2. **Treatment of hyperkalemia** is aimed at eliminating the cause, reversing membrane hyperexcitability, and removing potassium from the body (Table 8-15).

G. **Hypocalcemia (<8.5 mg·dl^{-1})** occurs as a result of parathyroid hormone deficiency (surgical parathyroid gland damage or removal, burns, or sepsis) or because of calcium chelation or precipitation (hyperphosphatemia as from cell lysis secondary to chemotherapy).
1. **The hallmark of hypocalcemia** is increased neuronal membrane irritability and tetany (Table 8-16).

TABLE 8-15. Severe Hyperkalemia:* Treatment

Reverse Membrane Effects
  Calcium (10% calcium gluconate, 10–30 ml iv, over 10
    minutes)

Transfer Potassium into Cells
  Glucose (D10W) and regular insulin (5–10 units regular
    insulin per 25–50 g of glucose)

Remove Potassium from Body
  Loop diuretics
  Potassium-exchange resins
  Hemodialysis (removes 25–50 mEq·h^{-1})

*>7 mEq·l^{-1}, electrocardiogram changes.

TABLE 8-16. Hypocalcemia: Clinical Manifestations

Cardiovascular
Cardiac dysrhythmias
Electrocardiogram changes (prolongation of the QT interval,
   T-wave inversion)
Hypotension
Congestive heart failure

Neuromuscular
Skeletal muscle spasm
Tetany
Skeletal muscle weakness
Seizures

Pulmonary
Laryngospasm
Bronchospasm
Hypoventilation

Psychiatric
Anxiety
Dementia

---

2. **Ionized hypocalcemia** is possible after multiple organ trauma and following cardiopulmonary bypass. Symptomatic hypocalcemia usually occurs when serum ionized calcium is <2.8 mg·dl^{-1}.
3. **The cornerstone of therapy** for confirmed, symptomatic ionized hypocalcemia is administration of calcium (Table 8-17).
4. In anesthesia practice, it is **important that ionized hypocalcemia not be overtreated** in patients recovering from cardiac surgery, especially in the presence of digitalis. Although administration of calcium may increase blood pressure, there is evi-

---

TABLE 8-17. Hypocalcemia: Acute Treatment

Administer Calcium
10 ml of 10% calcium gluconate iv over 10 minutes, followed
   by a continuous infusion
500–1000 mg of calcium orally every 6 hours

Administer Vitamin D

Monitor Electrocardiogram

---

dence that it attenuates beta-agonist effects of epinephrine and confers no benefit to patients who otherwise require inotropic or vasoactive drugs.

H. **Hypercalcemia** (>10.5 **mg·dl^{-1}**) occurs when calcium enters the ECF more rapidly than the kidneys can excrete the excess. Clinically, hypercalcemia most commonly results from an excess of bone resorption over bone formation, usually secondary to malignant disease, hyperparathyroidism, or immobilization.

1. Hypercalcemia causes a variety of pathophysiologic alterations that are most likely to occur when the serum calcium concentration is >11.5 mg·dl^{-1} (Table 8-18).

   a. **Urinary concentrating ability deteriorates** early in the presence of hypercalcemia.

   b. In response to hypovolemia, renal tubular reabsorption of sodium results in enhanced renal calcium reabsorption.

2. **A plasma calcium concentration >14 mg·dl^{-1} is a medical emergency** that requires aggressive therapy with saline infusion and furosemide to enhance calcium excretion (urinary output should be maintained at 200–300·ml·h^{-1}). **Mithramycin** (also called plicamycin), 25 µg·kg^{-1} iv, exerts a hypocalcemic effect in 12–24 hours. Toxic effects of mith-

---

TABLE 8-18. Hypercalcemia: Clinical Manifestations

Cardiovascular
  Hypertension
  Heart block
  Digitalis sensitivity

Neuromuscular
  Skeletal muscle weakness
  Hyporeflexia
  Sedation to coma

Renal
  Nephrolithiasis
  Polyuria (renal tubular dysfunction)
  Azotemia

Gastrointestinal
  Peptic ulcer disease
  Pancreatitis
  Anorexia

ramycin include thrombocytopenia, nephrotoxicity, and hepatotoxicity.

I. **Hypomagnesemia (<1.7 mg·dl^{-1})** is common in critically ill patients, most likely reflecting nasogastric suctioning and inability of the renal tubules to conserve magnesium.

1. **Clinical features of hypomagnesemia,** like hypocalcemia, are characterized by **increased neuronal irritability and tetany** (Table 8-19).

   a. Cardiac dysrhythmias following myocardial infarction or after cardiopulmonary bypass may be due to hypomagnesemia.

   b. Hypomagnesemia may cause hypokalemia as a result of renal potassium wasting, whereas hypomagnesemia and hypermagnesemia suppress parathyroid hormone secretion and can cause hypocalcemia.

3. **Treatment of magnesium deficiency** is with administration of magnesium supplements (Table 8-20).

   a. During magnesium repletion the **patellar reflexes** should be monitored frequently and magnesium withheld if they become suppressed.

   b. During intravenous infusion of magnesium, it is important to continuously monitor the electrocardiogram in order to detect cardiotoxicity.

TABLE 8-19. Hypomagnesemia: Clinical Manifestations

Cardiovascular
  Coronary vasospasm
  Cardiac dysrhythmias
  Refractory ventricular fibrillation
  Congestive heart failure

Neuromuscular
  Latent or overt tetany
  Skeletal muscle weakness
  Sedation
  Seizures

Miscellaneous
  Dysphagia
  Anorexia
  Nausea
  Hypokalemia
  Hypocalcemia

TABLE 8-20. Hypomagnesemia: Treatment

Administer magnesium*
Intravenous magnesium, 8–16 mEq over 1 hour, followed by
  2–4 mEq·h^{-1}
Intramuscular magnesium, 10 mEq every 4–6 hours
Oral magnesium, 70–105 mEq daily

*$MgSO_4$ 1 g = 8 mEq; $MgCl_2$ 1 g = 10 mEq.

TABLE 8-21. Hypermagnesemia: Clinical Findings

	Plasma Magnesium Concentration (mg·dl^{-1})
Normal	1.7–2.4
Therapeutic range (pre-eclampsia)	5–8
Hypotension	3–5
Deep tendon hyporeflexia	5
Somnolence	8.5
Deep tendon areflexia	12
Hypoventilation Heart block	18
Cardiac arrest	24

J. **Hypermagnesemia** (>2.5 mg·dl^{-1}) is usually iatrogenic (treatment of pregnancy-induced hypertension or premature labor).
  1. **Clinical features of hypermagnesemia** are evidenced in multiple organ systems (Table 8-21).
  2. Hypermagnesemia antagonizes the release and effect of **acetylcholine** at the neuromuscular junction, manifesting as potentiation of the action of nondepolarizing muscle relaxants.
  3. **Treatment** of neuromuscular and cardiac toxicity produced by hypermagnesemia can be promptly, but transiently, antagonized by calcium, 5–10 mEq iv.
    a. Urinary excretion of magnesium can be increased by expanding the ECF volume and inducing diuresis with a combination of furosemide and saline.
    b. In emergency situations, and in patients with renal failure, magnesium may be removed by dialysis.

9

Acid-Base Balance

Maintenance of the body's internal milieu is the major function of buffering systems, whereas oxygen transport and the successful preservation of aerobic metabolism are key components in maintaining cellular integrity (Smith H, Lumb PD: Acid-base balance. In: Barash PG, Cullen BF, Stoelting RK [eds]: Clinical Anesthesia, pp 237–250. Philadelphia, JB Lippincott, 1992). When normal aerobic metabolism is compromised or the ratio of buffering elements is altered, disturbances in acid-base homeostasis occur.

I. FUNDAMENTALS OF ACID-BASE BALANCE

A. The most important intravascular buffering system is the carbonic acid–bicarbonate buffer pair. The division of buffering between sodium bicarbonate and dissolved CO_2 leads to the commonly named metabolic and respiratory components of acid-base balance (Fig. 9-1).

B. The most commonly used values that impact directly on acid-base balance are Po_2, Pco_2, pH, hemoglobin oxygen saturation (So_2), bicarbonate ion (HCO_3) concentration, base excess (BE), and total oxygen content.

1. Blood-gas analyzers in clinical use perform all measurements (Po_2, Pco_2, pH) at a temperature of 37°C.

a. **Alpha-stat** management of blood gases uses values analyzed at 37°C and uncorrected for the patient's body temperature. This approach is based on the concept that maintenance of electrochemical neutrality (pH = pOH) requires the pH to change with alterations in body temperature.

b. **pH-stat** management of blood gases uses values corrected to the patient's body temperature (nomograms are available for this correction) at the time of sampling.

c. There is no universal agreement on the need to correct or not correct Pco_2 and pH for temperature. The decision is left to the clinician.

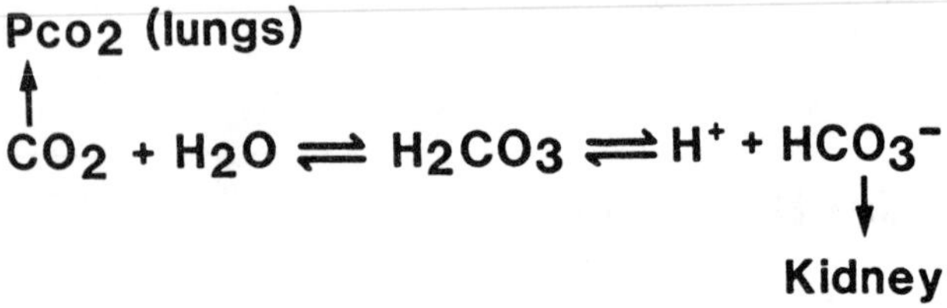

Pco2 (lungs)

$$\uparrow$$

$$CO_2 + H_2O \rightleftharpoons H_2CO_3 \rightleftharpoons H^+ + HCO_3^-$$

$$\downarrow$$

Kidney

Figure 9-1. Acid-base balance reflects the retention or elimination of carbon dioxide or bicarbonate ions by the lungs or kidneys, respectively.

    d. At the hypothermic temperature used in cardiopulmonary bypass, maintaining a temperature-corrected $Paco_2$ of 40 mm Hg may result in excessive amounts of CO_2 dissolved in the blood, leading to hyperperfusion of the brain.

  2. The **HCO_3 and BE values are calculated** from the measured Pco_2 and pH using a nomogram.

II. ACID-BASE CHEMISTRY

  A. Hydrogen ion (H^+) concentration is a function of the Pco_2 and HCO_3.

    1. A normal arterial pH of 7.4 has a H^+ of 40 $nmol \cdot l^{-1}$. From a pH of 7.2 to 7.5 the curve of H^+ concentration is relatively linear, and for each change of 0.01 pH unit from 7.40, the H^+ concentration can be estimated by a change of 1.

$$pH\ 7.40 = 40\ nmol \cdot l^{-1}$$
$$pH\ 7.39 = 41\ nmol \cdot l^{-1}$$
$$pH\ 7.41 = 39\ nmol \cdot l^{-1}$$

    2. Hydrogen ions are important in the performance of specific body functions (Table 9-1).

  B. Acute deviations in normal acid-base homeostasis are corrected by two processes, buffering and compensation.

    1. **Buffering** is the ability of certain substances in the blood to minimize variations in pH produced by acids by providing an available source of proton acceptors through a shift in the reaction between H^+ and H_2CO_3.

      a. Resulting CO_2 is eliminated *via* the lungs and as water through the kidneys.

      b. Without buffers, the addition of CO_2 and metabolic acids to the blood would produce unacceptable decreases in pH.

TABLE 9-1. Role of Hydrogen Ions in Body Functions

Distribution of potassium (a 0.1 unit change produces a 0.5–1.5 $mEq \cdot l^{-1}$ change)
Ability of hemoglobin to bind to oxygen
Enzyme activity

TABLE 9-2. Methods of Carbon Dioxide Transport in the Blood

Physical solution	5%–7%
Carbonic acid	<1%
Bicarbonate ion	90%
Carbamino compounds	5%

---

   2. **Compensation** is the process by which the magnitude of change in pH resulting from acid-base derangements is minimized by mechanisms that restore the HCO_3/CO_2 ratio (20:1). In this regard, acid-base homeostasis is dependent on the **symbiotic relationship between the kidneys (HCO_3) and the lungs (CO_2).**
      a. **Metabolic derangements** that alter pH by changes in HCO_3 evoke ventilatory compensation so as to increase or decrease Pa_{CO_2}. Ventilatory responses produce maximum compensatory effects in a matter of minutes or hours.
      b. **Ventilatory derangements** that alter pH by changes in P_{CO_2} stimulate renal compensation. For example, as Pa_{CO_2} increases, the kidneys conserve HCO_3. Renal compensation requires 3–5 days to become maximal.
      c. Restoration of pH to normal by renal compensatory mechanisms is unlikely, as this would remove the stimulus for compensation.
   C. CO_2 which is the normal waste product of cellular aerobic metabolism, is transported from the tissues in one of four forms (Table 9-2).
      1. CO_2 in **physical solution** (gaseous form) accounts for the partial pressure exerted by this gas (P_{CO_2}) and is the only form of CO_2 in the blood that can freely cross cell membranes, including the blood-brain barrier, and alter intracellular pH.

2. Carbonic anhydrase is a catalytic enzyme present in red blood cells and renal tubular cells; it accelerates the hydration of CO_2 to carbonic acid.

3. CO_2 production is relatively constant; thus the Pa_{CO_2} **is commonly used as a reflection of the adequacy of alveolar ventilation.**

III. ACID-BASE DISORDERS (Table 9-3)

A. **Metabolic alkalosis** (pH >7.45, HCO_3 >30 mEq·l^{-1}) is the most common metabolic disturbance in hospitalized patients, reflecting loss of H^+ *via* vomiting, nasogastric suction, and hypokalemia as a result of diuretics. Sudden correction of chronic respiratory acidosis, as may occur with injudicious mechanical hyperventilation of the lungs, may produce a metabolic alkalosis because excess HCO_3 (the compensatory mechanism for respiratory acidosis) cannot be immediately excreted by the kidneys.

1. Hypokalemia and alkalemia are associated with cardiac dysrhythmias and may potentiate the toxicity of cardiac glycosides.

2. Metabolic alkalosis shifts the oxyhemoglobin dissociation curve to the left, impairing peripheral unloading of oxygen.

3. **Treatment** of metabolic alkalosis is dependent on halting continuing H^+ losses and, if warranted, a trial of potassium chloride, acetazolamide (induces bicarbonaturia), or dilute hydrochloric acid (administered through a central vein).

B. **Metabolic acidosis** (pH <7.35, HCO_3 <20 mEq·l^{-1}) is produced by the accumulation of acids other than CO_2 (as occurs in ketoacidosis, lactic acidosis, renal failure, toxic dose of salicylates).

1. The **respiratory compensation** for metabolic acidosis is alveolar hyperventilation that results in a decrease of 1.2 mm Hg Pa_{CO_2} for every 1 mEq·l^{-1} decrease in HCO_3 concentration. Ultimately, **renal compensation** must occur to correct metabolic acidosis, as the lungs cannot excrete nonvolatile (fixed) acids. The kidneys' ability to increase acid excretion lags 12–24 hours behind the initial ventilatory response and may not reach its maximum for up to 5 days.

2. Blood lactate concentration is usually <2 nmol·l^{-1}, and increases reflect oxygen deficit and anaerobic metabolism (during shock, survival rate declines from 90% to 10% when the lactic acid concentration increases from 2 nmol·l^{-1} to 8 nmol·l^{-1}).

TABLE 9-3. Classification of Acid-Base Disturbances

	pH (7.35–7.45)	PaCO₂ (35–45 mm Hg)	HCO₃ (22–26 mEq·l⁻¹)
Metabolic Alkalosis			
Acute	↑↑	↑↑	↑↑
Chronic	↑↑	↑↑	↑↑
Metabolic Acidosis			
Acute	↓↓	↓↓	↓↓
Chronic	↓↓	↓↓	↓↓
Respiratory Acidosis			
Acute	↓ or NC	↑↑	↑↑
Chronic	↓ or NC	↑↑	↑↑
Respiratory Alkalosis			
Acute	↑ or NC	↓↓	↓↓
Chronic	↑ or NC	↓↓	↓↓

NC = No change.

3. Although HCO_3 therapy may increase lactate production, it usually is still warranted if metabolic acidosis is severe (pH <7.2).

   a. Full correction is never indicated because ongoing therapy should ameliorate the inciting event, and total correction initially leads rapidly to postresuscitation metabolic alkalosis, hypernatremia, hyperosmolarity, and cardiac dysrhythmias.

   b. An appropriate target pH is 7.25 (below this pH some enzymes do not function properly and the response of the heart and peripheral vasculature to catecholamines may be impaired).

   c. A common approach is to calculate the HCO_3 dose (BE × 0.2 × body weight in kilograms) and then administer one half this amount.

   d. In cardiopulmonary arrest, it is recommended that HCO_3 therapy be withheld for at least 10 minutes and then be given only as clinically necessary, with blood gas measurements as a guide. This recommendation is based on the observation that HCO_3 administration may produce arterial respiratory alkalosis and venous respiratory acidosis **(poor pulmonary blood flow renders the lungs unable to clear CO_2 dioxide resulting from HCO_3 therapy).**

4. Severe metabolic acidosis may be associated with decreased myocardial contractility, peripheral vasodilation, catecholamine release, and decreased threshold for ventricular fibrillation.

C. **Respiratory acidosis** (pH <7.35, $Paco_2$ >45 mm Hg) occurs from either decreased alveolar ventilation or increased carbon dioxide production (Table 9-4).

   1. **Compensation** by renal HCO_3 retention takes several days, such that acute respiratory acidosis is uncompensated, whereas in patients with chronic respiratory acidosis, the renal HCO_3 retention is sufficient to return pH to near normal.

   2. **In mixed acid-base disturbances,** respiratory acidosis is characterized by a $PaCO_2$ that is higher than would be expected from compensatory mechanisms correcting a primary alkalosis.

      a. Simple acute respiratory acidosis should have an HCO_3 concentration of between 24 and 32 $mEq \cdot l^{-1}$.

      b. If respiratory acidosis exists with an HCO_3 concentration <24 $mEq \cdot l^{-1}$, a coexisting metabolic acidosis is likely.

TABLE 9-4. Causes of Respiratory Acidosis

Decreased Alveolar Ventilation

Central nervous system depression (opioids, general anesthetics)

Peripheral muscle weakness (neuromuscular blockers, myasthenia gravis)

Chronic obstructive pulmonary disease

Acute respiratory failure

Increased CO_2 Production

Hypermetabolic states

    Sepsis

    Fever

    Multiple trauma

    Malignant hyperthermia

Hyperalimentation

---

    c. If respiratory acidosis exists with an HCO_3 concentration >32 mEq·l^{-1}, either chronic respiratory acidosis or coexisting metabolic alkalosis is likely.

  3. Treatment of acute respiratory acidosis consists of elimination of the precipitating factor and, if necessary, mechanical breathing assistance to increase alveolar ventilation. Abrupt correction of the Pa_{CO_2} in a patient with chronic respiratory acidosis results in a persistent elevation in the HCO_3 concentration until the kidneys can appropriately compensate.

 D. Respiratory alkalosis (pH >7.45, Pa_{CO_2} <35 mm Hg) occurs when alveolar ventilation exceeds CO_2 production (Table 9-5).

  1. There is no significant renal compensation in acute respiratory alkalosis; therefore it can be corrected rapidly. In contrast, with chronic respiratory alkalosis, abrupt correction of Pa_{CO_2} results in a persistently low HCO_3 concentration until the kidneys can appropriately compensate.

  2. The expected metabolic compensation for a primary chronic respiratory alkalosis is a 1 mEq·l^{-1} decrease in HCO_3 for every 2 mm Hg decrease in Pa_{CO_2}.

IV. OXYGENATION

 A. Mitochondrial oxygen utilization accounts for about 90% of total cellular oxygen consumption, which re-

TABLE 9-5. Causes of Respiratory Alkalosis

Spontaneous Hyperventilation
  Pain
  Anxiety
  Hypoxemia
  Sepsis
  Central nervous system disease
  Impending congestive heart failure

Mechanically Induced Hyperventilation
  Treat increased intracranial pressure
  Neuroanesthesia

Decreased CO_2 Production
  General anesthesia
  Hypothermia

sults in the production of potential energy in the form of adenosine triphosphate (ATP). The critical level of oxygen required in the mitochondria for oxidative phosphorylation to proceed normally is about 1 mm Hg.

B. **Arterial oxygen content** (see Appendix A). Oxygen present in arterial blood is bound to hemoglobin (Sao_2) or dissolved in plasma (Po_2). The partial pressure of oxygen determines the gradient to drive oxygen to tissues.

1. **The oxyhemoglobin dissociation curve** describes the influence of Po_2 on Sao_2 (see Fig. 7-2). The sigmoid shape of the curve is such that a Pao_2 <60 mm Hg produces substantial decreases in Sao_2 (decreased transfer of oxygen to tissues), whereas a Pao_2 >60 mm Hg produces only modest increases in Sao_2.

   a. A normal Pao_2 (80–100 mm Hg) represents an Sao_2 of 97%, whereas a normal Pvo_2 (40 mm Hg) represents an Svo_2 of 75%.

   b. The position of the oxyhemoglobin dissociation curve is often expressed as the P_{50} (Po_2 when Sao_2 is 50%) (Table 9-6) (see Fig. 7-2).

2. The normal **arterial to venous oxygen content difference** is 5 ml·dl^{-1}.

3. At sea level, the inspired Po_2 is about 150 mm Hg, and this is decreased to about 100 mm Hg in the alveoli (Pao_2), principally reflecting uptake of alveolar oxygen by pulmonary blood flow.

4. Any difference between the Pao_2 and the Pao_2 is most likely a reflection of the influence of **shunt** or **ventilation-to-perfusion (V/Q) inequality.**

TABLE 9-6. Factors That Alter the Position of the Oxyhemoglobin Dissociation Curve

Left Shift (P_{50} <26 mm Hg)	Right Shift (P_{50} >26 mm Hg)
Temperature <37°C	Temperature >37°C
pH >7.4	pH <7.4
Decreased 2,3-DPG*	Increased 2,3-DPG
Hemoglobin F	

*2,3-DPG-2,3-diphosphoglycerate.

TABLE 9-7. Causes of Arterial Hypoxemia

Decreased Inspired Oxygen Concentration
  Anesthetic machine/circuit malfunction
  Altitude
Hypoventilation
Ventilation-to-Perfusion Inequality
  (most likely cause; treatment is supplemental oxygen; see Fig. 10-4)
Absolute Shunt (refractory to correction with supplemental oxygen; see Fig. 10-4)
  Endobronchial intubation
  Atelectasis
  Anatomic
Diffusion Impairment (usually manifests only with exercise)

TABLE 9-8. Classification of Tissue Hypoxia

Anemic hypoxia (decrease in the quantity or quality of hemoglobin)
Hypoxemic hypoxia (low Pa_{O_2})
Circulatory hypoxia (shock, inadequate tissue perfusion)
  Hypovolemic (massive hemorrhage)
  Cardiogenic (myocardial infarction)
  Distributive (sepsis, anaphylaxis)
  Obstructive (pulmonary embolus, aortocaval compression)
Histotoxic hypoxia (cyanide poisoning)

C. **Hypoxemia** is defined as a resting PaO_2 that is more than 2 standard deviations below the normal mean resting PaO_2 for that patient's age and the inspired concentration of oxygen (Table 9-7).

D. **Hypoxia** is defined as inadequate tissue oxygenation (Table 9-8).

10

Hemostasis and Hemotherapy

Bleeding as a result of a defect in hemostasis may have numerous causes (Ellison N: Hemostasis and hemotherapy. In Barash PG, Cullen BF, Stoelting RK [eds]: Clinical Anesthesia, pp 251–264. Philadelphia, JB Lippincott, 1992). Treatment of bleeding requires an understanding of available blood products.

I. HEMOSTASIS

A. **Normal physiology.** When a leak in the circulatory system develops, a **primary hemostatic plug** will form within 5 minutes of injury, requiring only an interaction between the injured vessel and platelets. Formation of a **definitive hemostatic plug** requires an additional 1–2 hours and involves **activation of the coagulation mechanism** (converts fibrinogen to fibrin to form a loose **fibrin clot**) and **activation of Factor XIII** (results in formation of a **firm fibrin clot,** which retracts into a definitive hemostatic plug under the influence of platelets). **Fibrinolysis** is subsequently activated to localize the clot (Fig. 10-1).

B. The **coagulation mechanism** is essential to prevent bleeding from damaged blood vessels <1 mm in diameter. **Activation of coagulation factors** is surface-oriented, with activation normally prevented by physiologic anticoagulants such as **plasma antithrombin III** and dilutional effects on local concentrations of coagulation factors provided by blood flow (Table 10-1).

C. **Platelets** are necessary for all phases of coagulation, beginning with the stimulus that initiates **platelet adhesion** to nonplatelet endothelial surfaces. **Adenosine diphosphate** released from platelets is a potent stimulus for subsequent platelet aggregation. Substances released from platelets cause contraction of the injured vessel wall. Activated platelet membranes act as a surface for the action of coagulation factors. **Clot retraction,** which is the final step in clot formation, is due to a platelet protein, **thrombosthenin.**

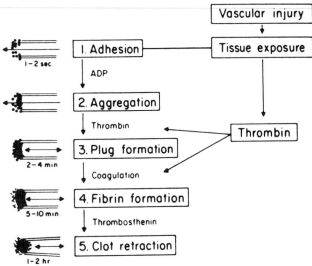

Figure 10-1. Schematic depiction of steps in clot formation.

TABLE 10-1. Classification of Coagulation Factors

Factor	Synonym	Minimal Level for Surgical Hemostasis (% of normal)
I	Fibrinogen	50–100
II	Prothrombin	20–40
III	Tissue thromboplastin	
IV	Calcium	
V	Labile factor	5–20
VII	Stable factor	10–20
VIII	Antihemophilia factor	30
IX	Antihemophilia factor B	20–25
X	Stuart-Prower factor	10–20
XI	Plasma thromboplastin antecedent	20–30
XII	Hageman factor	0
XIII	Fibrin stabilizing factor	1–3

D. **Fibrinolysis** is necessary to localize fibrin deposition to the area of injury as well as to remove the secondary hemostatic plug (recanalize) during healing. For example, radial arteries that occlude after catheter removal almost always recanalize. Activation of the **plasminogen system** by tissue plasminogen activator results in the formation of **plasmin,** which digests fibrin to form fibrin split products. **Disseminated intravascular coagulation** (DIC) is a pathologic form of fibrinolysis in response to increased thrombogenesis.

II. TESTS OF HEMOSTASIS

A screening coagulation profile is recommended in patients scheduled for major surgery as well as those with a bleeding history (Table 10-2).

A. **History** is especially important to elicit information about the hemostatic response to prior surgical procedures (dental extraction) and ingestion of drugs considered to be anticoagulants (aspirin).

B. **Tests of coagulation mechanisms**

1. **Activated coagulation time (ACT, 90–120 seconds)** evaluates the intrinsic system and the final common pathway. ACT is widely used to monitor heparin therapy.

2. **Partial thromboplastin time (PTT, <35 seconds)** evaluates the intrinsic system and the final common pathway. This test detects deficiencies of coagulation factors below 25% of normal levels except for Factors VII and XIII.

3. **Prothrombin time (PT)** (compared with laboratory control for interpretation of normal value) evaluates the extrinsic system and the final common pathway. This test is widely used to monitor coumarin anticoagulation.

4. **Thrombin time (20–35 seconds)** evaluates the final stage of fibrin formation. Prolongation occurs when plasma fibrinogen concentrations are below 90 $mg \cdot dl^{-1}$ or in the presence of heparin.

C. **Tests of platelet function**

1. **Platelet count.** Bleeding rarely occurs unless the platelet count is <50,000 $cells \cdot mm^{-3}$. The platelet count is a quantitative test only and does not measure platelet function.

2. **Bleeding time (3–8 minutes)** measures both the quality and quantity of platelets.

3. **Clot retraction** is a qualitative test of platelet function, with some clot retraction at 37°C in 2–4 hours being considered a positive response.

TABLE 10-2. Screening Tests for Coagulation Disorders

	Partial Thromboplastin Time	Prothrombin Time	Platelet Count	Bleeding Time
Liver disease	I/NC	I	D/NC	NC
Oral anticoagulants	I/NC	I	NC	NC
Thrombocytopenia	NC	NC	D	—
Aspirin	NC	NC	NC	NC
Heparin	I	I/NC	NC	NC
Hemophilia	I	NC	NC	—
Von Willebrand's disease	I/NC	NC	NC	—
DIC	I/NC	I/NC	D	—

I = increased; D = decreased; NC = no change.

D. **Tests of fibrinolysis**
   1. **Clot lysis.** A clot should not lyse at 37°C for up to 48 hours.
   2. **Fibrin split products** are formed from the breakdown of fibrin or fibrinogen and are elevated in patients with DIC.
E. **Thrombelastography** (TEG) evaluates clot formation from initial procoagulant activation and fibrin formation to eventual clot lysis. The diagnosis of coagulation factor activity deficiency, platelet abnormalities, and DIC is possible from a single blood sample. Use of fresh frozen plasma and platelets should be reserved for patients with documented defects in coagulation as confirmed by a thrombelastogram. Indeed, patients experiencing moderate to massive blood loss with replacement, including crystalloid solutions, do not experience dilutional coagulopathy as confirmed by thrombelastography.

III. PATHOLOGY

A. **Congenital defects** are relatively rare.
   1. **Hemophilia A (Factor VIII deficiency)** is transmitted as a sex-linked recessive trait that affects males and accounts for 85% of the hemophilias.
      a. **Surgery.** Factor VIII:C levels should be maintained >30% at all times by administration of Factor VIII concentrates (cryoprecipitate from one donor or lyophilized products prepared from pooled plasma) starting 1.5 hours before surgery (Table 10-1). The elimination half-time of Factor VIII (10–12 hours) necessitates treatment every 8–12 hours. The magnitude of the operation influences duration of treatment (24 hours for minor dental surgery versus several weeks following orthopedic reconstructive operations).
      b. Blood-transmitted diseases (hepatitis, acquired immunodeficiency syndrome) often accompany treatment of hemophilia A with cryoprecipitate or pooled plasma.
      c. Antibodies to or inhibitors of Factor VIII develop in 7–10% of treated patients.
   2. **Von Willebrand's disease** may affect up to 1% of the population; it is a milder bleeding disorder than hemophilia A. Cryoprecipitate is the blood product of choice for treatment because Factor VIII concentrates lack Factor VIII:vWF. Depending on the type of von Willebrand's disease, Factor VIII concentrates or vasopressin may also be used to raise Factor VIII:C levels.

B. Acquired defects

1. **Anticoagulants.** Coumarin-like drugs inhibit vitamin K–dependent factors (Factors II, VII, IX, and X) and prolong the PT. Vitamin K is a specific antidote but requires 3–6 hours to work. For emergency surgery, the effects of coumarin can be reversed with administration of banked blood, which contains all the vitamin K–dependent factors in adequate amounts.

2. **Liver failure.** In advanced cases, bleeding may be caused by decreased production of clotting factors, thrombocytopenia due to hypersplenism, fibrinolysis, or esophageal varices. Synthesis of clotting factors decreases in proportion to the loss of hepatocytes, and PT is a good prognostic indicator. Vitamin K is not effective because Factors I, V, and XI are not vitamin K–dependent factors. Vitamin K is effective when malabsorption due to lack of bile salts or intestinal sterilization is the cause of a prolonged PT.

3. **Disseminated intravascular coagulation** is a pathologic response involving simultaneous and diffuse thrombogenesis. This response may accompany trauma, sepsis, shock, hemolytic transfusion reactions, burns, cancer, and intrauterine death.

   a. **Diagnosis** of DIC requires a high index of suspicion plus the presence of abnormal laboratory values. In addition, plasma fibrinogen levels are usually decreased; and fibrin split products can be detected.

   b. **Treatment** of DIC is correction of the primary triggering disorder. Cryoprecipitate to provide fibrinogen and Factor VIII and platelet concentrates may be required. Heparin, although a controversial therapy (40–80 $\mu g \cdot kg^{-1}$ every 4–6 hours), may be considered in an attempt to halt clot formation, which is responsible for consumption of coagulation factors and platelets.

4. **Thrombocytopenia** may occur in massive transfusions, liver failure, or DIC. Massive transfusions do not usually lower concentrations of coagulation factors to levels that result in bleeding (see Section II E).

IV. HEMOTHERAPY

A. Red blood cells (RBCs) versus whole blood administration. Treatment of deficient oxygen-carrying capacity (anemia) requires only RBCs, whereas acute blood loss with concomitant loss of cells and plasma is logically treated with whole blood. Objections to using packed RBCs to treat surgical blood loss are a slow infusion rate due to high viscosity, inadequate volume replacement, and deficiency of coagulation factors. Reconstitution with saline overcomes the problems of slow infusion and inadequate volume replacement. Ca^{2+}-containing solutions should not be used to reconstitute packed RBCs. A suggested compromise is that patients who lose more than 25% of their blood volume and who are continuing to bleed should receive whole blood. Platelets may be required regardless of whether packed RBCs or whole blood is used to replace blood loss.

B. **Fresh frozen plasma.** The value of fresh frozen plasma to provide coagulation factors for patients with liver failure or massive transfusions is not proved. PT and PTT probably do not possess sufficient specificity to justify administration of fresh frozen plasma. Prophylactic use of fresh frozen plasma is not recommended. Furthermore, 10 units of platelet concentrates may contain as much as 500 ml of plasma, which has the same amount of coagulation factors as 2 units of fresh frozen plasma.

C. **Platelets.** One unit of platelets for every 10 kg body weight is recommended to treat bleeding due to thrombocytopenia. Platelets should be administered rapidly to maximize hemostatic efficacy.

V. COMPLICATIONS OF TRANSFUSIONS
(Table 10-3)

A. Recognition of an **acute hemolytic transfusion reaction** in an anesthetized patient may be difficult. **Hematuria** as a reflection of free plasma hemoglobin may be the first sign. Hypotension is likely, and DIC may occur before or after the diagnosis is made. Treatment is immediate discontinuation of the incompatible blood transfusion and support of blood pressure to maintain renal blood flow, combined with diuretic therapy to maintain urine flow. Monitoring of coagulation status is indicated. Hemodialysis is required if acute renal failure occurs.

B. A temperature increase of $>1°C$ in association with a transfusion signals a **febrile reaction.** This is the most common type of reaction and rarely is associated with hypotension. Although benign, it may be difficult to differentiate from a hemolytic reaction or sepsis. Until the diagnosis is proved, the blood transfusion must be halted. Treatment is with antipyretics.

TABLE 10-3. Complications of Transfusion

Acute hemolytic transfusion reaction (ABO-Rh incompatibility; immediate versus delayed)

Febrile reaction

Allergic reaction

Disease transmission (hepatitis, cytomegalovirus, acquired immunodeficiency syndrome)

Bacterial contamination

Depletion of procoagulants and platelets

Immunosuppression

Microaggregates

Circulatory overload

Metabolic complications (hypothermia, citrate toxicity, altered plasma potassium concentration)

    C. During anesthesia the appearance of **hives** in a patient receiving blood may be the only manifestation of an **allergic reaction.** Hypotension is unlikely to occur. Treatment is with an **antihistamine** (diphenhydramine, $0.5-1.0$ mg·kg^{-1} iv). When it is due to **immunoglobulin A antibodies,** the reaction may be life threatening and may require treatment with epinephrine.

    D. After 3–5 days of storage, **microaggregates** consisting of platelets and leukocytes accumulate in whole blood. Micropore filters (10–40 μm) remove this debris, although the clinical significance of infused microaggregates is unproved. Regardless of the decision to use or not use micropore filters, it is always mandatory to administer blood through a 170-μm filter.

VI. MASSIVE BLOOD TRANSFUSIONS

    A. Transfusion of one or more blood volumes in a 24-hour period is defined as a massive blood transfusion. In an adult, the blood volume is estimated as about 5000 ml (60–70 ml·kg^{-1}); thus, transfusion of 10 or more units of whole blood is considered massive. **Dilutional coagulopathy** is a possible side effect of massive blood transfusion. Nevertheless, administration of coagulation factors (fresh frozen plasma) or platelets should be based on appropriate coagulation tests rather than preestablished formulas (e.g., the infusions of these components after a fixed number of units of blood administration).

TABLE 10-4. Changes in Citrate-Phosphate-Dextrose Blood During Storage

	Day 1	Day 7	Day 14	Day 21
Blood pH	7.1	7.0	7.0	6.9
Blood P_{CO_2} (mm Hg)	48	80	110	140
Blood lactate (mEq·l^{-1})	41	101	145	179
Plasma potassium (mEq·l^{-1})	3.9	12	17	21
Plasma glucose (mg·dl^{-1})	345	312	282	231
Plasma hemoglobin (mg·dl^{-1})	1.7	7.8	13	19
2,3-DPG (μM·ml^{-1})	4.8	1.2	1.0	<1.0
Platelets (%)	10	0	0	0
Factors V and VIII (%)	70	50	40	20

2,3-DPG- 2,3-diphosphoglycerate.

TABLE 10-5. Content of Crystalloid Solutions

Solution	Glucose ($mg \cdot dl^{-1}$)	Na^+ ($mEq \cdot l^{-1}$)	Cl^- ($mEq \cdot l^{-1}$)	K^+ ($mEq \cdot l^{-1}$)	Mg^{2+} ($mEq \cdot l^{-1}$)	Ca^{2+} ($mEq \cdot l^{-1}$)	Lactate ($mEq \cdot l^{-1}$)	pH	$mOsm \cdot l^{-1}$
Extracellular fluid	100	140	108	4.5	2.0	5.0	5.0	7.4	290
5% Dextrose in water	5000							5.0	253
Lactated Ringer's solution		130	109	4.0		3.0	28	6.7	273
5% Dextrose in lactated Ringer's solution	5000	130	109	4.0		3.0	28	5.3	527
Normal saline		154	154					5.7	308
5% Dextrose in normal saline	5000	154	154					4.2	561
Normosol-R		140	98	5.0	3.0		*	7.4	295

*Contains acetate, 27 $mEq \cdot l^{-1}$, and gluconate, 13 $mEq \cdot l^{-1}$.

TABLE 10-6. Colloids Available for Maintaining Intravascular Fluid Volume
Albumin (5% or 25%)
Plasma protein fraction
Dextran
Hydroxyethyl starch

B. Changes in blood during storage may become an important consideration when massive blood transfusions are administered (Table 10-4). Newer preservatives (e.g., CPD-A1) allow longer periods of storage of red blood cells (21 versus 35 days).

VII. BLOOD SUBSTITUTES

A. **Autologous blood** is the safest form of blood and the best substitute for homologous blood. Patients may **predeposit** their own blood before surgery, assuming the preoperative hematocrit is >30%. Alternatively, **acute isovolemic hemodilution** and collection of 1–2 units of blood immediately before surgery may be considered. Intraoperative scavenging also provides blood for autologous blood transfusion.

B. **Type and screen** denote blood that has been typed for A, B, and Rh antigens and screened for antibodies. This blood is also available to other patients in the likely event it is not needed during surgery.

C. **Crystalloid infusion** is used to maintain normovolemia in a patient who is losing blood (Table 10-5). Because these solutions leave the intravascular space, it is often recommended that 2–4 ml of crystalloid solution be administered for each milliliter of blood loss. The hematocrit below which crystalloid replacement of blood loss is no longer acceptable must be individualized but probably is in the range of 25–30%.

D. **Colloid** used in lieu of crystalloid to replace blood loss has the advantage that it may be used in a 1:1 ratio because it stays intravascular (Table 10-6). It has the disadvantage of being more expensive, however. Heating of albumin and plasma protein fraction to 60°C removes the risk of hepatitis. There is no evidence that outcome is improved in patients receiving colloid rather than crystalloid solutions to replace blood loss.

BASIC PRINCIPLES
OF PHARMACOLOGY
IN ANESTHESIA
PRACTICE

11

Autonomic Nervous System Physiology and Pharmacology

Anesthesiology is the practice of autonomic nervous system (ANS) medicine (Lawson NW: Autonomic nervous system physiology and pharmacology. In Barash PG, Cullen BF, Stoelting RK [eds]: Clinical Anesthesia, pp 319–384. Philadelphia, JB Lippincott, 1992). The ANS is principally responsible for maintaining internal homeostasis. Drugs used during anesthesia as well as painful stimulation and disease states often produce ANS-related side effects.

I. FUNCTIONAL ANATOMY

The ANS is divided into the **sympathetic nervous system** (SNS, adrenergic system) and the **parasympathetic nervous system** (PNS, cholinergic system). The SNS and PNS produce complementary effects on the activity of organ systems (Table 11-1).

A. **Central autonomic nervous system organization.** The principal site of ANS organization is the **hypothalamus** (blood pressure control, temperature regulation, stress responses). Vital centers for hemodynamic and ventilatory control are in the medulla oblongata and pons.

B. **Peripheral autonomic nervous system organization** (Fig. 11-1)

1. The cell body of the preganglionic neuron originates in the central nervous system (CNS) and synapses in an autonomic ganglion (an exception is the adrenal medulla). Postganglionic neurons arise from the autonomic ganglia and are distributed to effector organs. There are 22 pairs of SNS (paravertebral) ganglia that are located nearer the spinal cord than the innervated organ. In con-

TABLE 11-1. Homeostatic Balance Between Divisions of the Autonomic Nervous System

	Sympathetic Nervous System	Parasympathetic Nervous System
Heart		
Sinoatrial node	Tachycardia	Bradycardia
Atrioventricular node	Enhanced conduction	Slowed conduction
His-Purkinje system	Increased automaticity	Minimal effect
Myocardium	Increased contractility	Minimal decrease in contractility
Blood vessels		
Skin and mucosa	Constriction	Dilation
Skeletal muscle	Constriction (alpha)	Dilation
	Dilation (beta)	
Pulmonary	Constriction	Dilation
Bronchial smooth muscle	Relaxation	Contraction
Gastrointestinal tract		
Gallbladder	Relaxation	Contraction
Gut motility and secretions	Decreased	Increased
Bladder		
Detrusor	Relaxation	Contraction
Trigone	Contraction	Relaxation
Glands (nasal, lacrimal, salivary, pancreatic)	Vasoconstriction and reduced secretion	Stimulation of secretions
Sweat glands	Diaphoresis	No effect
Apocrine glands	Thick and odiferous secretions	No effect
Eye		
Pupil	Mydriasis	Miosis
Ciliary	Relaxation for far vision	Contraction for near vision

130

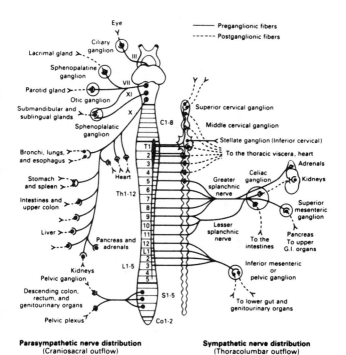

Figure 11-1. Schematic distribution of the efferent autnomic nervous system.

       trast, PNS ganglia are located in or near the innervated organ.

2. **Preganglionic fibers** are myelinated (rapid conduction), whereas **postganglionic fibers** are nonmyelinated.

3. Activation of the SNS produces a diffuse physiologic response **(mass reflex),** whereas activation of the PNS produces more **discrete responses.** For example, vagal stimulation may produce bradycardia with no effect on intestinal motility.

4. **Autonomic nervous system innervation.** The heart is well supplied by the SNS and PNS, but vagal fibers have little or no distribution to the ventricles. The peripheral circulation is principally under the control of the SNS. Basal ANS tone maintains arteriolar diameter at about 50%

TABLE 11-2. Classification of Adrenergic Receptors

	Agonist	Antagonist	Location	Action
Alpha₁	Norepinephrine	Prazosin Phentolamine* Labetalol*	Smooth muscle (blood vessels, sphincters)	Vasoconstriction Increased cardiac automaticity
Alpha₂	Clonidine Norepinephrine	Yohimbine Phentolamine*	Presynaptic and postsynaptic sites in the CNS	Inhibit release of norepinephrine
Beta₁	Isoproterenol* Epinephrine* Norepinephrine* Dopamine* Dobutamine*	Metoprolol Esmolol Propranolol* Timolol* Labetalol*	Heart	Increased heart rate, contractility, conduction, and automaticity
Beta₂	Isoproterenol* Epinephrine* Norepinephrine* Terbutaline Ritodrine Albuterol	Propranolol* Timolol* Labetalol*	Liver Smooth muscle (skeletal and coronary arteries) Pancreas	Glycogenolysis Bronchodilation Uterine relaxation Vasodilation Insulin secretion
Dopamine₁	Dopamine	Droperidol	Renal vasculature	Vasodilation
Dopamine₂	Dopamine	Domperidone	Presynaptic	Inhibit release of norepinephrine

*Nonselective.

of maximum, thus permitting the potential for further vasoconstriction or vasodilation. By functioning as a reservoir for about 80% of the blood volume, small changes in venous capacitance produced by the SNS produce large changes in venous return.

C. **Autonomic nervous system transmission** of impulses across terminal junctional sites of the peripheral ANS depends on liberated chemicals (neurotransmitters).

    1. **Acetylcholine (ACh)** is the neurotransmitter at preganglionic nerve endings of the SNS and PNS and postganglionic nerve endings of the PNS.

    2. **Norepinephrine (NE)** is the neurotransmitter at postganglionic nerve endings of the SNS (exception in sweat glands, where ACh is the neurotransmitter).

    3. Chromaffin cells of the adrenal medulla take the place of SNS postganglionic neurons and release NE and **epinephrine (EPI)** (predominates) into the circulation as neurotransmitter hormones.

D. **Receptors** appear to be macromolecules on cell membranes, which when activated by an agonist (NE or ACh) lead to a response by an effector cell. An **antagonist** is a substance that interferes with elicitation of a response at a receptor site by an **agonist.**

    1. **Cholinergic receptors** are subdivided into **muscarinic** (postganglionic nerve endings) and **nicotinic** (autonomic ganglia and neuromuscular junction) receptors. ACh is the neurotransmitter. Atropine is a specific antagonist at muscarinic receptors. ACh is not taken up by the presynaptic nerve terminals and, in contrast to NE, must be continuously synthesized.

    2. **Adrenergic receptors** are subdivided into **alpha, beta,** and **dopaminergic,** with subtypes for each category. NE is the neurotransmitter at alpha and beta receptors (Table 11-2).

E. **Adrenergic-receptor number or sensitivity** is inversely related to the ambient concentration of catecholamines **(up-regulation or down-regulation).** For example, chronic treatment of asthma with beta agonists can result in tachyphylaxis due to down-regulation. Denervation or chronic treatment with a beta antagonist results in up-regulation.

II. MOLECULAR PHARMACOLOGY AND EFFECTOR RESPONSE

Receptors are only the first link in a series of reactions that summate in the cellular response. A chemical mes-

senger **(first messenger)** (neurotransmitter or drug) inter-
acts with a receptor (stimulatory or inhibitory) that influences the activity of the enzyme **adenyl cyclase.** Adenyl
cyclase catalyzes the conversion of **adenosine triphosphate to cyclic adenosine monophosphate (second messenger).** The interaction of the receptor with adenyl cyclase is determined by **guanine nucleotide** regulatory (G)
proteins. G proteins act as transducers of information
across cell membranes. Ca^{2+} functions as the **third messenger.**

III. AUTONOMIC NERVOUS SYSTEM REFLEXES

A. **Arterial baroreceptors,** located in the carotid sinus
   and aortic arch, react to alterations in stretch caused
   by changes in blood pressure. Increased sensory traffic from the baroreceptors owing to increased blood
   pressure inhibits SNS traffic. The resulting relative
   increase in vagal tone produces vasodilation, slowing
   of the heart rate, and lowering of blood pressure. Volatile anesthetics interfere with baroreceptor function;
   thus, anesthetic-induced reductions in blood pressure may not evoke reflex heart rate changes.
B. **Venous baroreceptors,** located in the right atrium and
   great veins, produce an increased heart rate when the
   right atrium is stretched by increased filling pressure
   (Bainbridge reflex). Slowing of the heart rate during
   spinal anesthesia may reflect activation of venous
   baroreceptors as a result of reduced venous return.

IV. CLINICAL AUTONOMIC NERVOUS SYSTEM PHARMACOLOGY

The ultimate response evoked by a drug depends on the
(1) plasma concentration achieved, (2) number of receptors occupied and strength of binding, and (3) reflex adjustments in response to drug effects.

A. **Ganglionic antagonists. Trimethaphan** produces ganglionic blockade by competition with ACh receptors.
   Rapid hydrolysis by plasma cholinesterase necessitates administration of trimethaphan by continuous
   intravenous infusion (500 mg diluted in 250–500 ml;
   start infusion at 10–20 $\mu g\ kg^{-1}\cdot min^{-1}$) so as to titrate
   blood pressure to the desired level. Tachyphylaxis
   and mydriasis (the latter obscures eye signs for neurosurgery) detract from the use of this drug for controlled hypotension.
B. **Anticholinesterases** inhibit activity of acetylcholinesterase, which normally destroys ACh by hydrolysis.

As a result of this inhibition, there is accumulation of ACh at muscarinic and nicotinic receptors.

1. **Reversible cholinesterase inhibitors (neostigmine, pyridostigmine, edrophonium)** delay hydrolysis of ACh for 1–8 hours. Muscarinic activity is evoked by lower concentrations of ACh than necessary to produce desired **nicotinic effects** (reversal of nondepolarizing muscle relaxants). Simultaneous administration of an **anticholinergic drug** protects patients from undesired muscarinic effects (bradycardia, salivation, bronchospasm, hypermotility) without preventing nicotinic effects of ACh.

2. **Nonreversible cholinesterase inhibitors** (organophosphate compounds, such as insecticides and nerve gases) produce signs of ACh toxicity that necessitate treatment with intravenous administration of atropine, 35–70 $\mu g \cdot kg^{-1}$ every 3–10 minutes, until muscarinic symptoms abate. Atropine has no detectable impact on ACh-induced skeletal muscle paralysis (nicotinic effect), and mechanical support of ventilation may be necessary.

   a. **Pralidoxime** reactivates acetylcholinesterase activity and may be useful in treatment of organophosphate poisoning.

   b. **Echothiophate** eye drops administered for treatment of glaucoma produce prolonged inhibition of acetylcholinesterase. Responses to succinylcholine may be prolonged for 2–3 weeks after cessation of topical therapy.

C. An **anticholinergic** is any drug that interferes with the muscarinic actions of ACh as a neurotransmitter by competitive inhibition at cholinergic postganglionic nerves.

   1. There are marked variations in sensitivity to anticholinergic drugs at different muscarinic sites (see Table 3-8).

   2. **Central anticholinergic syndrome** is characterized by symptoms that range from sedation to delirium, presumably reflecting inhibition of muscarinic CNS receptors in the CNS by anticholinergics.

      a. The diagnosis is confirmed by peripheral signs of antimuscarinic activity (dry mouth, mydriasis, flushed skin).

      b. **Treatment** is intravenous administration of **physostigmine** in 1-mg doses, not to exceed a total of about 3 mg. The duration of action of physostigmine may be shorter than that of the offending drug, requiring repeated injection should symptoms recur. Physostigmine is effective because its tertiary amine structure allows it to cross the blood-brain barrier readily. Other anticholinesterases are quaternary ammonium compounds that lack lipid solubility necessary to gain prompt entrance into the CNS.

D. **Adrenergic agonists** include drugs characterized as **vasopressors (sympathomimetics)** and **inotropes (catecholamines).** Most adrenergic agonists activate both alpha and beta receptors, with the predominant dose-related pharmacologic effect being the expression of this mixed receptor activation (Table 11-3).

  1. **Hemodynamic effects** evoked by adrenergic agonist drugs include changes in heart rate **(chronotropism),** cardiac output **(inotropism),** conduction velocity of the cardiac impulse **(dromotropism),** cardiac rhythm, and systemic vascular resistance (SVR). Effects of these drugs on capacitance veins (venous return) may be as important as inotropic actions and more important than arteriolar effects (Table 11-4).

  2. **Side effects** reflect excessive alpha or beta receptor activity.

  3. **Methoxamine** is a pure arterial vasoconstrictor that increases SVR and decreases cardiac output even though blood pressure is elevated. Few clinical indications remain, although a single intravenous dose may convert paroxysmal atrial tachycardia reflexly through baroreceptor stimulation.

  4. **Phenylephrine** is considered a pure alpha agonist, but unlike methoxamine, this drug produces greater venoconstriction than arterial constriction. As a result, venous return and blood pressure are increased.

     a. **Side effects.** Excessive vasoconstriction produced by phenylephrine can elicit baroreceptor-mediated bradycardia with associated decreases in cardiac output. Increased SVR may further contribute to decreases in cardiac output and increases in myocardial oxygen requirements.

     b. **Clinical uses.** Phenylephrine is administered as a single intravenous dose (50–100 µg) to treat anesthetic-induced reductions in blood pressure, hypotension during cardiopulmonary bypass, and as a continuous infusion to maintain perfusion pressure during cerebral and peripheral vascular procedures. Use of

TABLE 11-3. Doses and Principal Sites of Action of Adrenergic Agonists

	Dose (iv, adults)		Alpha₁ (Arterial)	Alpha₂ (Venous)	Beta₁	Beta₂	Dopamine₁
	Bolus	Continuous Infusion					
Methoxamine	5–10 mg		++++	+/−	0	0	0
Phenylephrine	50–100 µg	0.15 µg·kg⁻¹·min⁻¹ (10 mg in 250 ml; 40 µg·ml⁻¹)	++++	+++++	0	0	0
Norepinephrine		0.1 µg·kg⁻¹·min⁻¹ (4 mg in 250 ml; 16 µg·ml⁻¹)	+++	+++	++++	+	0
Metaraminol		0.5 µg·kg⁻¹·min⁻¹ (100 mg in 250 ml; 400 µg·ml⁻¹)	++	++	+++	0	0
Epinephrine	2–8 µg* 300–500 µg†	0.015 µg·kg⁻¹·min⁻¹ (1 mg in 250 ml; 4 µg·ml⁻¹)	+++	+++	++++	++++	0
Ephedrine	5–10 mg		++	+++	+++	++	0
Mephentermine	15–30 mg		++	+	+++	+	0
Dopamine		4 µg·kg⁻¹·min (500 mg in 250 ml; 2000 µg·ml⁻¹)	+	++++	+++	+++++	++++
Dobutamine		2–30 µg·kg⁻¹·min⁻¹ (250 mg in 250 ml; 1 mg·ml⁻¹)	+/−	?	++++	++	0
Isoproterenol		1–5 µg·min⁻¹ (1 mg in 250 ml; 4 µg·ml⁻¹)	0	0	++++	++++	0

*dose to treat hypotension
†dose for cardiac arrest

TABLE 11-4. Hemodynamic Effects of Adrenergic Agonists

	Heart Rate	Cardiac Output	Systemic Vascular Resistance	Venous Return	Renal Blood Flow
Methoxamine	D	D	I	NC	D
Phenylephrine	D	D	I	I	D
Norepinephrine	D	D	I	I	D
Metaraminol	D	D	I	I	D
Epinephrine	I	I	I	I	D
Ephedrine	I	I	I	I	I/D
Mephentermine	I	I	I	I(?)	I/D
Dopamine	NC	I	D/NC	I	I
Dobutamine	I(?)	I	NC/D	?	I/NC
Isoproterenol	I	I	D	D	I/NC

D = decrease; I = increase; NC = no change.

138

phenylephrine to maintain perfusion pressures during vascular procedures must be done cautiously, as this practice can evoke myocardial ischemia in susceptible patients.

5. **Norepinephrine and metaraminol** produce similar dose-related hemodynamic effects characterized by greater alpha than beta effects. Vasoconstriction elevates blood pressure but may also reduce tissue blood flow (especially renal blood flow) and increase myocardial oxygen requirements. Continuous infusions to maintain systolic blood pressure above 90–100 mm Hg require invasive monitoring and attention to fluid management.

6. **Epinephrine.** Alpha effects of EPI predominate in renal and cutaneous vasculature to decrease blood flow, whereas beta effects increase blood flow to skeletal muscles.

   a. **Side effects.** Cardiac dysrhythmias are a hazard of excess beta stimulation. Volatile anesthetics, especially halothane, sensitize the myocardium to circulating catecholamines. For this reason, the subcutaneous or submucosal dose of EPI administered during halothane anesthesia should be limited to about 1 $\mu g \cdot kg^{-1}$ (2–3 $\mu g \cdot kg^{-1}$ is probably acceptable during enflurane or isoflurane anesthesia). In contrast to adults, children seem to tolerate higher doses of subcutaneous EPI without developing cardiac dysrhythmias.

   b. **Clinical uses.** EPI is administered to (1) treat asthma (0.3–0.5 mg subcutaneously), (2) cardiac arrest or life-threatening allergic reactions (0.3–0.5 mg iv), (3) produce hemostasis (1:200,000 or 5 $\mu g \cdot ml^{-1}$ injected subcutaneously or submucosally), (4) to prolong regional anesthesia (0.2 mg added to local anesthetic solutions for spinal block or as a 1:200,000 concentration for epidural block), or (5) maintain cardiac output, such as a continuous iv infusion to maintain cardiac output, such as following cardiopulmonary bypass.

7. **Ephedrine** produces cardiovascular effects that resemble those produced by EPI; however, its potency is greatly reduced, although its duration of action is about 10 times longer than that of EPI. Venoconstriction is greater than arterial constriction; thus, venous return and cardiac output are improved. A beta effect increases heart rate and further facilitates cardiac output. The alpha and

beta effects of ephedrine result in a modest and predictable increase in blood pressure.

   a. **Side effects.** Tachycardia and cardiac dys-rhythmias are possible but less likely to occur than after administration of EPI.

   b. **Clinical uses.** Ephedrine is the most commonly used vasopressor (5–10 mg iv) to treat reductions in blood pressure produced by anesthesia (especially regional blocks) and is considered the drug of choice in obstetrics because uterine blood flow directly parallels ephedrine-induced increases in blood pressure. It is appropriate to administer ephedrine as a temporizing measure to restore perfusion pressure while the underlying cause of hypotension is corrected.

8. **Mephentermine** is a vasopressor with hemodynamic effects similar to those of ephedrine.

9. **Dopamine** is an agonist at dopaminergic (2–5 μg kg^{-1}·min^{-1}), beta (2–10 μg·kg^{-1}·min^{-1}), and alpha (>10 μg·kg^{-1}·min^{-1}) receptors. Infusion rates >10 μg·kg^{-1}·min^{-1} may produce sufficient vasoconstriction to offset desirable dopaminergic (increased renal blood flow) and beta (increased cardiac output) receptor stimulation.

   a. **Side effects.** Tachycardia and cardiac dys-rhythmias occur infrequently. Extravasation of dopamine can produce gangrene. Pulmonary artery pressure may be increased, detracting from the use of dopamine in patients with right-sided heart failure. Insulin secretion is inhibited, explaining the common occurrence of hyperglycemia during infusion of dopamine.

   b. **Clinical uses.** Dopamine is most commonly administered as a continuous intravenous infusion (2–10 μg·kg^{-1}·min^{-1}) for its inotropic and diuretic effects in patients with poor myocardial contractility, such as following cardiopulmonary bypass.

10. **Dobutamine** is a synthetic catecholamine derived from isoproterenol. It produces a positive inotropic effect with minimal effects on heart rate and SVR (an advantage over isoproterenol). Increases in cardiac output may not be accompanied by changes in blood pressure, emphasizing the weak to absent alpha effects of this drug.

   a. **Side effects.** Increases in automaticity of the sinoatrial node and increases in conduction of cardiac impulses through the atrioventricular node and ventricles occur, emphasizing the need for caution in administering this drug to patients with atrial fibrillation or other tachydysrhythmias.

    b. Clinical uses. Dobutamine is most commonly administered as a continuous intravenous infusion (2–30 $\mu g \cdot kg^{-1} \cdot min^{-1}$) for its inotropic effects in patients with poor myocardial contractility, such as following cardiopulmonary bypass.

11. **Isoproterenol** is a nonspecific beta agonist that lacks alpha effects. Cardiac output is increased by virtue of elevations in heart rate as well as enhanced myocardial contractility, whereas reductions in SVR contribute to decreased afterload.

    a. Side effects. Myocardial oxygen requirements are increased owing to elevations in heart rate and contractility, whereas myocardial oxygen delivery may be concomitantly reduced as a reflection of vasodilation and decreased diastolic blood pressure (coronary perfusion pressure). For these reasons, myocardial ischemia may be evoked in vulnerable patients. Increases in cardiac output may be diverted to nonvital tissues such as skeletal muscles.

    b. Clinical uses. Isoproterenol is most commonly administered as a continuous intravenous infusion (0.015 $\mu g \cdot kg^{-1} \cdot min^{-1}$) for the treatment of congestive heart failure associated with bradycardia, asthma, or pulmonary hypertension. This catecholamine acts as a **chemical cardiac pacemaker** in the presence of complete heart block.

12. **Combination therapy** is theoretically intended to maximize inotropic effects and minimize vasoconstrictive actions. Invasive monitoring is necessary to guide therapy.

    a. Dopamine-nitroprusside or nitroglycerin results in increases in cardiac output that are greater than with either drug along.

    b. Dopamine-dobutamine results in preferential distribution of cardiac output to the kidneys.

    c. Norepinephrine-phentolamine. A 250-ml solution of NE (4 mg) plus phentolamine (5–10 mg) is designed to maximize the beta effects and mask the alpha effects of NE.

13. **Ritodrine** is a predominant beta$_2$ agonist that is administered to stop premature labor **(tocolytic**

effect). Side effects include hyperglycemia, hypokalemia, and tachycardia. Tachycardia may be sufficient to produce pulmonary edema in some parturients.

14. Nonadrenergic sympathomimetic drugs

    a. Aminophylline is administered as a single iv injection (5 mg·kg^{-1} slowly) or as a continuous iv infusion (0.5–1.0 mg·kg^{-1}·h^{-1}) to produce bronchodilation and increased cardiac output. Aminophylline produces beta effects owing to its inhibition of phosphodiesterase and an antiadenosine effect. Cardiac dysrhythmias are a hazard, especially during general anesthesia with halothane.

    b. Amrinone is administered as a single intravenous injection over 2–3 minutes (0.75 mg·kg^{-1}) followed by a continuous intravenous infusion (5–10 μg·kg^{-1}·min^{-1}). This drug is a phosphodiesterase inhibitor that improves cardiac output by positive inotropic effects as well as vasodilation with resultant decreases in SVR.

    c. Enoximone is a phosphodiesterase inhibitor that is a more potent inotrope than amrinone and also produces pulmonary and systemic arterial vasodilation.

    d. Digoxin is administered principally to treat congestive heart failure and control supraventricular cardiac dysrhythmias such as atrial fibrillation. A therapeutic effect occurs within 10 minutes after an intravenous injection of 0.25–1.0 mg to adults. Signs of **digitalis toxicity** (cardiac dysrhythmias, gastrointestinal disturbances) must be inquired about when evaluating patients preoperatively. Digitalis toxicity is enhanced by hypokalemia or injections of Ca^{2+}. Iatrogenic hyperventilation of the lungs with associated hypokalemia should be avoided during anesthesia. Most recommend continuation of digitalis therapy in the perioperative period, especially when the drug is being administered for control of heart rate. Prophylactic preoperative administration of digitalis is controversial but may be of unique value in elderly patients undergoing thoracic surgery.

E. Alpha antagonists produce orthostatic hypotension, tachycardia, and miosis.

    1. Phentolamine is a nonselective and competitive antagonist at alpha$_1$ and alpha$_2$ receptors; it is usually administered intravenously in doses of 2–5 mg until adequate control of blood pressure is achieved. Tachycardia reflects continued presynaptic release of NE owing to alpha$_2$ receptor blockade.

2. **Prazosin** is a selective postsynaptic alpha$_1$ antagonist that leaves intact the negative feedback mechanism for NE release that is mediated by presynaptic alpha$_2$ activity. This drug is useful in the preoperative preparation of patients with pheochromocytoma.

F. **Beta antagonists** are distinguished by differing pharmacokinetic and pharmacodynamic characteristics (Table 11-5).

1. **Side effects** of beta antagonists include heart block, worsening of congestive heart failure, bronchospasm, vasoconstriction (coronary arteries), and inhibition of insulin release. Excessive SNS activity (hypertension, angina) often accompanies abrupt withdrawal of beta antagonists, presumably reflecting prior up-regulation of beta receptors due to chronic suppression of agonist activity.

2. **Beta$_1$ selectivity (cardioselective)** implies greater safety in treatment of patients with obstructive pulmonary disease, diabetes mellitus, or peripheral vascular disease because beta$_2$ agonist effects (bronchodilation, vasodilation) are presumably maintained. The clinical significance of membrane-stabilizing activity (a local anesthetic effect on myocardial cells at high doses) or intrinsic sympathomimetic activity (partial beta agonist activity at low doses) is not documented.

3. **Propranolol** is a nonselective beta antagonist that may be administered in single intravenous doses of 0.1–0.5 mg (maximum dose about 2 mg) to slow heart rate during anesthesia. Additive negative inotropic or chronotropic effects with inhaled or injected anesthetics are likely to occur but have not been a significant clinical problem.

4. **Timolol** is administered as a topical preparation for treatment of glaucoma. There may be sufficient systemic absorption to cause bradycardia and hypotension that is resistant to reversal with atropine.

5. **Esmolol** is a cardioselective beta$_1$ antagonist administered as a single intravenous bolus (0.5 mg·kg^{-1}) or as a continuous intravenous infusion (50–200 μg·kg^{-1}·min^{-1}) to produce rapid and short-term

TABLE 11-5. Pharmacokinetics of Beta Antagonists

	Relative Beta$_1$ Selectivity	Membrane-Stabilizing Activity	Intrinsic Sympathomimetic Activity	Elimination Half-Time (hours)	Lipid Solubility	Route of Elimination
Propranolol	0	+	0	3–4	+++	Hepatic
Nadolol	0	0	0	14–24	0	Renal
Timolol	0	0	0	4–5	+	Hepatic/renal
Pindolol	0	+	++	3–4	+	Hepatic/renal
Esmolol	++	0	0	0.16	?	Plasma esterase
Acebutolol	+	+	+	3–4	0	Hepatic
Atenolol	++	0	0	6–9	0	Renal
Metoprolol	++	0	0	3–4	+	Hepatic

reductions in heart rate and blood pressure. A unique feature is rapid hydrolysis by plasma esterases, allowing precise control of drug effect during continuous intravenous infusion.

G. **Mixed antagonists. Labetalol** produces selective alpha$_1$- and nonselective beta-antagonist effects. Administered as a single intravenous dose over 2 minutes (0.05–0.15 mg·kg^{-1}), this drug is useful in controlling excessive blood pressure and heart rate elevations in response to painful stimulation during general anesthesia. Although the magnitude is less than with beta antagonists, worsening of congestive heart failure or bronchospasm may follow the administration of labetalol.

V. CALCIUM ENTRY BLOCKERS

Calcium entry blockers interact with the cell membranes to interfere with movement of Ca^{2+} into cells through ion-specific channels. These channels are referred to as slow channels because their transition between the resting, activated, and inactivated states is delayed compared with fast Na^+ channels.

A. Calcium entry blockers are a heterogenous group of drugs with dissimilar structures and different electrophysiologic and pharmacologic properties. These drugs are most useful for the treatment of supraventricular tachydysrhythmias and coronary vasospasm (Table 11-6).

B. **Verapamil** is the drug of choice for **termination of supraventricular dysrhythmias,** and it is also effective in slowing the heart rate in patients with atrial fibrillation and atrial flutter. There is a dose-dependent increase in the PR interval and delay in conduction of the cardiac impulse through the atrioventricular node. Caution must be exercised when treating patients with Wolff-Parkinson-White syndrome, as verapamil may increase conduction velocity in the accessory tract. Verapamil, when combined with propranolol and digitalis, may result in excessive bradycardia. Unlike beta antagonists, verapamil does not increase airway resistance in patients with obstructive pulmonary disease.

C. **Nifedipine** is more effective than nitroglycerin for treatment of angina pectoris due to coronary vasospasm. Vasodilation results in compensatory tachycardia, and cardiac output may increase as a result of afterload reduction. Administration of nifedipine is

TABLE 11-6. Comparative Effects of Calcium Entry Blockers			
	Verapamil	Nifedipine	Diltiazem
Dose			
Intravenous ($\mu g \cdot kg^{-1}$)	75–150	5–15	75–150
Oral (mg every 8 hours)	80–160	10–20	60–90
Negative inotropic	+	0	0/+
Negative chronotropic	+	0	0/+
Negative dromotropic	+ + + +	0	+ +
Coronary vasodilation	+ +	+ + + +	+ + +
Systemic vasodilation	+ +	+ + + +	+ +
Bronchodilation	0/+	0/+	
Elimination half-time (hours)	2–7	4–5	4
Route of elimination	Renal	Renal	Hepatic

146

useful during anesthesia when there is evidence of myocardial ischemia associated with hypertension.

D. Diltiazem is an effective coronary vasodilator but a poor peripheral vasodilator; it often produces bradycardia.

E. Nicardipine produces vasodilation of coronary arteries without altering activity of the sinus node or conduction of cardiac impulses through the atrioventricular node.

F. Nimodipine is a highly lipophilic drug that produces somewhat selective vasodilation of cerebral arteries, resulting in a favorable effect on the severity of neurologic deficits caused by cerebral vasospasm following subarachnoid hemorrhage.

G. Calcium entry blockers may exhibit additive myocardial depressant effects with volatile anesthetics, which may also interfere with inward Ca^{2+} movement. Opioids do not seem to alter the response to calcium entry blockers. Calcium entry blockers seem to augment the effects of both depolarizing and nondepolarizing muscle relaxants in a manner similar to that of mycin antibiotics.

VI. SYMPATHOLYTICS

Sympatholytics block central SNS outflow or NE release from presynaptic neurons, resulting in an antihypertensive effect. These drugs also reduce anesthetic requirements for inhaled and injected drugs.

A. Clonidine. Stimulation of $alpha_2$ receptors in the vasomotor center of the medulla oblongata is thought to decrease SNS activity and enhance vagal tone.

1. **Side effects.** Sedation, bradycardia, and dry mouth are common. Abrupt discontinuation of clonidine, as before surgery, may result in rebound hypertension. This hypertension may be confused with anesthesia emergence symptoms, but it is usually delayed for about 18 hours. Withdrawal hypertension is more likely in patients receiving more than 1.2 mg·day^{-1}. Transdermal administration of clonidine is an alternative to the oral route because an intravenous preparation is not available. Life-threatening withdrawal hypertension may be treated with nitroprusside.

2. **Clinical uses.** In addition to its antihypertensive effect, clonidine administered preoperatively (5 µg·kg^{-1} orally) attenuates SNS reflex responses such as those associated with direct laryngoscopy or surgical stimulation and greatly reduces anes-

thetic requirements (40% or more) for volatile drugs or opioids. Placed in the subarachnoid or epidural space, this drug produces analgesia that may be accompanied by sedation and bradycardia but not depression of ventilation. More selective alpha$_1$ agonists administered to animals produce dose-related and stereospecific (receptor mechanism) reductions in anesthetic requirements (MAC).

B. **Dexmedetomidine** is a more selective alpha$_2$ agonist than clonidine.

VII. CONVERTING ENZYME INHIBITORS

A. Inhibitors of angiotensin-converting enzyme **(captopril, enalapril, lisinopril)** prevent the conversion of angiotensin I to angiotensin II. These drugs are highly effective in the treatment of congestive heart failure and essential hypertension as well as renovascular and malignant hypertension.

B. Side effects are minor, with the principal cardiovascular effect being decreased SVR.

VIII. VASODILATORS

Vasodilators decrease blood pressure by dose-related direct effects on vascular smooth muscle independent of alpha or beta receptors (Table 11-7). These drugs often evoke baroreceptor-mediated increases in heart rate. Combination with a beta antagonist (intravenous propranolol or esmolol) may be necessary to offset this reflex tachycardia (maintain heart rate < 100 beats·min^{-1}).

A. **Hydralazine** in doses of 5–10 mg administered intravenously every 10–20 minutes is useful to control perioperative hypertension.

B. **Nitroprusside** is administered as a continuous intravenous infusion (starting dose is 0.25–0.5 µg·kg^{-1}·min^{-1}) using an infusion pump and continuous monitoring of blood pressure. The dose is increased slowly as needed to **control hypertension** or to **produce controlled hypotension.** Rarely is more than 3–5 µg·kg^{-1}·min^{-1} of nitroprusside required in an anesthetized patient. Acute hypertensive responses can be treated with single intravenous injections of 50–100 µg.

1. The hypotensive effect of nitroprusside reflects direct relaxation of arterial and venous smooth muscle, causing decreases in preload and afterload. Hypotensive effects of nitroprusside are potentiated by volatile anesthetics and blood loss.

TABLE 11-7. Doses and Sites of Action of Vasodilators

	Dose (iv, adults)		Site of Action	Onset	Duration
	Bolus	*Continuous Infusion*			
Hydralazine	5–10 mg		Arterial	15–20 minutes	4–6 hours
Nitroprusside	50–100 μg	0.25–5.0 μg·kg^{-1}·min^{-1} (50 mg in 250 ml; 200 μg·ml^{-1})	Arterial and venous	1–2 minutes	2–5 minutes
Nitroglycerin		0.25–3.0 μg·kg^{-1}·min^{-1} (50 mg in 250 ml; 200 μg·ml^{-1})	Venous and arterial	2–5 minutes	3–5 minutes
Diazoxide	300 mg		Arterial	3–5 minutes	5–12 hours
Trimethaphan		10–20 μg·kg^{-1}·min^{-1} (500 mg in 250 ml; 2 mg·ml^{-1})	Ganglia	1 minute	2–4 minutes

2. **Side effects.** The ferrous iron of nitroprusside reacts with sulfhydryl groups in red blood cells and releases cyanide, which is reduced to thiocyanate in the liver. High doses of nitroprusside (>10 $\mu g \cdot kg^{-1} \cdot min^{-1}$) may result in **cyanide toxicity.** There is no evidence that renal or hepatic diseases increase the likelihood of cyanide toxicity.

   a. **Diagnosis.** Tachyphylaxis, elevated venous oxygen tension, and metabolic acidosis signal the development of cyanide toxicity (cyanide binds to cytochrome oxidase, causing cellular hypoxia) and the need to discontinue the infusion of nitroprusside immediately.

   b. **Treatment** of cyanide toxicity is with sodium thiosulfate (150 $mg \cdot kg^{-1}$ in 50 ml of water) administered intravenously over 15 minutes to speed the conversion of cyanide to thiocyanate.

C. **Nitroglycerin** is administered as a continuous intravenous infusion ($0.25-3.0$ $\mu g \cdot kg^{-1} \cdot min^{-1}$) to treat myocardial ischemia. Its predominant action is on venules, causing increased venous capacitance and decreased venous return. Control of hypertension with nitroglycerin is less reliable than with nitroprusside, emphasizing the minimal effect of this drug on arterial smooth muscle. Unlike nitroprusside, nitroglycerin poses no risk of cyanide toxicity. For this reason, nitroglycerin may be chosen over nitroprusside to control hypertension associated with pre-eclampsia (cyanide can cross the placenta).

D. **Diazoxide** is administered as a single intravenous dose ($3-5$ $mg \cdot kg^{-1}$ every 5 minutes) to treat hypertensive emergencies. It has a greater effect on resistance than capacitance vessels, thus decreasing afterload with little or no effect on preload. Ability to titrate blood pressure to a given level, as with nitroprusside, is not possible with diazoxide.

12

Nonopioid Intravenous Anesthetics

Nonopioid drugs can be injected intravenously as a bolus to induce anesthesia, or they can be administered by continuous infusion (especially propofol) for partial or complete maintenance of anesthesia (Fragen RJ, Avram MJ: Nonopioid intravenous anesthetics. In Barash PG, Cullen BF, Stoelting RK [eds]: Clinical Anesthesia, pp 385–412. Philadelphia, JB Lippincott, 1992) (Table 12-1).

I. CHEMISTRY AND FORMULATION

A. **Barbiturate solutions** are alkaline (pH 10–11), and mixing with acidic solutions (lactated Ringer's solution, other drugs) results in precipitation of barbiturates as free acids.

B. **Diazepam** is not available as a water-soluble salt. The solution contains propylene glycol and will precipitate when mixed with other drug solutions.

C. **Midazolam** is water-soluble (pH 3.5) and compatible with other solutions.

D. **Etomidate** (formulated with propylene glycol), ketamine (pH 3.5–5.5), and propofol should not be mixed with other drugs.

E. **Propofol** should be drawn into a sterile syringe, taking appropriate precautions to avoid contamination because the liquid preparation may act as a culture medium. Each ampule is intended for single patient use and should be discarded at the end of the patient's anesthetic.

II. STRUCTURE-ACTIVITY RELATIONSHIPS

Structure-activity relationships describe how modifications in chemical structure of prototypical drugs affect physicochemical properties of derivatives.

TABLE 12-1. Doses of Nonopioid Drugs Administered Intravenously for Anesthesia

	Bolus	Continuous Infusion
Barbiturates		
Thiopental	3–5 mg·kg^{-1}	
Thiamylal	3–5 mg·kg^{-1}	
Methohexital	1.0–1.5 mg·kg^{-1}	0.1–0.3 mg·kg^{-1}·min^{-1}
Benzodiazepines		
Diazepam	0.3–0.5 mg·kg^{-1}	
Midazolam	0.1–0.2 mg·kg^{-1}	2–5 μg·kg^{-1}·min^{-1}
Etomidate	0.2–0.3 mg·kg^{-1}	
Ketamine	1–2 mg·kg^{-1}	
Propofol	1.5–2.5 mg·kg^{-1}	0.1 mg·kg^{-1}·min^{-1}

A. Replacement of an oxygen atom in position two of barbituric acid with a sulfur atom produces **thiobarbiturates (thiopental, thiamylal)**, which have a more rapid onset and shorter duration of action than their corresponding oxybarbiturate analogues (pentobarbital, secobarbital). **Methylation** on the one position of barbituric acid produces methohexital, which has a rapid onset and short duration of action at the expense of an increased incidence of excitatory side effects.

B. The fused imidazole ring allows midazolam to be water-soluble and stable in acidic aqueous solution yet lipophilic at physiologic pH.

C. Pharmacologic activity may be limited to the + or − **stereoisomer,** as determined by the presence of one or more carbon atoms with an asymmetric center.

III. MECHANISMS OF ACTION

Mechanisms of action of nonopioid induction drugs are not understood, but proposed theories invoke actions of cell membranes **(biophysical theories)** or interactions with neurotransmitters **(transmitter theories).**

A. Modulation of **GABAminergic transmission** may be important in actions of barbiturates, benzodiazepines, etomidate, and propofol. Gamma-aminobutyric acid (GABA) is an inhibitory neurotransmitter, and activation of postsynaptic GABA receptors increases **chloride conductance** through ion channels, resulting in **hyperpolarization** (inhibition) of the postsynaptic neuron.

B. **Ketamine** may interact with (1) central nervous system muscarinic receptors as an antagonist, (2) opioid receptors as an agonist (analgesia at mu receptors and dysphoria at sigma receptors), and (3) an antagonist at N-methyl-D-aspartate **(NMDA)** receptors that respond to L-glutamate.

C. **Flumazenil** is a specific benzodiazepine receptor antagonist, whereas **physostigmine** is a nonspecific cortical stimulant.

IV. PHARMACOKINETICS (Table 12-2)

A. The hypnotic action of **standard induction doses** of nonopioid drugs is terminated by **redistribution of drug to inactive tissue sites**; thus, the concentration at active receptor sites is diluted.

B. **Clearance** becomes a dominant influence on the plasma drug concentration versus time relationship only after the end of the rapid decline in plasma drug concentration characterizing the distribution phase.

   1. Hepatic clearance of methohexital greatly exceeds that of thiopental, contributing to a shorter duration of action if repeated doses are administered.

   2. Rapid clearance of propofol facilitates the use of this drug by continuous intravenous infusion for partial or complete maintenance of anesthesia.

C. **Elimination half-time ($T_{1/2\beta}$)** is directly dependent on volume of distribution and inversely related to clearance. The wide range of $T_{1/2\beta}$ for nonopioid drugs principally reflects differences in clearance.

D. **Redistribution (versus clearance)** in the termination of drug effects becomes more prominent when inactive tissue sites for redistribution are saturated by single high doses, multiple doses, or continuous infusions.

E. **Volatile anesthetics and pharmacokinetics**

   1. Reductions in hepatic blood flow or metabolism produced by volatile anesthetics could delay clearance and prolong $T_{1/2\beta}$ of large or repeated doses of nonopioid induction drugs, especially those most dependent on hepatic extraction (methohexital, etomidate, ketamine).

   2. Nonspecific stimulation of drug-metabolizing enzymes by volatile anesthetics is unlikely to alter clearance of induction drugs.

F. **Age and pharmacokinetics.** Elderly patients require lower induction doses of nonopioid anesthetics, a phenomenon that could reflect slowed passage of drug into peripheral compartments (intercompartmental clear-

TABLE 12-2. Pharmacokinetics of Nonopioid Intravenous Anesthetics

	Volume of Distribution at Steady State $(l \cdot kg^{-1})$	Clearance $(ml \cdot kg^{-1} \cdot min^{-1})$	Elimination Half-Time (hours)	Hepatic Extraction Ratio	Protein Binding (%)
Thiopental	2.3	3.4	11.4	0.15	85
Methohexital	2.2	10.9	3.9	0.50	73
Diazepam	1.1	0.4	46.6	0.03	98
Midazolam	1.1	7.5	2.7	0.51	94
Etomidate	2.5	17.9	2.9	0.90	77
Ketamine	3.1	19.1	3.1	0.90	12
Propofol	2.8	59.4	0.9	0.90	97

ance) or altered distribution of cardiac output to organs
necessary for drug elimination.

V. EFFECTS ON ORGAN SYSTEMS

A. **Central nervous system.** In addition to decreased levels
of consciousness, clinically desirable effects of nonopioid drugs include reductions in cerebral blood flow, cerebral metabolic oxygen requirements, and intracranial
pressure (ICP), as well as a sleep pattern on the electroencephalogram. Many of these responses are uniquely
helpful in the management of patients with intracranial
pathology and increased ICP (Table 12-3).

1. Thiopental and etomidate can produce maximum
decreases in cerebral metabolic oxygen requirements (flat electroencephalogram) that are deemed
necessary for drug-induced **brain protection.** A similar effect on the electroencephalogram produced
with high doses of methohexital is not recommended, as refractory postdrug seizures may occur.

2. Thiopental in low doses does not affect somatosensory evoked potentials. Etomidate can alter the
waveform to mimic ischemia.

3. Ketamine increases cerebral blood flow and is unacceptable for administration to patients at risk for
increased ICP.

B. **Respiratory effects.** Depression of ventilation is characteristic of all these drugs. Differences are apparent

	Cerebral Blood Flow	Cerebral Metabolic Requirements for Oxygen	Intracranial Pressure
TABLE 12-3. Effects of Nonopioid Intravenous Anesthetics in the Central Nervous System			
Thiopental	– –	– –	– –
Methohexital	– –	– –	– –
Diazepam	–	–	–
Midazolam	–	–	–
Etomidate	– –	– –	– –
Ketamine	+ +	+	+
Propofol	– –	– –	– –

when nonopioid drugs are used as sedatives or hypnotics in spontaneously breathing patients (Table 12-4).

1. Apnea may follow intravenous administration of nonopioid induction drugs. For this reason, equipment must always be available to provide assisted ventilation of the lungs.

2. Airway instrumentation in a lightly anesthetized patient with hyper-reactive airways (from asthma or cigarette smoking) may result in bronchoconstriction. It is incorrect to attribute this response to increased airway sensitivity produced by thiopental.

3. Methohexital is associated with a greater incidence of hiccups and coughing than other nonopioid induction drugs.

4. Prior opioid administration, as in premedication, accentuates the ventilatory depressant effects of nonopioid induction drugs.

5. Ketamine is associated with increased airway secretions, and its sympathomimetic effects are presumed to be responsible for **bronchodilation** (may relieve bronchospasm in asthmatics).

C. **Cardiovascular effects.** All nonopioid induction drugs produce depressant or stimulant effects on the cardiovascular system (Table 12-5).

1. **Hypovolemia** exaggerates the hypotensive effects of barbiturates, benzodiazepines, and propofol.

2. **Ketamine** produces **central sympathetic nervous system stimulation** to increase blood pressure, heart rate, and myocardial contractility. This response is **blunted** by concomitant administration of various drugs (barbiturates, benzodiazepines, inhaled anesthetics) and may be **enhanced** by pancuronium.

TABLE 12-4. Effects of Nonopioid Intravenous Anesthetics on Ventilation

	Depression of Ventilation	Airway Resistance
Thiopental	+ +	0
Methohexital	+ +	0
Diazepam	+	0
Midazolam	+	0
Etomidate	+	0
Ketamine	0	− −
Propofol	+ +	0

TABLE 12-5. Effects of Nonopioid Intravenous Anesthetics on the Cardiovascular System

	Mean Arterial Pressure	Heart Rate	Cardiac Output	Systemic Vascular Resistance	Venodilation
Thiopental	–	+	–	0/+	+
Methohexital	–	+ +	–	?	+
Diazepam	0/–	–/+	0	–/+	+
Midazolam	0/–	–/+	0/–	0/–	+
Etomidate	0	0	0	0	0
Ketamine	+ +	+ +	+	+	0
Propofol	–	+	0/–	–	+

     a. Increased myocardial oxygen requirements produced by ketamine are undesirable in patients with coronary artery disease.

     b. In critically ill patients, the autonomic nervous system may be impaired and ketamine may act as a cardiovascular depressant.

     c. Ketamine may be advantageous for intravenous induction of anesthesia (1–2 mg·kg^{-1}) in hypovolemic patients or in the presence of cardiac failure, as it is the only induction drug that stimulates the cardiovascular system.

3. Etomidate (0.2–0.3 mg·kg^{-1} iv) produces the least detrimental cardiovascular changes of all the nonopioid induction drugs. This drug may be considered as an alternative to ketamine for induction of anesthesia in hypovolemic patients.

4. Benzodiazepines administered intravenously for the induction of anesthesia (diazepam, 0.3–0.5 mg·kg^{-1}; midazolam, 0.1–0.2 mg·kg^{-1}) produce modest depressant effects on the heart and systemic vasculature. Opioids may accentuate the blood pressure-lowering (vasodilating) effects of benzodiazepines.

5. Barbiturates (thiopental, 3–5 mg·kg^{-1}; methohexital, 1.0–1.5 mg·kg^{-1}) have more cardiovascular effects than benzodiazepines when administered intravenously for the induction of anesthesia. Thiopental's principal effect is to decrease cardiac output (Table 12-6).

     a. Baroreceptor reflex activity is probably responsible for the increased heart rate produced in response to thiopental-induced reductions in cardiac output and blood pressure. Myocardial depressant effects of thiopental may be exaggerated when the baroreflex is blunted by volatile anesthetics or beta antagonists.

     b. Methohexital is associated with a greater increase in heart rate than occurs after induction of anesthesia with thiopental.

TABLE 12-6. Mechanisms of Barbiturate-Induced Reductions in Cardiac Output

Decreased venous return
Direct myocardial depression
Reduced sympathetic outflow from the central nervous system

6. **Propofol** $(1.5-2.5 \text{ mg·kg}^{-1})$, administered intravenously for induction of anesthesia, produces reductions in blood pressure similar to those produced by thiopental.

7. **Cardiac dysrhythmias** are not commonly observed after administration of nonopioid anesthetics.

D. **Hepatorenal effects.** Direct adverse effects do not occur, although nonopioid anesthetics that reduce blood pressure can decrease hepatic blood flow and urine output.

E. **Endocrine effects.** The **adrenocortical response to stress** is decreased for 5–8 hours after induction of anesthesia with etomidate but not with other nonopioid anesthetics. The clinical significance, if any, of this effect is not known.

F. **Allergic effects**
   1. **Histamine release** may occur after rapid intravenous administration of thiopental but does not seem to occur with other nonopioid anesthetics.
   2. Life-threatening allergic reactions are a rare possibility after administration of barbiturates.

VI. USES DURING CLINICAL ANESTHESIA

A. **Induction of anesthesia**
   1. Differences in rapidity of onset for comparable induction doses depend on speed of injection, volume of distribution, and cardiac output. Most of the nonopioid anesthetics act in one arm–brain circulation time (exceptions are benzodiazepines and ketamine). Opioids administered as premedication or given intravenously (fentanyl 50–150 μg, sufentanil 10–20 μg) shortly before induction facilitate the onset of unconsciousness, especially that produced by benzodiazepines.
   2. Normal induction doses of barbiturates, etomidate, and propofol last 3–5 minutes.
   3. Midazolam $(0.05-0.1 \text{ mg·kg}^{-1})$ and ketamine $(2-4 \text{ mg·kg}^{-1})$ can be administered intramuscularly, and methohexital $(20-30 \text{ mg·kg}^{-1})$ has been administered rectally in uncooperative patients, often children.
   4. Doses for induction should be reduced in elderly and hypovolemic patients, recognizing that a slowed circulation time may delay the onset of unconsciousness.
   5. **Pain on injection** is least likely after intravenous injection of thiopental, midazolam, and ketamine and most likely after diazepam, etomidate, and propofol.

The likelihood of painful intravenous injection is less when the drug is injected into a larger vein in the forearm than a small vein in the hand. Opioid administration or lidocaine injected into the vein preceding or mixed with the induction drug may reduce the incidence of this reaction.

6. **Excitatory phenomena** (myoclonus, hiccups) are most likely to occur with induction of anesthesia using methohexital or etomidate.

B. Maintenance

1. Ketamine can be used by infusion to maintain both unconsciousness and analgesia, but the other nonopioid drugs are most suitable for maintaining unconsciousness in combination with an inhaled anesthetic (most often nitrous oxide).

2. Drugs with the most rapid elimination times (propofol) are least likely to cause prolonged drowsiness when given by infusion.

3. Availability of a benzodiazepine antagonist (flumazenil) facilitates the use of continuous intravenous infusion of midazolam ($2-5 \ \mu g \cdot kg^{-1} \cdot min^{-1}$).

C. Recovery

1. Assuming that equivalent doses are administered, time to recovery is fastest with propofol, followed in sequence by methohexital, etomidate, thiopental, midazolam, ketamine, and diazepam. Patients receiving propofol return to a clearheaded state sooner and exhibit a lower incidence of nausea and vomiting than with the other nonopioid induction anesthetics.

2. Emergence delirium during recovery from ketamine may be lessened by giving a benzodiazepine or thiopental before or with ketamine.

3. Venous thrombosis or phlebitis is most likely after intravenous administration of diazepam or etomidate, both of which are dissolved in propylene glycol.

13

Opioids

Opioid is an inclusive term that describes all drugs (natural or synthetic) that bind to morphine receptors (Murphy MR: Opioids. In Barash PG, Cullen BF, Stoelting RK [eds]: Clinical Anesthesia, pp 413–438. Philadelphia, JB Lippincott, 1992). This term includes drugs that are **agonists** (morphine, fentanyl), **agonist-antagonists** (butorphanol, nalorphine), and **antagonists** (naloxone). *Opiate* is often used interchangeably with *opioid* but historically designates only drugs derived from opium (morphine, codeine). *Narcotic* is a nonspecific designation applicable to any drug that produces sleep.

I. PHARMACOLOGY

A. Receptors and endogenous opioid peptides

1. Opioids interact with specific receptors in the central nervous system (CNS) and other areas such as the gastrointestinal tract (Table 13-1).

2. Mu receptors are subdivided into **mu$_1$ (analgesia)** and **mu$_2$ (ventilatory depression).** This suggests it may be possible to separate opioid-induced analgesia from depression of ventilation.

3. Receptors involved in mediating analgesia are found in greatest density in the **periaqueductal gray area** of the midbrain and the **substantia gelatinosa** of the spinal cord.

B. Estimated Relative Potencies and Dosages of Opioids (Table 13-2)

C. Central nervous system effects (Table 13-3)

1. Opioid-induced analgesia leaves intact other sensory and motor modalities. A patient may be aware of the stimulus but describes it as less or not painful.

2. **Dysphoria** rather than euphoria may occur when opioids are administered to pain-free patients.

3. **Unconsciousness** (anesthesia) is not predictably produced even with high doses of opioids, espe-

TABLE 13-1. Classification of Opioid Receptors		
Receptor Subtype	Prototype Drug	Proposed Actions
Mu$_1$	Opioid agonists (morphine)	Supraspinal analgesia
Mu$_2$	Opioid agonists (morphine)	Depression of ventilation Gastrointestinal effects Cardiovascular effects
Delta	Enkephalins	Spinal analgesia
Kappa	Dynorphin	Spinal analgesia Sedation
Epsilon	β-Endorphin	Hormones(?)
Sigma	Ketamine(?)	Psychomimetic effects

cially in young patients. In critically ill patients, an opioid may be used as the sole "anesthetic," but more often these drugs are supplemented (inhaled anesthetics, benzodiazepines) to ensure total amnesia.

4. **Seizures** are unlikely in humans even with high doses of opioids. The exception is meperidine, which is metabolized to a CNS stimulant, normeperidine.

5. **Emesis** reflects opioid-induced stimulation of the chemoreceptor trigger zone, especially in ambulatory patients, suggesting a vestibular component. At equianalgesic doses, the incidence of emesis is similar for all opioid agonists. High doses of opioids depress the vomiting center and may overcome the chemoreceptor trigger zone–stimulating effect.

D. **Cardiovascular effects** (Table 13-4)
   1. Stability of cardiovascular and myocardial responses with high doses of opioids (an exception is meperidine, which has a significant negative inotropic effect at doses as low as 2.0–2.5 mg·kg^{-1}) is the reason these drugs are used for anesthesia in patients who would not tolerate cardiovascular depression produced by volatile anesthetics.

   2. Histamine release may accompany rapid administration of high doses of morphine but not the injection of fentanyl or sufentanil.

Drug	Potency Ratio	Analgesic Dose	Anesthetic Dose
Morphine	1	10 mg	1–5 mg·kg^{-1}
Meperidine	0.1	100 mg	—
Fentanyl	100	100 μg	50–150 μg·kg^{-1}
Sufentanil	500–1000	10–20 μg	5–20 μg·kg^{-1}
Alfentanil	10–20	500–1000 μg	100–200 μg·kg^{-1}
Pentazocine	0.3–0.5	30–50 mg	—
Butorphanol	5	2–3 mg	—
Nalbuphine	1	10 mg	—
Buprenorphine	30	0.3 mg	—
Dezocine	1	10 mg	—

TABLE 13-2. Estimated Relative Potencies and Dosages of Opioids*

*Potency ratios and doses are estimates relative to morphine and are intended only as guidelines. Anesthetic doses of opioids may not reliably produce amnesia/unconsciousness.

163

TABLE 13-3. Central Nervous System Effects of Opioids	
Analgesia	Depressed cough reflex
Euphoria	Nausea and vomiting
Sedation	Seizures (high doses?)
Miosis (diagnostic of opioid administration	

TABLE 13-4. Cardiovascular Effects of Opioids
Bradycardia (reflects stimulation of vagal nucleus in the medulla)
Arteriolar and venous dilation (orthostatic hypotension)
Histamine release (morphine)

E. **Ventilatory effects**
1. All opioid agonists produce a dose-dependent depression of ventilation (Table 13-5).
   a. It is likely that equianalgesic doses of opioids produce equivalent depression of ventilation, but the peak effects and durations are determined by the pharmacokinetics of each drug. For example, fentanyl produces peak depression of ventilation following intravenous injection in 5–10 minutes compared with 30–60 minutes for morphine.
   b. Short-acting opioids such as fentanyl are more acceptable as intraoperative opioids because they do not produce prolonged depression of ventilation.
2. Depression of ventilation is accentuated in older patients and by concomitant administration of other CNS depressant drugs. Opioid-induced depression of ventilation is antagonized by pain or movement, as is associated with "stir-up" regimens. Hypoventilation may appear in the early postoperative period because of an absence of these stimuli.
F. **Hepatorenal and gastrointestinal effects**
1. In humans, opioids do not evoke the release of antidiuretic hormone. Conversely, surgical stimulation does evoke the release of antidiuretic hormone, with a resultant decrease in urine output.

TABLE 13-5. Ventilatory Effects of Opioids

Increased arterial carbon dioxide tension
Decreased breathing rate
Increased tidal volume
Decreased minute ventilation
Decreased ventilatory response to carbon dioxide (brain stem depression)

2. Opioids increase ureteral and detrusor muscle tone, resulting in the possibility of urinary retention.

3. **Spasm of the sphincter of Oddi** induced by opioids may produce pain that mimics angina pectoris (see Chapter 28). In this regard, naloxone reverses biliary colic but not angina, whereas nitroglycerin relieves pain of both origins. Opioid-induced sphincter spasm can also prevent visualization of contrast material in the duodenum during cholangiography, resulting in the erroneous conclusion that the common bile duct is blocked by a stone.

4. Decreased gastrointestinal motility delays gastric emptying and increases the risk of aspiration.

G. **Endocrine effects.** High doses of opioids used for anesthesia modify or block the metabolic stress response to surgery **(stress-free anesthesia).**

H. **Reproductive effects.** Opioids are not teratogenic. Morphine produces more neonatal depression than does meperidine, presumably reflecting increased permeability of the neonatal blood-brain barrier to morphine. Metabolites of meperidine are likely to be trapped in an acidotic distressed fetus because of their pK_a.

I. **Neuromuscular junction and skeletal muscle effects**

1. All opioids (especially fentanyl and its analogues) given intravenously in high doses (fentanyl, 8 $\mu g \cdot kg^{-1}$) have the ability to produce **rigidity of skeletal muscles, particularly in the chest and abdomen.** Skeletal muscle rigidity has been reported to occur both intraoperatively and postoperatively.

2. The incidence and severity of skeletal muscle rigidity may be increased by rapid infusion of the opioid or addition of nitrous oxide (N_2O).

3. Truncal rigidity may make ventilation of the lungs difficult to impossible, requiring the administration of a muscle relaxant. Application of high

levels of positive airway pressure in attempts to ventilate the lungs in the presence of opioid-induced skeletal muscle rigidity may cause gastric distention, impede venous return, and result in hypotension.

II. TOXICOLOGY

A. Opioid overdose is associated with coma, miosis, and depression of ventilation. Death is unlikely if depression of ventilation and associated arterial hypoxemia are prevented. Treatment of overdose is ventilation of the lungs with oxygen and administration of naloxone, 0.2–0.4 mg iv every 2–3 minutes, until the patient is breathing and responsive. Pulmonary edema and seizures may accompany an opioid overdose.

B. **Allergic reactions** to opioids are unlikely, perhaps reflecting their similarity to endogenous endorphins. Flushing, wheals, and urticaria in the area of the injection site are not uncommon and reflect localized drug-induced histamine release rather than an allergic reaction.

III. PHARMACOKINETICS AND PHARMACODYNAMICS (Table 13-6)

A. **Morphine**

1. The large volume of distribution of relatively lipid-insoluble morphine suggests extensive tissue uptake into hydrophilic tissues, especially skeletal muscles.

2. Clearance of morphine is primarily the result of hepatic metabolism to **morphine glucuronide,** with less than 15% of a dose eliminated unchanged in the urine. Plasma concentrations of morphine are low, reflecting the large volume of distribution. The high hepatic extraction ratio ensures that little orally administered morphine reaches the circulation, owing to enterohepatic first-pass metabolism.

3. The pK_a of morphine is such that less than 10% is non-ionized in plasma. It is this non-ionized lipid-soluble fraction that can cross the blood-brain barrier.

4. Morphine is considered to be a relatively long-acting opioid on the basis of its analgesic effects. Nevertheless, its elimination half-time ($T_{1/2\beta}$) is shorter than that of fentanyl.

TABLE 13-6. Pharmacokinetics and Pharmacodynamics of Opioids

	Elimination Half-Time (h)	Volume of Distribution (l·kg^{-1})	Clearance (ml·kg^{-1}·min^{-1})	Protein Binding (%)	pK$_a$
Morphine	1.7–2.2	3.2–3.4	15–23	26–36	7.9
Meperidine	3.2–7.9	2.8–4.2	5–17	58–82	8.5
Fentanyl	3.1–7.9	3.5–5.9	8–21	79–87	8.4
Sufentanil	2.7	1.7	13	93	8.0
Alfentanil	1.2–1.9	0.3–1.0	2.8–7.9	89–92	6.5

    5. Plasma concentrations of morphine do not consistently correlate with the intensity of analgesia or depression of ventilation.

    6. A maximum decrease in inhaled anesthetic requirements (MAC) of about 67% is produced by morphine (5 mg·kg^{-1}) administered to animals, suggesting that this drug does not provide complete anesthesia.

B. Meperidine

    1. Hepatic metabolism is rapid, with the production of **normeperidine,** meperidinic acid, and normeperidinic acid. Normeperidine is an active metabolite possessing twice the convulsive properties of meperidine with only half the analgesic effect. Less than 10% of meperidine appears unchanged in the urine.

    2. Meperidine is more lipid-soluble than morphine, as reflected by a more rapid onset of analgesia.

    3. Unlike morphine, there is a reasonable correlation between the plasma concentration of meperidine and the intensity of its effects (0.7 µg·ml^{-1} produces pain relief in 95% of patients). Administration of 100 mg of meperidine intramuscularly every 4 hours results in plasma concentrations above the minimal analgesic level only 35% of the time. A correlation between plasma concentrations and analgesia allows the use of continuous intravenous infusion regimens to maintain constant therapeutic (analgesic) plasma levels of meperidine.

C. Fentanyl

    1. Extreme lipid solubility accounts for the rapid onset of CNS effects (depression of ventilation occurs within 2 minutes) and a large volume of distribution of fentanyl, which results in a relatively long $T_{1/2\beta}$.

    2. Hepatic metabolism (N-dealkylation) is extensive, with less than 10% of fentanyl being excreted unchanged in the urine.

    3. The pK$_a$ of fentanyl is such that less than 10% of the drug is non-ionized at physiologic pH and is available to readily cross the blood-brain barrier.

    4. **Biphasic depression of ventilation** postoperatively, after apparent recovery, may reflect increased perfusion of skeletal muscles associated with movement during awakening from anesthesia. Later, when patients are unstimulated (often in the postanesthesia care unit), a second period of depressed ventilation becomes obvious.

5. In animals, a maximum reduction in MAC of 66% is produced by plasma fentanyl concentrations of 30 ng·ml^{-1}. In patients, a plasma concentration of 15 ng·ml^{-1} is produced by intravenous administration of 50 μg·kg^{-1} as a loading dose, followed by an infusion of 0.5 μg·kg^{-1}·min^{-1}.

6. The short duration of action of fentanyl is because of its rapid redistribution from the CNS to inactive tissue sites. High or repeated doses of fentanyl saturate these inactive tissue sites and convert fentanyl to a long-acting opioid. It is probably not rational to give patients increasing doses of fentanyl after all opioid receptors are occupied, because this will prolong the effect but not increase its intensity.

D. Sufentanil

1. Sufentanil is the most potent opioid available for clinical use, being approximately five to ten times more potent than fentanyl. Despite its increased potency, sufentanil is probably not more efficacious than fentanyl as a complete anesthetic and, like other opioids, requires the concomitant use of adjuvant drugs (inhaled anesthetics, benzodiazepines) to produce complete anesthesia.

2. A smaller volume of distribution combined with a clearance similar to that of fentanyl accounts for the shorter $T_{1/2\beta}$ of sufentanil compared with that of fentanyl.

E. Alfentanil

1. The rapid onset of action of alfentanil (1–2 minutes) reflects its pK$_a$ of 6.5. As a result, 89% is nonionized at physiologic pH and available to cross lipid barriers.

2. A small volume of distribution (alfentanil is less lipid-soluble than fentanyl) means that there is more alfentanil in the plasma for elimination by the liver. Only about 0.4% is excreted unchanged in the urine.

3. Alfentanil clearance is about one half that of fentanyl, but the greater decrease in alfentanil's volume of distribution relative to the decrease in its clearance results in a significantly shorter $T_{1/2\beta}$.

4. Alfentanil is a useful drug for **continuous intravenous infusion** because its small volume of distribution and short $T_{1/2\beta}$ preclude significant accumulation in the body. High intravenous doses for induction of anesthesia (150 μg·kg^{-1}) in combination with N$_2$O rapidly establish levels sufficient for

tracheal intubation while the subsequent plasma concentration is maintained by a continuous intravenous infusion. Intermittent intravenous bolus doses are effective in supplementing the continuous infusion if surgical stimulation changes abruptly. Because alfentanil does not accumulate to any significant degree in the body, the intravenous infusion can be turned off 15–20 minutes before the end of the procedure, with the likely expectation of rapid patient awakening.

5. Alfentanil produces a maximum 70% reduction in MAC.

IV. DRUG INTERACTIONS

A. Because opioids are not complete anesthetics, they are often used in combination with other drugs (inhaled anesthetics, benzodiazepines, muscle relaxants). The combination of opioids and other CNS depressants seems to produce additive anesthetic effects.

1. The combination of even low to moderate doses of benzodiazepines and opioids may create an increased risk for ventilatory depression.

2. Propranolol decreases the first pass uptake of fentanyl in the lungs.

3. N_2O in combination with opioids may produce negative inotropic effects, especially in patients with poor left ventricular function. Addition of benzodiazepines to opioids (or vice versa) may cause decreases in cardiac output, blood pressure, and systemic vascular resistance that do not occur with either drug alone. The mechanism seems to be a decrease in sympathetic nervous system outflow from the CNS.

4. Pancuronium offsets the heart rate–slowing effects of opioids, whereas vecuronium and presumably atracurium do not alter the vagotonic effects of opioids.

B. **Cimetidine** may prolong the $T_{1/2\beta}$ of fentanyl by directly or indirectly decreasing hepatic blood flow.

C. **Monoamine oxidase inhibitors and tricyclic antidepressants** may exaggerate and prolong the effects of opioids. Hyperpyrexia, severe depression of ventilation, and seizures have occurred in patients who are treated with monoamine oxidase inhibitors and then receive meperidine.

V. IMPACT OF PRE-EXISTING DISEASES

A. **Age.** Although variability is great, the elderly tend to demonstrate decreases in clearance and increased intensity and prolongation of the effects of opioids.

B. **Renal disease**
   1. Only a small amount of most opioids is excreted unchanged by the kidneys, and renal failure would be expected to have limited impact on dosage requirements, especially with fentanyl.
   2. Normeperidine, the major metabolite of meperidine, may accumulate and result in prolonged depression of ventilation and seizures.
   3. Naloxone-reversible opioid effects may occur in patients with renal failure up to 7 days after the last dose of morphine. Morphine glucuronide, the major metabolite of morphine, has opioid effects but is usually limited in its ability to cross the blood-brain barrier. However, it is possible that continued high plasma concentrations of this metabolite and an altered blood-brain barrier associated with uremia could facilitate entrance into the CNS.

C. **Liver disease**
   1. **Clearance** of opioids is heavily dependent on the liver, and a prolonged $T_{1/2\beta}$ is predictable in patients with severe liver disease.
   2. Initial doses of opioids usually produce the expected intensity of effect in patients with liver disease. Subsequent doses should be greatly reduced or delayed because clearance is slowed and significant accumulation can occur.

D. **Obesity**
   1. Excessive adipose tissue might increase the volume of distribution and prolong the $T_{1/2\beta}$ of lipid-soluble opioids, especially fentanyl.
   2. When opioids are administered in doses based on ideal body weight, the initial response is likely to be normal. Accumulation may occur with high or repeated doses or continuous infusions of opioids to obese patients.

E. **Neurologic problems**
   1. Opioid-induced miosis, vomiting, and mental depression may mask important clinical signs of CNS pathology.
   2. In patients with increased intracranial pressure, opioids are not specifically contraindicated if ventilation of the lungs is mechanically supported to prevent drug-induced elevations in Pa_{CO_2}.

TABLE 13-7. Clinical Uses of Opioids

Premedication
Induction of anesthesia (sole drug or adjuvant)
Intraoperative analgesia
Postoperative pain relief (patient-controlled analgesia, neuraxial, parenteral)
Adjuvant to facilitate mechanical ventilation and tolerance to tracheal tube

---

VI. CLINICAL USES OF OPIOIDS (Table 13-7)

A. Opioids may be used as the sole drug for induction and maintenance of anesthesia in severely ill patients, such as those with severe left ventricular dysfunction. The negative inotropic effects of volatile anesthetics can be avoided when opioids are selected.

B. Fentanyl, sufentanil, and alfentanil are the most commonly used opioids for induction and maintenance of anesthesia (alone or as adjuvants) because of their rapid onset and more predictable duration of action. Morphine should be administered slowly (5 mg·min^{-1}) to avoid histamine release. Meperidine is rarely used for induction and maintenance of anesthesia because of its detrimental negative inotropic effects.

VII. OPIOID AGONIST-ANTAGONISTS AND PARTIAL AGONISTS

Opioid agonist-antagonists and partial antagonists are presumed to bind to mu receptors, where they exert limited actions **(partial agonists)** or no effect **(competitive antagonist).** Those opioids that are antagonists at mu receptors often exert agonist activity at kappa or sigma receptors.

A. **Pentazocine**

1. Analgesic effects reflect agonist activity at kappa receptors, with a potency about one fourth that of morphine.

2. Maximum analgesia and depression of ventilation are produced by doses of 30–50 mg **(ceiling effect).**

3. Dysphoric effects (at high doses) and adverse cardiac effects (increased systolic blood pressure and

pulmonary artery pressure, catecholamine release) limit the usefulness of this drug.

B. Butorphanol

1. Butorphanol is a potent analgesic (2–3 mg equivalent to 10 mg of morphine), with weak antagonist effects at mu receptors.

2. Like pentazocine, there is a ceiling effect with a maximum reduction in MAC of about 11%. Dysphoria may occur, although the incidence seems less than following administration of pentazocine.

C. Nalbuphine

1. Nalbuphine is an agonist at kappa receptors (10 mg equivalent to 10 mg of morphine) and antagonist at mu receptors.

2. A ceiling effect occurs, but unlike pentazocine or butorphanol, adverse cardiac and CNS effects are unlikely.

3. Nalbuphine is an effective drug (15 μg·kg^{-1} iv up to a total dose of 10 mg) to reverse ventilatory depression of mu agonists (morphine, fentanyl) while maintaining acceptable analgesia.

VIII. ANTAGONISTS

A. Naloxone and naltrexone are pure competitive antagonists at mu, delta, kappa, and sigma receptors. All opioid effects, including analgesia and depression of ventilation, are reversed in parallel.

B. **Naloxone** is administered intravenously (20–40-μg increments) to surgical patients to reverse unwanted opioid-induced depression of ventilation or sedation while still preserving acceptable analgesia.

1. Peak effects of naloxone occur 1–2 minutes after intravenous injection and last 1–4 hours. Persistent opioid-induced depression of ventilation may require a repeat dose of naloxone when the effects of the antagonist wane.

2. A continuous intravenous infusion of naloxone (3–10 μg·kg^{-1}·h^{-1}) may be useful for production of prolonged antagonist effects following high doses of opioids or administration of neuraxial opioids.

3. High doses of naloxone that abruptly reverse analgesia in postoperative patients may result in pain-induced activation of the sympathetic nervous system manifesting as hypertension, cardiac dysrhythmias, pulmonary edema, and cardiac arrest.

C. Naloxone can be used to reverse agonist-antagonist opioids, but high doses generally are necessary because naloxone has a greater affinity for mu receptors than for kappa and sigma receptors.

D. **Naltrexone** is a long-acting competitive antagonist ($T_{1/2\beta}$ 10 hours) that is available for oral administration to patients with opioid addiction.

14

Inhalation Anesthesia

The role of inhalation drugs in general anesthesia is changing, with an increased use of intravenous drugs (opioids, benzodiazepines) as adjuvants to reduce the required dose of inhaled anesthetic or to minimize side effects of inhaled drugs (Stevens WC, Kingston HGG: Inhalation anesthesia. In Barash PG, Cullen BF, Stoelting RK [eds]: Clinical Anesthesia, pp 439–465. Philadelphia, JB Lippincott, 1992). Inhaled anesthetics of greatest importance today are the weakly potent inorganic gas nitrous oxide (N_2O) and the fluorinated hydrocarbon volatile anesthetics, halothane, enflurane, isoflurane, sevoflurane, and desflurane (Fig. 14-1 and Table 14-1).

I. PHARMACOKINETICS OF INHALED ANESTHETICS

A. Uptake, distribution, and elimination

1. **Induction of anesthesia** occurs when an anesthetizing partial pressure has been achieved in the brain (Pbr). The brain can be considered as the final site for a series of concentration gradients in anesthetic partial pressures that begins with the concentration of anesthetic delivered from the anesthesia machine (Table 14-2).

2. **The goal of inhalation anesthesia is to maintain an optimal and unchanging Pbr as reflected by the alveolar partial pressure (PA).** The ability to clinically measure and monitor the PA (mass spectrometry) allows anesthesiologists to control the depth of anesthesia (Pbr).

3. **The rate of induction of anesthesia** is determined by the rate of rise of the PA. During induction of anesthesia, blood returning to the lungs from tissues has a lower partial pressure (tissue uptake) than that in the alveoli. As a result, uptake of anesthetic occurs

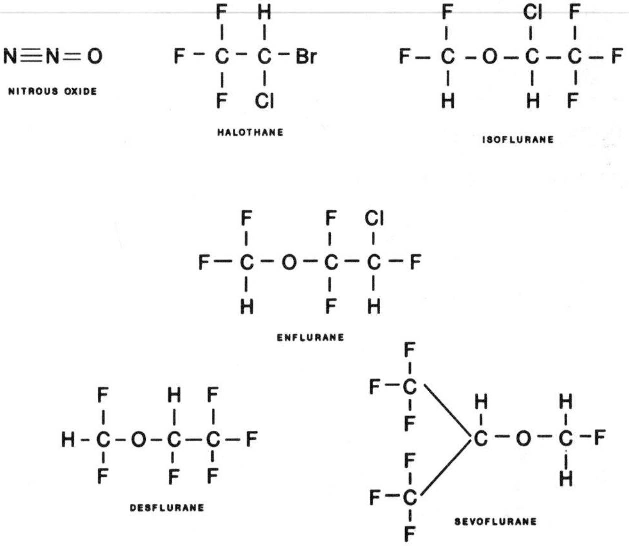

Figure 14-1. Chemical structure of inhaled anesthetics.

from alveoli and creates an **inspired-to-alveolar partial pressure difference.**

4. **Solubility (partition coefficients)** of anesthetics in blood and tissues determines the time necessary for equilibration between two phases to occur (Table 14-3).

   a. **Blood:gas solubility** determines uptake from the alveoli into the blood and thus the rate of induction.

   b. **Brain:blood solubility** determines the time necessary for equilibration of partial pressures between the blood and brain.

5. **Concentration effect.** The higher the inspired partial pressure (PI), the more rapid the increase in PA.

6. **Second gas effect.** Administration of high concentrations of N_2O accelerates the rate of uptake of concomitantly inhaled gases (isoflurane, oxygen).

7. **Emergence from anesthesia** reflects reversal of the concentration gradients established during its induction. In contrast to induction of anesthesia, the rate of recovery from anesthesia may be influenced by **metabolism** of the inhaled anesthetic. Recovery is most

TABLE 14-1. Physical Characteristics of Inhaled Anesthetics

	Molecular Weight (g)	Boiling Point (°C)	Vapor Pressure at 20°C (mm Hg)	Chemical Stabilizer Necessary	Flammability Limits
N_2O	44	−88			No*
Halothane	197.4	50.2	241	Yes	No
Enflurane	184.5	56.5	175	No	No
Isoflurane	184.5	48.5	238	No	No
Sevoflurane	200	58.5	160		11% in O_2
Desflurane	168	23.5	664	No	20.8% in O_2

*Supports combustion.

TABLE 14-2. **Concentration Gradients Developed During General Anesthesia**

Delivered	> Inspired	> Alveolar	> Arterial	> Brain
	(P_I)	(P_A)	(P_a)	(P_{br})

TABLE 14-3. **Partition Coefficients at 37°C**

	Blood: Gas	Brain: Blood	Muscle: Blood	Fat: Blood	Oil: Gas
N_2O	0.47	1.1	1.2	2.3	1.4
Halothane	2.3	2.9	3.5	60	224
Enflurane	1.91	1.4	1.7	36	98.5
Isoflurane	1.4	2.6	4.0	45	90.8
Sevoflurane	0.6	1.7	3.1	47.5	53.4
Desflurane	0.42	1.3	2.0	27.2	18.7

TABLE 14-4. **Anesthetic Requirements (MAC) for Inhaled Anesthetics**

	MAC (%)	MAC % with 60–70% N_2O
N_2O	104	
Halothane	0.77	0.29
Enflurane	1.70	0.60
Isoflurane	1.15	0.50
Sevoflurane	1.71	0.66
Desflurane	6.0	2.83

rapid following short-duration administration of inhaled anesthetics that are poorly soluble in blood and tissues.

B. **The requirement for anesthetics—MAC**

   1. **MAC** is the minimum alveolar concentration of inhaled anesthetic at 1 atmosphere that prevents movement in 50% of subjects in response to a painful (surgical incision) stimulus. MAC reflects P_{br} because the P_A is in equilibrium with the brain. Clinically, it is necessary to establish a MAC of 1.2–1.3 to prevent movement in at least 95% of patients. Combinations

**TABLE 14-5. Factors That Influence
Anesthetic Requirements (MAC)**

Decrease MAC

Increasing age
Hypothermia
Other CNS depressants (opioids, benzodiazepines)
Decreased CNS neurotransmitter (antihypertensives)
Acute ethanol intoxication
Alpha$_2$ agonists (clonidine)
Pregnancy

Increase MAC

Hyperthermia
Chronic ethanol abuse
Increased CNS neurotransmitter levels (monoamine oxidase
inhibitors)

No Change in MAC

Duration of anesthesia
Gender
Paco$_2$ 21–95 mm Hg

of inhaled anesthetics have additive effects on MAC
(1% reduction in MAC for every 1% N$_2$O).

2. Comparison of effects of inhaled anesthetics on various organ systems is based on evaluation of equally potent MACs of each drug (Table 14-4).

3. Various physiologic and pharmacologic factors influence MAC (Table 14-5).

II. EFFECTS OF INHALED ANESTHETICS ON ORGANS AND SYSTEMS

A. Central nervous system

1. Volatile anesthetics produce drug-specific and dose-dependent increases in cerebral blood flow by virtue of their cerebral vasodilating effects (Fig. 14-2).

   a. N$_2$O is a cerebral vasodilator, but its limited potency is associated with only modest increases in cerebral blood flow.

   b. Increases in cerebral blood flow produced by volatile anesthetics tend to normalize with time. For example, cerebral blood flow normalizes after 2 hours of halothane administration.

2. Volatile anesthetics decrease cerebral metabolic oxygen requirements, with the greatest reduction pro-

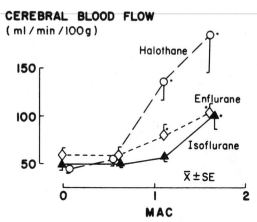

Figure 14-2. Dose-dependent effects of volatile anesthetics on cerebral blood flow.

duced by isoflurane (flat electroencephalogram [EEG] at about 2 MAC). The cerebral blood flow at which EEG evidence of ischemia occurs is lower with isoflurane than with halothane, suggesting a possible cerebral protecting effect of isoflurane. Isoflurane is associated with better maintenance of the relationship between cerebral metabolic oxygen requirements and cerebral blood flow, perhaps explaining the lower increase in cerebral blood flow produced by this drug.

3. In patients with decreased intracranial compliance, drug-induced increases in cerebral blood flow produce parallel increases in cerebral blood volume and intracranial pressure. Volatile anesthetics can alter production and reabsorption of cerebrospinal fluid, but as with cerebral blood flow, these effects normalize with time. In the presence of modest hypocapnia, isoflurane appears less likely to produce potentially dangerous increases in intracranial pressure than enflurane or halothane.

4. Enflurane is unique in producing dose-dependent spike-wave activity on the EEG, which is exaggerated by hypocapnia.

5. Volatile anesthetics and N_2O produce decreased amplitude and increased latency in the cortical components of somatosensory evoked potentials.

B. Respiratory system

1. **Ventilatory volumes and frequency of breathing.** Volatile anesthetics produce drug-specific and dose-

dependent depression of ventilation, as evidenced by increases in $P_{a}CO_2$ (Fig. 14-3).

   a. Decreases in tidal volume are incompletely offset by increases in rate of breathing **(rapid, shallow breathing characteristic of the anesthetic state)** such that alveolar ventilation is reduced.

   b. Substitution of N_2O for a portion of the volatile anesthetic results in less elevation of $P_{a}CO_2$ at the same total MAC as with the volatile anesthetic alone.

2. **Effects on the intercostal muscles and diaphragm.** Loss of intercostal muscle function with increasing doses of volatile anesthetics results in the characteristic **rocking boat appearance of ventilation** (chest collapses and abdomen protrudes as the diaphragm descends during inspiration) during deep anesthesia.

3. **Chemical control of breathing.** Volatile anesthetics produce dose-dependent decreases in the ventilatory response to carbon dioxide, whereas even subanesthetic concentrations (0.1 MAC) of these drugs block the ventilatory response to hypoxemia. The absence of hyperpnea during arterial hypoxemia means that a useful clinical sign of hypoxia cannot be relied on during anesthesia.

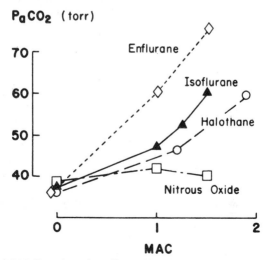

Figure 14-3. Dose-dependent effects of inhaled anesthetics on $P_{a}CO_2$ (mm Hg).

     a. Assisted ventilation of the lungs to offset anes-
thetic-induced increases in Pa_{CO_2} is of limited
value because apnea occurs when Pa_{CO_2} is lowered by about 5 mm Hg.

     b. Surgical stimulation sufficiently increases venti-
lation to lower Pa_{CO_2} about 5 mm Hg.

4. Airway caliber. Volatile anesthetics are equally effective in decreasing airway resistance by causing bronchodilation. All volatile anesthetics are equally effective for patients with asthma, although halothane
may be preferable to isoflurane because the latter has
a pungent odor that can cause airway irritation.

5. Hypoxic pulmonary vasoconstriction. Volatile anesthetics in doses administered clinically do not seem
to interfere with diversion of blood flow away from
poorly ventilated or unventilated alveoli (see Chapter 20).

C. Circulatory system

  1. Hemodynamics. Volatile anesthetics produce drug-
specific and dose-dependent **decreases in blood
pressure** as a result of decreases in cardiac output
(halothane and enflurane) or decreases in systemic
vascular resistance (isoflurane) (Figs. 14-4 and 14-5).

    a. Increased heart rate during administration of iso-
flurane may reflect maintenance of baroreceptor
activity in response to reductions in blood pressure. Minimal to absent changes in heart rate during halothane-induced reductions in blood pressure suggest impairment of baroreceptor activity.

    b. Distribution of cardiac output is altered by anes-
thetics, with increased flow to the brain (halothane), skeletal muscles (isoflurane), and skin and
decreased blood flow to the kidneys, liver, and
gastrointestinal tract.

    c. Substitution of N_2O for a portion of the volatile an-
esthetic results in less reduction in blood pressure
at the same total MAC as with the volatile anesthetic alone.

    d. N_2O produces a **mild sympathomimetic effect**
manifesting as increases in systemic vascular resistance and pulmonary vascular resistance. When
added to high doses of opioids, N_2O can decrease
blood pressure and cardiac output.

  **2. Cardiac dysrhythmias, conduction, and drug inter-
actions.** Isoflurane and enflurane are less likely than
halothane to produce cardiac dysrhythmias in the
presence of increased plasma concentrations of epinephrine (Fig. 14-6).

    a. Children are less likely than adults to develop epi-
nephrine-induced cardiac dysrhythmias.

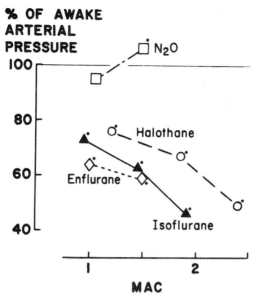

Figure 14-4. Dose-dependent effects of inhaled anesthetics on blood pressure.

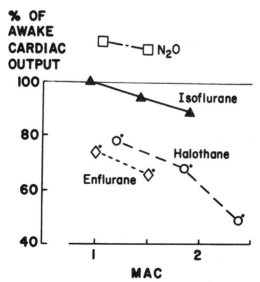

Figure 14-5. Dose-dependent effects of inhaled anesthetics on cardiac output.

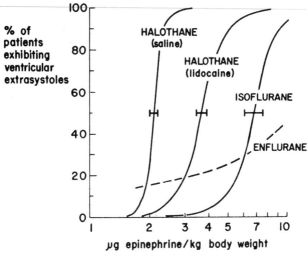

Figure 14-6. Dose-response curves for epinephrine in the presence of volatile anesthetics.

           b. Volatile anesthetics exert a direct depressant effect on the sinoatrial node. Cardiac conduction is preserved through normal pathways better by isoflurane than by enflurane or halothane.

           c. Myocardial depression produced by volatile anesthetics may be enhanced by calcium entry blockers and beta antagonists.

      3. Coronary circulation. Isoflurane may uncouple the generally close relationship between coronary blood flow and myocardial oxygen requirements more than other volatile anesthetics. Isoflurane-induced dilation of intramyocardial arterioles, particularly in the presence of reduced coronary perfusion pressure and critical anatomic location of coronary artery stenosis, could divert blood flow away from areas of myocardium supplied by pressure-dependent collaterals **(coronary artery "steal")** (see Chapter 21).

  D. **Renal effects** of volatile anesthetics are mainly a reflection of changes in blood flow to the kidneys. Anesthesia is typically associated with a decrease in renal blood flow, glomerular filtration rate, and urine output.

  E. Volatile anesthetics have inherent **muscle relaxant properties** and also potentiate the effects of nondepolarizing muscle relaxants. The mechanism of potentiation may involve desensitization of the postjunctional membrane or changes in skeletal muscle blood flow. Potentiation of nondepolarizing muscle relaxants is greatest with isoflurane and enflurane, intermediate with halothane, and least with N_2O.

F. **Uterine relaxation** accompanies administration of all the volatile anesthetics and can contribute to uterine blood loss when gravid patients are anesthetized. Inhaled drugs delivered to a pregnant patient also cross the placenta and similarly affect her fetus.

15

Muscle Relaxants

Drugs that primarily and specifically interfere with the physiologic sequence of neuromuscular transmission are classified as muscle relaxants (neuromuscular blocking drugs) (Bevan DR, Donati F: Muscle relaxants. In: Barash PG, Cullen BF, Stoelting RK [eds]: Clinical Anesthesia, pp 481–508. Philadelphia, JB Lippincott, 1992). Muscle relaxants are not anesthetics and should not be used to mask skeletal muscle movement in inadequately anesthetized patients. The decision to include a muscle relaxant as part of the general anesthetic is based on many factors (Table 15-1).

I. PHYSIOLOGY AND PHARMACOLOGY

   A. The process of skeletal muscle contraction originates at the neuromuscular junction (NMJ) with the release of acetylcholine (ACh). Anatomically, the NMJ is the synapse between the presynaptic membrane of the motor nerve ending and the postsynaptic membrane of the skeletal muscle fiber (Fig. 15-1).
   B. **Release of acetylcholine.** Sites for release of ACh from the nerve terminal occur in nerve membrane projections in close proximity to folds in the synaptic membrane, thus favoring rapid receptor activation. Activation of the postsynaptic nicotinic receptor requires simultaneous occupation of the receptor's two alpha subunits by ACh (Fig. 15-2).
   C. ACh is hydrolyzed by **acetylcholinesterase** to choline (reused for synthesis of new ACh) and acetate.
   D. **Postsynaptic events.** Skeletal muscle contraction occurs when ACh-induced changes in the muscle cell's transmembrane permeability result in inward movement of sodium sufficient to decrease intracellular negativity (depolarization) and cause an **action potential.** Propagation of the action potential initiates release of calcium from the sarcoplasmic reticulum into the sarcoplasm, where activation of myosin adeno-

---

TABLE 15-1. Factors That Influence Inclusion of Muscle Relaxants as Part of General Anesthesia

Surgical Procedure
  Anatomic location
  Patient position

Anesthetic Technique
  Inhalation vs. injection
  Airway management (mask vs. endotracheal tube)
  Ventilation management (spontaneous vs. controlled)

Patient Factors
  Body habitus (lean vs. obese)
  American Society of Anesthesiologists' physical status
    parameters
  Age

---

sine triphosphate leads to excitation-contraction coupling of the myofilaments.

E. **Presynaptic events.** There is growing evidence that presynaptic receptors have a regulatory role in the release of ACh that is reflected by fade on the electromyogram at high stimulation frequencies.

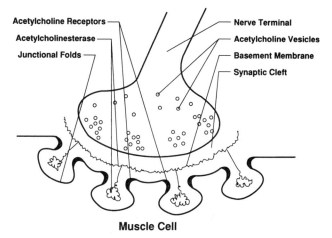

Muscle Cell

Figure 15-1. Diagram of the neuromuscular junction.

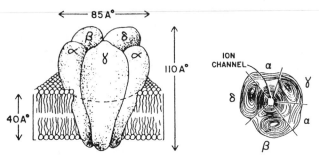

Figure 15-2. The nicotinic acetylcholine receptor consists of five glycoprotein subunits arranged to form an ion channel. The alpha subunits carry a recognition site for agonists and antagonists.

II. NEUROMUSCULAR PHARMACOLOGY

Neuromuscular blocking drugs are characterized as **depolarizing** (mimic action of ACh at binding sites) or **nondepolarizing** (compete with ACh for binding sites) (Table 15-2).

III. DEPOLARIZING BLOCKING DRUGS: SUCCINYLCHOLINE

A. **Succinylcholine (SCh)** still enjoys great popularity because it is the only rapid-onset, short-duration neuromuscular blocking drug available.
B. **Neuromuscular effects.** SCh binds to postsynaptic nicotinic receptors, where it exhibits ACh-like activity. SCh also binds to extrajunctional receptors located on the muscle fiber and presynaptic receptors.
   1. The net effect of SCh-induced depolarization is uncoordinated skeletal muscle activity that manifests clinically as **fasciculations.**
   2. A transient increase in the plasma potassium concentration ("hyperkalemia") is probably the result of the large number of open ACh receptors that allow potassium to flow from the inside to the outside of the skeletal muscle cells.
   3. Nonparalyzing doses of nondepolarizing drugs **(pretreatment)** block visible evidence of SCh-induced depolarization, suggesting that presynaptic receptors are principally involved in the production of fasciculations.

TABLE 15-2. Classification of Muscle Relaxants

Depolarizing
  Succinylcholine

Nondepolarizing
  Long-acting
    d-Tubocurarine
    Metocurine
    Pancuronium
    Doxicurium
    Pipecuronium
  Intermediate-acting
    Atracurium
    Vecuronium
  Short-acting
    Mivacurium
    Rocuronium

   4. The blocking effect of SCh at the NMJ is probably owing to **desensitization** (prolonged exposure to an agonist leads to a state characterized by a lack of responsiveness of the receptors).
 C. **Characteristics of depolarizing blockade.** SCh initially produces features characterized as phase I block (Table 15-3).
   1. **Phase II block.** After prolonged exposure to SCh, the characteristics of the block change, and features of nondepolarizing blockade appear (Table 15-4).
   2. The onset of phase II block coincides with **tachyphylaxis.**

TABLE 15-3. Characteristics of Phase I Depolarizing Blockade

Decreased twitch amplitude
Absence of fade with continuous (tetanic) stimulation
Similar decreases in the amplitude of all twitches in the train-of-four (ratio >0.7)
Absence of post-tetanic potential
Fasciculations
Antagonism by nondepolarizing muscle relaxants
Augmentation by anticholinestrase drugs

TABLE 15-4. Characteristics of Nondepolarizing Neuromuscular Blockade

Decreased twitch amplitude
Fade with continuous (tetanic) stimulation
Train-of-four ratio <0.7
Post-tetanic potentiation
Absence of fasciculations
Antagonism by anticholinesterase drugs
Augmentation by other nondepolarizing muscle relaxants

    D. Pharmacology of succinylcholine. SCh is rapidly metabolized (elimination half-time estimated to be 2–4 minutes) by **plasma cholinesterase (pseudocholinesterase)** to choline and succinylmonocholine.
        1. The ED_{95} of SCh in the presence of opioid–nitrous oxide anesthesia is 0.30–0.35 $mg \cdot kg^{-1}$.
        2. The onset of neuromuscular blocking effect is usually within 1 minute following high doses of SCh (1–2 $mg \cdot kg^{-1}$ iv), and the time until full recovery of the electromyographic response is 10–12 minutes after a dose of 1 $mg \cdot kg^{-1}$ iv.
        3. A small proportion of patients (1:1500 to 1:3000) have a genetically determined **(atypical plasma**

TABLE 15-5. Side Effects of Succinylcholine

Bradycardia (especially in children; more likely in adults with second dose)
Allergic reactions
Fasciculations
Muscle pains (relationship to fasciculations not firmly established)
Increased intragastric pressure (offset by even greater increase in lower esophageal sphincter pressure)
Increased intraocular pressure (not reliably blunted by pretreatment)
Increased intracranial pressure
Transient increase in plasma potassium concentration (normal increase of 0.5–1.0 $mEq \cdot l^{-1}$ is enhanced by denervation injuries, burns, and extensive trauma)
Trigger for malignant hyperthermia (masseter muscle spasm may be an early sign)

---

cholinesterase) inability to metabolize SCh (1–1.5 mg·kg^{-1} iv lasts 3–6 hours).

E. **Side Effects** (Table 15-5)

F. **Clinical uses.** The main indication for SCh is to facilitate tracheal intubation (1 mg·kg^{-1} iv is the usual dose, increased to 1.5–2.0 mg·kg^{-1} iv if pretreatment is used). Children are slightly more resistant to the effects of SCh than adults and higher doses may be recommended for them (pretreatment is not necessary in patients <10 years of age because fasciculations are uncommon before this age).

IV. NONDEPOLARIZING DRUGS

A. **Effects at the neuromuscular junction.** Nondepolarizing neuromuscular blocking drugs bind to postsynaptic receptors (must bind to one of the alpha subunits) in a competitive fashion to produce neuromuscular blockade. An excess of ACh, as occurs with the administration of an anticholinesterase drug, can tilt the balance in favor of neuromuscular transmission.

B. **Characteristics of nondepolarizing blockade** (Table 15-4)

C. **Pharmacokinetics** (Table 15-6)
   1. The pharmacokinetic variables derived from measurements of the plasma concentrations of nondepolarizing muscle relaxants depend on the dose administered, the sampling schedule used, and the accuracy of the assay.
   2. All nondepolarizing muscle relaxants have a volume of distribution that is approximately equal to extracellular fluid volume.

D. **Onset and duration of action** (Table 15-7)
   1. Although peak plasma concentrations of nondepolarizing muscle relaxants occur within 1–2 minutes of injection, the **onset of maximum blockade** is reached only after 5–7 minutes, reflecting the effect of cardiac output, distance of the skeletal muscle from the heart, and skeletal muscle blood flow.
   2. The **duration of action** of nondepolarizing drugs is determined by the time required for plasma concentrations to decrease below a critical level.

E. **Individual Nondepolarizing Relaxants** (Tables 15-6, 15-7, 15-8, and 15-9).
   1. *d*-**Tubocurarine** has been replaced by drugs that exhibit minimal cardiovascular activity (*d*-tubocurarine causes dose-related histamine release),

(*Text continues on pg 194*)

TABLE 15-6. Typical Pharmacokinetic Data for Nondepolarizing Muscle Relaxants

	Volume of Distribution ($l \cdot kg^{-1}$)	Clearance ($ml \cdot kg^{-1} \cdot min^{-1}$)	Elimination Half-Time (minutes)
d-Tubocurarine	0.3–0.6	1–3	90–350
Metocurine	0.4	1.3	220
Pancuronium	0.3	1–2	100–130
Doxicurium	0.2	2.5	95
Pipecuronium	0.3	2.4	140
Atracurium	0.2	5.5	20
Vecuronium	0.4	4.5	110
Mivacurium	0.2*	75*	2.2*
Rocuronium	0.3	4.0	130

*approximate values

TABLE 15-7. Comparative Pharmacology of Nondepolarizing Muscle Relaxants

	ED_{95} $(mg \cdot kg^{-1})$	Onset (minutes)	Recovery Index (minutes)	T90 (minutes)
d-Tubocurarine	0.51	6	25–35	70–90
Metocurine	0.28	5	30–40	80–90
Pancuronium	0.07	5–7	25	60
Doxacurium	0.025	10–14	NA	80–100
Pipecuronium	0.05–0.06	5–6	30–40	80–90
Atracurium	0.2	5–6	10–15	30
Vecuronium	0.05	5–6	10–15	30
Mivacurium	0.08	3–6	6–8	25
Rocuronium	0.3	3–4	10–15	30

NA = data not avaliable.

TABLE 15-8. Autonomic and Histamine-Releasing Effect of Muscle Relaxants

	Nicotonic Receptors at Autonomic Ganglia	Cardiac Muscarinic Receptors	Histamine Release
Succinylcholine	Stimulates	Stimulates	Rare
d-Tubocurarine	Blocks + +	No effect	+ + +
Metocurine	Blocks	No effect	+ +
Pancuronium	No effect	Blocks +	None
Doxacurium	No effect	No effect	None
Pipecuronium	No effect	No effect	None
Atracurium	No effect	No effect	+
Vecuronium	No effect	No effect	None
Mivacurium	No effect	No effect	+

although it is still occasionally used for pretreatment (3 mg·70 kg^{-1}).

2. **Atracurium**

a. **Metabolism** is by the Hofmann reaction (nonenzymatic degradation at body temperature and pH) and by ester hydrolysis. It has been estimated that two thirds of atracurium undergoes ester hydrolysis and one third is degraded by the Hofmann reaction. A metabolite of atracurium is laudanosine, which is a cerebral stimulant. Nevertheless, with the doses of atracurium administered clinically, it is doubtful that this metabolite is of any clinical significance.

b. **Hypotension and tachycardia** may accompany atracurium doses >0.4 mg·kg^{-1} (>2 × ED$_{95}$), reflecting dose-related histamine release (attenuated by injection of the muscle relaxant over 1–3 minutes). Similar effects occur after the use of d-tubocurarine or metocurine but at much lower doses.

c. **Dose requirements** are similar in all age groups, presumably reflecting the organ independence of atracurium's elimination.

d. The short duration of action, rapid recovery, and absence of significant cardiovascular and hemodynamic effects have encouraged the use of atracurium as a continuous infusion or as intermittent injections in several situations, in-

TABLE 15-9. Mechanisms for Clearance of Nondepolarizing Muscle Relaxants

	Renal Excretion (% Unchanged)	Biliary Excretion (% Unchanged)	Hepatic Degradation	Hydrolysis in Plasma
d-Tubocurarine	45	10–40	Insignificant	0
Metocurine	43	<2	Insignificant	0
Pancuronium	80	5–10	10–40%	0
Doxacurium	70	?	?	Minimal
Pipecuronium	70	20	10%	0
Atracurium	Insignificant	Insignificant	Modest (?)	Spontaneous Enzymatic
Vecuronium	15–25	40–75	20–30%	0
Mivacurium	Insignificant	Insignificant	Insignificant	Enzymatic

cluding ambulatory surgery, and in patients
with renal and hepatic disease.

3. **Doxacurium** is a long-acting nondepolarizing muscle relaxant that is devoid of histamine releasing or cardiovascular side effects. This drug may be most useful in patients with ischemic heart disease who are undergoing prolonged anesthesia or long-term mechanical ventilation of the lungs.

4. **Mivacurium** is a short-acting nondepolarizing neuromuscular blocking drug that is hydrolyzed by plasma cholinesterase.
   a. At 2 × ED_{95} the onset of mivacurium is 2.5 minutes, and recovery to 95% twitch height occurs in about 30 minutes.
   b. **Recovery time** after discontinuing an infusion of mivacurium is similar to that of SCh.
   c. The cardiovascular response to mivacurium is minimal at doses up to 2 × ED_{95} (rapid intravenous injection of 3 × ED_{95} may evoke sufficient histamine release to transiently lower mean arterial pressure by about 15%).
   d. The effect of anticholinesterase drugs is additive to the rapid rate of spontaneous recovery from mivacurium-induced neuromuscular blockade.

5. **Pancuronium** is a long-acting nondepolarizing neuromuscular blocking drug with a steroid structure but lacking any endocrine effects.
   a. The drug is metabolized to a 3-OH compound that has one half the neuromuscular blocking activity of the parent compound.
   b. Pancuronium is associated with modest (usually <15%) increases in heart rate, blood pressure, and cardiac output.
   c. Pancuronium does not release histamine.
   d. The use of pancuronium to provide muscle relaxation may offer some advantage over the use of cardiovascularly neutral muscle relaxants in patients anesthetized with high doses of opioids.

6. **Pipecuronium** is a long-acting aminosteroid nondepolarizing neuromuscular blocking drug that is devoid of histamine-releasing or cardiovascular side effects.

7. **Vecuronium** is an intermediate-acting aminosteroid nondepolarizing muscle relaxant with no cardiovascular side effects.
   a. Vecuronium is a nonquaternary ammonium compound produced by demethylation of the pancuronium molecule. This demethylation de-

creases the ACh-like characteristics of the molecule and increases its lipophilicity, which encourages hepatic uptake.

b. Vecuronium undergoes spontaneous deacetylation. The most potent of the resulting metabolites, 3-OH vecuronium, has about 60% of the activity of vecuronium, is excreted by the kidneys, and may contribute to prolonged paralysis.

c. The cardiovascular neutrality and intermediate duration of action make vecuronium a suitable drug for use in patients with ischemic heart disease or those undergoing short ambulatory surgery.

V. DRUG INTERACTIONS (Table 15-10)

VI. DISEASES THAT ALTER THE RESPONSE TO MUSCLE RELAXANTS (Table 15-11)

VII. MONITORING NEUROMUSCULAR BLOCKADE (see Chapter 7, Section VI)

A. Why Monitor? The margin of safety is narrow because blockade occurs over a narrow range of receptor occupancy. Furthermore, there is considerable interindividual variability in response to the same dose of

---

TABLE 15-10. Drug Interactions Involving Muscle Relaxants

Volatile anesthetics (dose-dependent potentiation of all muscle relaxants)

Local anesthetics (potentiate effects of all muscle relaxants)

Nondepolarizing muscle relaxants (depending on combination, produce additive or synergistic effects; clinical significance doubtful)

Nondepolarizing-depolarizing muscle relaxants (response depends on sequence; nondepolarizer before SCh interferes with SCh blockade; nondepolarizer after SCh is potentiated)

Antibiotics (aminoglycosides and polymyxins most likely to potentiate muscle relaxants)

Anticonvulsants (resistance to nondepolarizing muscle relaxants)

TABLE 15-11. Diseases That Alter the Response to
Muscle Relaxants

Myasthenia gravis (usually slightly resistant to succinylcholine
and highly sensitive to nondepolarizing muscle relaxants)

Myotonia (sustained contracture in response to
succinylcholine; normal response to nondepolarizing muscle
relaxants)

Muscular dystrophy (avoid succinylcholine)

Neurologic diseases (isolated reports of hyperkalemia in
response to succinylcholine)

Hemiplegia/paraplegia (hyperkalemia in response to
succinylcholine; resistant to nondepolarizing muscle
relaxants)

Burn injury (hyperkalemia in response to succinylcholine;
resistant to effects of nondepolarizing muscle relaxants)

neuromuscular blocking drug. To test the function of
the NMJ, a peripheral nerve is stimulated electrically
with a peripheral nerve stimulator, and the response
of the skeletal muscle is assessed (see Table 7-16).

B. **Stimulator characteristics.** The response of the nerve
to electrical stimulation depends on three factors: the
current applied, the duration of the current, and the
position of the electrodes.

C. **Monitoring Modalities** (see Table 7-17)

D. **Recording the Response**
   1. **Visual and tactile evaluation** is the easiest and
      least expensive way to assess the response to elec-
      trical stimulation applied to a peripheral nerve.
      The disadvantage of this technique is the subjec-
      tive nature of its interpretation.
   2. **Measurement of force** using a force transducer
      provides accurate assessment of the response elic-
      ited by electrical stimulation of a peripheral nerve.
   3. **Electromyography** measures the electrical rather
      than mechanical response of the skeletal muscle.

E. **Choice of Muscle**
   1. The **adductor pollicis** supplied by the ulnar nerve
      is the most common skeletal muscle monitored
      clinically. This muscle is relatively sensitive to
      nondepolarizing muscle relaxants, and during re-
      covery it is blocked more than some respiratory
      muscles such as the diaphragm and laryngeal ad-
      ductors.
   2. Stimulation of the **facial nerve** produces contrac-
      tion of the obicularis oculi muscle. Onset of block-
      ade is more rapid, and recovery occurs sooner than

TABLE 15-12. Assessment of the Adequacy of Reversal
of Neuromuscular Blockade

Responses to electrical stimulation of a peripheral nerve
Head lift for 5 seconds
Tongue protrusion
Hand grip strength
Maximum negative inspiratory pressure >minus 25 cm H_2O

at the adductor pollicis muscle. In this regard, the
time course of blockade correlates well with that
of other resistant muscles such as the diaphragm.

F. Clinical Applications (see Table 7-16)
  1. **Monitoring onset.** After induction of anesthesia,
     the intensity of neuromuscular blockade must be
     assessed to determine the time for tracheal intu-
     bation (maximum relaxation of laryngeal and res-
     piratory muscles). Single-twitch stimulation is
     often utilized to monitor the onset of neuromus-
     cular blockade.
  2. **Surgical relaxation** is usually adequate when
     fewer than two or three visible twitches of the
     train-of-four are observed in response to stimula-
     tion of the adductor pollicis muscle.
  3. **Monitoring recovery** is useful in determining
     whether spontaneous recovery has progressed to a
     degree that allows reversal agents to be given (pref-
     erably four twitches visible) and to assess the ef-
     fect of these drugs (supplement with other clinical
     observations) (Table 15-12).
  4. **Factors Affecting the Monitoring of Neuromuscu-
     lar Blockade**
     a. If the monitored hand is cold, the degree of pa-
        ralysis will appear to be increased.
     b. If the monitored limb is characterized by nerve
        damage (stroke, spinal cord transection, pe-
        ripheral nerve trauma), there is inherent resis-
        tance to the effects of muscle relaxants, and the
        degree of skeletal muscle paralysis will be
        underestimated.

VIII. ANTAGONISM OF NEUROMUSCULAR BLOCKADE

A. Anticholinesterase pharmacology. The pharmacologic
   principle involved in drug-enhanced antagonism of
   muscle relaxants is the reduction of the effect of com-

TABLE 15-13. Pharmacokinetics of Anticholinesterase Drugs

	Patient Status	Volume of Distribution $(l \cdot kg^{-1})$	Clearance $(ml \cdot kg^{-1} \cdot min^{-1})$	Elimination Half-Time (minutes)
Edrophonium	Normal	1.1	9.6	110
	Renal failure	0.7	2.7	206
Neostigmine	Normal	0.7	9.2	77
	Renal failure	1.6	7.8	181
Pyridostigmine	Normal	1.1	8.6	112
	Renal failure	1.0	2.1	379

petitive blocking drugs by increasing the concentration of ACh at the NMJ.

1. **Inhibition of acetylcholinesterase** by anticholinesterase drugs (neostigmine, edrophonium, pyridostigmine) results in an increase in the amount of ACh that reaches the receptor.
2. Anticholinesterase drugs may also have presynaptic effects.
3. **Potency** ratios are difficult to determine because the slopes of the edrophonium and neostigmine dose-response curves are not parallel.
4. The **pharmacokinetics** of anticholinesterase drugs reflect the dependence of these drugs on renal clearance (Table 15-13).
5. **Pharmacodynamics.** The onset of action of edrophonium to peak effect (1–2 minutes) is much more rapid than that of neostigmine (7–11 minutes) or pyridostigmine.
   a. Recovery of neuromuscular activity reflects spontaneous recovery plus augmented (accelerated) recovery induced by the anticholinesterase drug.
   b. **Recurarization** should not be expected as long as the duration of the anticholinesterase drug exceeds that of the muscle relaxant.
B. **Factors Affecting Reversal** (Table 15-14)
   1. The dose of anticholinesterase drug selected and the time to effective recovery are directly related to the intensity of blockade at the time of reversal (Table 15-15).
      a. Neostigmine is more effective than edrophonium or pyridostigmine in antagonizing intense neuromuscular blockade.

TABLE 15-14. Factors Affecting Reversal

Block intensity (time to drug-augmented recovery is directly proportional to intensity of blockade present at the time of reversal; see Table 15-15)

Anticholinesterase dose

Choice of relaxant

Age

Renal failure

Acid-base balance (impairment of reversal by acidosis is difficult to document)

TABLE 15-15. Recommended Doses of
Anticholinesterase Drugs Based
on Train-of-Four Stimulation

Visible Twitches	Fade	Dose (mg·kg^{-1})
<2	+ + + +	Neostigmine, 0.07
3–4	+ + +	Neostigmine, 0.04
4	+ +	Edrophonium, 0.5
4	±	Edrophonium, 0.25

    b. Because of the ceiling effect, there is little benefit in administering more than 0.07 mg·kg^{-1} of neostigmine.

  2. The overall rate of recovery (spontaneous plus drug-enhanced) is more rapid from atracurium or vecuronium than from pancuronium.

  3. Recovery of neuromuscular activity occurs more rapidly with lower doses of anticholinesterase drugs in infants and children than in adults.

C. Cardiovascular effects. Anticholinesterase drugs evoke profound vagal stimulation that can be prevented by concomitant administration of an anticholinergic drug.

  1. Because of its rapid onset (1 minute), atropine is appropriate for use in combination with edrophonium, whereas glycopyrrolate (onset 2–3 minutes) may be more suitable for use with neostigmine or pyridostigmine.

  2. Atropine requirements are less when combined with edrophonium (7–10 μg·kg^{-1}) than with neostigmine (15–20 μg·kg^{-1}).

D. Other cholinergic effects of anticholinesterase drugs include increased salivation, enhanced bowel motility (concern about increase in bowel anastomatic leakage), and an alleged increased incidence of nausea and vomiting after ambulatory surgery.

16

Local Anesthetics

Local anesthetics are drugs that block the generation and propagation of impulses in excitable tissues, most notably the spinal cord, spinal nerve roots, and peripheral nerves, but also skeletal muscle, cardiac muscle, and the brain (Carpenter RL, Mackey DC: Local anesthetics. In Barash PG, Cullen BF, Stoelting RK [eds]: Clinical Anesthesia, pp 509–541. Philadelphia, JB Lippincott, 1992).

I. CHEMISTRY OF LOCAL ANESTHETICS

A. The local anesthetic molecule consists of **three building blocks** (Fig. 16-1).

B. The intermediate chain connecting the lipophilic head and the hydrophilic tail contains an ester or amide linkage, thus subdividing the clinically useful local anesthetic into **aminoesters** or **aminoamides** (Table 16-1).

C. Structure-activity relationships

1. Local anesthetics are prepared as hydrochloride salts, which in aqueous solution dissociate into an **ionized (charged and hydrophilic quaternary amine)** and a **non-ionized (uncharged and lipophilic tertiary amine)** form (Table 16-2).

2. Both the non-ionized and ionized forms of the local anesthetic molecule are involved in the blockade of nerve impulses. Non-ionized molecules most likely interact with Na^+ channels by passing through the lipid environment of the axon membrane. Ionized molecules probably gain access to specific receptors on the interior of the Na^+ channel through the aqueous pathway of the Na^+ channel pore.

D. Commercial preparations

1. The hydrochloride salt solution is acidified to pH 4.4–6.4 to favor existence of the water-soluble ionized form of the local anesthetic molecule.

2. **Epinephrine (EPI)-containing solutions** must be acidified because alkaline solutions promote oxidation of catecholamines.

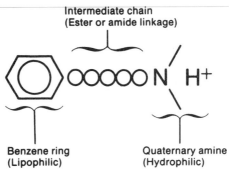

Figure 16-1. General structure of local anesthetics.

3. **Antioxidants** (sodium metabisulfite, sodium ethylenediaminetetra-acetic acid [EDTA]) may be added to local anesthetic solutions to retard their breakdown.

4. **Antimicrobial preservative (parabens derivatives)** are added to local anesthetic solutions contained in multidose vials. Parabens are potent allergens and may be responsible for allergic reactions falsely attributed to the local anesthetic. Potential **cytotoxicity** of preservatives dictates against use of preservative-containing solutions for spinal, epidural, or intravenous regional anesthesia.

II. MECHANISM OF ACTION OF LOCAL ANESTHETICS

A. **Anatomy of the peripheral nerve** (Table 16-3)

B. **Physiology of the nerve fiber.** Information is transmitted by electrical signals generated and conducted by neurons. The propagation of rapid changes in membrane potential is known as the **action potential.** Electrical excitability occurs because of the presence in the axolemma of **voltage-sensitive ion channels** that are specific for Na^+, K^+, and Ca^{2+}.

1. In response to voltage fluctuations, these channels open and close sequentially in gatelike fashion to allow the rapid diffusion of specific ions down their concentration gradients. The resultant ionic current flux across the cell membrane depolarizes and repolarizes it. Although Na^+, K^+, and Ca^{2+} channels are each important for initiation and propagation of

the action potential in neurons, the **properties of the Na⁺ channel (exists in one of three states)** are the most important (Fig. 16-2).

2. Transmission of a signal by propagation of an action potential is an **all-or-none phenomenon.** This is characterized by a wave of depolarization that spreads at a constant speed, activating the Na^+ channels of each successive membrane segment as it travels along the axon.

3. **Myelinization** of nerve fibers increases the speed of neural transmission as the action potential jumps from one node of Ranvier to the next (saltatory conduction).

C. **Electrophysiologic effects of local anesthetics.** The accepted mechanism of action through which all local anesthetics produce blockade of nerve impulses is **inhibition of ion flux across the channels that specifically conduct Na⁺.** The ion gradient and resting membrane potential are unchanged, but the increase in Na^+ permeability associated with the nerve impulse is inhibited.

D. **Minimum blocking concentration (C_m)** is defined as the lowest concentration of local anesthetic that blocks impulse conduction along a given nerve fiber. This concentration provides a measure of relative potency of local anesthetics and is analogous to minimum alveolar concentration (MAC) for inhaled anesthetics.

E. **Differential block** describes blockade of the components of a peripheral nerve that proceeds at different rates with loss of sympathetic function first, followed by loss of pinprick sensation, touch and temperature discrimination, and, finally, loss of motor function. The exact mechanism of differential blockade has not been conclusively demonstrated.

III. PHARMACOKINETICS

A. **Local disposition.** The amount of local anesthetic that reaches a nerve depends to a large extent on the proximity of injection to the nerve **(intraneural injection is painful and may result in nerve damage).** A **minimum volume** is necessary to provide adequate spread of local anesthetic around the nerves, and a **minimum concentration (total mass)** is necessary to provide an adequate diffusion gradient for penetrance into the nerve.

1. Connective tissue and adipose tissue barriers vary among different nerves in the body. Spinal nerve roots are floating free in cerebrospinal fluid, and

(*Text continues on pg 208*)

TABLE 16-1. Classification and Uses of Local Anesthetics

	Clinical Uses	Usual Concentration (%)	Usual Onset	Usual Duration (hours)	Maximum Single Dose (mg)*	pH of Solution†	Unique Characteristics
Aminoesters							
2-Chloroprocaine	Infiltration	1	Fast	0.5–1.0	1000 + EPI	2.7–4.0	Lowest systemic toxicity
	PNB	2	Fast	0.5–1.0	1000 + EPI		Intrathecal route may be neurotoxic
	Epidural	2–3	Fast	0.5–1.5	1000 + EPI		Used for differential spinal
Procaine	Infiltration	1	Fast	0.5–1.0	1000	5.0–6.5	
	PNB	1–2	Slow	0.5–1.0	1000		
	Spinal	10	Moderate	0.5–1.0	200		
Tetracaine	Topical	2	Slow	0.5–1.0	80	4.5–6.5	
	Spinal	0.5	Fast	2–4	20		
Aminoamides							
Lidocaine	Topical	4	Fast	0.5–1.0	500 + EPI	6.5	
	Infiltration	0.5–1.0	Fast	1–2	500 + EPI		
	IV regional	0.25–0.5			500		
	PNB	1.0–1.5	Fast	1–3	500 + EPI		
	Epidural	1–2	Fast	1–2	500 + EPI		
	Spinal	5	Fast	0.5–1.5	100		

Drug	Route	Concentration	Onset	Duration	Max dose (mg)	pH†	Comments
Prilocaine	IV regional	0.25–0.5			600		Least toxic amide
	PNB	1.5–2.0	Fast	1.5–3.0	600		Methemoglobinemia possible when ≥600 mg
	Epidural	1–3	Fast	1.0–2.5	600	4.5	
Mepivacaine	PNB	1.0–1.5	Fast	2–3	500 + EPI		Duration of plain solutions longer than lidocaine without EPI, useful when EPI contraindicated
	Epidural	1–2	Fast	1.0–2.5	500 + EPI	4.5	
Bupivacaine	PNB	0.25–0.5	Slow	4–12	200 + EPI		Exaggerated cardiotoxicity with accidental iv injection
	Epidural	0.25–0.75	Moderate	2–4	200 + EPI		
	Spinal	0.5–0.75	Fast	2–4	20	4.6–6.0	
Etidocaine	PNB	0.5–1.0	Fast	3–12	300 + EPI		Low doses produce sensory > motor blockade
	Epidural	1.0–1.5	Fast	2–4	300 + EPI	4.5	Motor > sensory blockade
Ropivacaine (same as bupivacaine)							

*Use only as a guide, as influenced by many factors.
†EPI-containing solutions have a pH 1.0–1.5 units lower than plain solutions.
EPI = epinephrine; PNB = peripheral nerve block.

TABLE 16-2. Effect of pH on Local Anesthetic Dissociation

| | | % of Total Drug in Non-ionized Form | | |
	pK_a	pH 7.4	pH 7.0	pH 7.8
2-Chloroprocaine	9.1	2	0.8	5
Procaine	8.9	3	1	7
Tetracaine	8.6	14	6	28
Lidocaine	7.9	24	11	48
Mepivacaine	7.6	39	20	61
Bupivacaine	8.1	17	7	33
Etidocaine	7.7	24	11	44
Ropivacaine	8.1			

small amounts of local anesthetic produce profound blockade. In contrast, the brachial plexus and sciatic nerves are surrounded by fascial sheaths and adipose tissue, and the application of large amounts of drug is necessary to provide reliable anesthesia. Furthermore, during diffusion to the nerve, the local anesthetic is diluted by absorption into tissues, blood, and lymph.

2. The rapidity and extent of diffusion depend primarily on the pK_a of the local anesthetic, the concentration of local anesthetic injected, and its lipid solubility. Because the pK_a of all local anesthetics is higher than physiologic pH, most of the injected anesthetic is in the ionized (less lipid-soluble) form. This may explain, in part, the relatively poor ability of tetracaine to spread and penetrate tissues (brachial plexus block), whereas it is very effective when injected into the subarachnoid space, where diffusion barriers are minimal. Acidosis from local infection retards diffusion of local anesthetics because of increased ionization. Lipid solubility enhances the ability of local anesthetics to penetrate lipid barriers around nerves, but this may be offset by increased nonspecific binding with lipid components of nonneural tissues.

3. **Kinetics of nerve block.** When local anesthetic is deposited near the brachial plexus, the onset of motor blockade often precedes the onset of sensory blockade. This reflects the peripheral location of motor

TABLE 16-3. Classification and Anatomy of Nerve Fibers

Classification	Anatomic Location	Myelin	Diameter (μm)	Rate of Conduction (m·s⁻¹)	Function
A Fibers					
A alpha	Afferent to and efferent from muscles and joints	Yes	6–22	30–85	Motor Proprioception
A beta					
A gamma	Efferent to muscle spindles	Yes	3–6	15–35	Muscle tone
A delta	Sensory roots and afferent peripheral nerves	Yes	1–4	5–25	Pain Temperature Touch
B-Fibers	Preganglionic sympathetic	Yes	3	3–15	Vasomotor Pilomotor
C-Fibers					
sC	Postganglionic sympathetic	No	0.3–1.3	0.7–1.3	Vasomotor Pilomotor
drC	Sensory roots and afferent peripheral nerves	No	0.4–1.2	0.1–2.0	Pain Temperature Touch

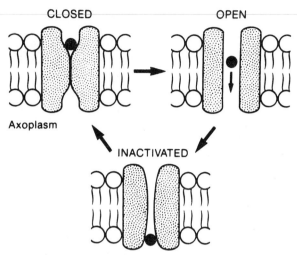

Figure 16-2. The Na$^+$ channel exists in one of three states.

fibers in the nerve bundle compared with the central (core) location of sensory fibers. A similar sequence would not be expected for spinal anesthesia, in which diffusion barriers are minimal.

B. **Systemic absorption** influences the amount of local anesthetic remaining at the perineural injection site and thus the duration of anesthesia. **Peak blood levels (Cmax)** of local anesthetics that follow perineural injection are influenced by several factors (Table 16-4).

1. The **maximum safe dose of a local anesthetic** is based on the likely Cmax that will occur after perineural injection. These doses are not absolute and must be **considered only as imprecise guidelines** that will be altered by many complex and often unpredictable events (Table 16-1).

2. Although the maximum safe dose of a local anesthetic is frequently stated in terms of mg·kg^{-1}, there is no correlation between the patient's body weight and peak plasma levels.

C. **Distribution and elimination**

1. Local anesthetic that is absorbed into the venous circulation is initially distributed to the lungs, where substantial uptake occurs so as to limit the drug that reaches the systemic circulation for distribution

TABLE 16-4. Determinants of Local Anesthetic Blood Levels

Total dose of local anesthetic
Site of injection (intercostal>epidural>brachial plexus)
Addition of vasoconstrictors (more effective with lidocaine than bupivacaine)
Drug-induced local vasodilation (bupivacaine>lidocaine)
Local tissue binding as influenced by lipid solubility
Tissue perfusion
Concomitant drug therapy
Renal disease
Hepatic disease

to tissues, especially highly perfused (vessel-rich group) organs such as the brain and heart.

2. **Protein binding** determines the amount of drug available to produce a pharmacologic effect, because only the unbound fraction is pharmacologically active. The extent of protein binding varies among patients (up to eightfold) and depends on the specific local anesthetic and the concentration (Table 16-5).

3. **Clearance**

a. **Aminoamides** are cleared from the plasma by hepatic metabolism. Monoethylglycinexylidide is an active metabolite of lidocaine that can contribute to toxicity even when plasma levels of lidocaine are in a therapeutic range.

b. **Aminoesterases** are rapidly cleared from the plasma by plasma and liver cholinesterases. Plas-

TABLE 16-5. Protein Binding of Local Anesthetics

Anesthetic	Protein Binding (%)
2-Chloroprocaine	—
Procaine	5
Tetracaine	85
Lidocaine	65
Mepivacaine	75
Bupivacaine	95
Etidocaine	95
Ropivacaine	94

ma levels of these local anesthetics in patients with deficient or atypical cholinesterase enzyme may be elevated.

4. **Physical and pathophysiologic factors**
   a. **Decreased cardiac output** impairs removal of local anesthetics from the plasma, presumably reflecting decreased hepatic blood flow. The rate of intravenous infusion of lidocaine to treat cardiac dysrhythmias may need to be reduced in patients with congestive heart failure in order to avoid potentially toxic plasma levels.
   b. **Liver disease** prolongs the elimination half-time ($T_{1/2\beta}$) of lidocaine and presumably of all aminoamides.
   c. **Age** does not consistently alter the initial dose of local anesthetic, but subsequent doses should be modified to avoid cumulative drug effects in elderly patients. The $T_{1/2\beta}$ of aminoamides is prolonged two to three times in neonates but resembles adult values after about 6 months of age.
   d. **Acid-base.** Fetal acidosis appears to result in greater transfer of local anesthetic from a mother to her fetus, but there is no evidence that an acidotic fetus is more susceptible to local anesthetic-induced toxicity.

D. **Drug actions and interactions**
   1. Volatile anesthetics, cimetidine, and propranolol may alter clearance of local anesthetics through inhibition of mixed function oxidases or decreases in hepatic blood flow.
   2. There is no evidence that diazepam can displace bupivacaine from its binding sites. Therefore, use of diazepam to treat a toxic reaction will not increase the unbound fraction of bupivacaine.

E. **Combinations of local anesthetics.** A mixture of an aminoester (2-chloroprocaine) and an aminoamide (bupivacaine) in an attempt to produce a block of rapid onset and long duration seems logical but has not been demonstrated to be advantageous. Toxicity from mixtures of local anesthetics seems to be additive rather than synergistic.

IV. TOXICITY OF LOCAL ANESTHETICS

A. **Allergic reactions** are rare (especially with aminoamides), but when they do occur they can be life-threatening. Aminoesters are more allergenic than aminoamides because of their relationship to p-aminobenzoic acid. Parabens are present in multidose local anesthetic solutions, other drugs, cosmetics, and foods. Prior exposure to parabens may sensitize patients to subsequent administration of local anesthetic solutions containing these materials, resulting in an allergic reaction unrelated to the local anesthetic.

B. **Local tissue toxicity** is rare when proper concentrations of local anesthetics are used. 2-Chloroprocaine has been implicated in neurotoxicity and is not recommended for subarachnoid injection. This toxicity may be more related to the low pH of the solution and to the preservative, sodium bisulfite, than to the local anesthetic molecule. Newer preparations of chloroprocaine contain EDTA rather than bisulfite.

C. **Systemic toxicity** most frequently results from **accidental intravascular injection,** producing a concentration-dependent continuum of effects manifesting principally at the brain and heart (Fig. 16-3).

   1. **Central nervous system (CNS) toxicity** manifesting as seizures probably results from selective depression of inhibitory fibers or centers in the CNS, allowing excessive excitatory input. Seizures appear to originate in the **amygdala,** with subsequent spread leading to tonic-clonic seizures. CNS toxicity is in-

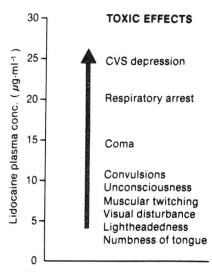

Figure 16-3. Dose-dependent symptoms of local anesthetic toxicity. CVS = cardiovascular system.

creased by an elevated Pa_{CO_2}. Accidental injection of a low dose of local anesthetic (bupivacaine, 2.5 mg) into the vertebral artery during performance of a stellate ganglion block can result in tonic-clonic seizures. CNS toxicity is decreased by barbiturates, benzodiazepines, and inhaled anesthetics.

2. **Cardiovascular system toxicity**
   a. High systemic concentrations of local anesthetics (usually four to seven times those that cause seizures) can produce **decreased myocardial contractility, refractory cardiac dysrhythmias, and vasodilation,** resulting in cardiovascular collapse that is resistant to treatment.
   b. Local anesthetics produce a dose-dependent delay in the transmission of cardiac impulses by their action on cardiac Na^+ channels. **Bupivacaine is more cardiotoxic than lidocaine,** presumably because the time for dissociation of bupivacaine from Na^+ channels during the diastolic time present with a heart rate of 60–150 beats·min^{-1} is insufficient, leading to persistent Na^+ channel blockade. In this regard, bupivacaine is about 70 times more potent than lidocaine in blocking cardiac conduction at physiologic heart rates.
   c. **Ropivacaine** has a potency and duration of action that resemble bupivacaine, but it lacks significant cardiovascular toxicity (dissociates from sodium channels more rapidly than bupivacaine).
   d. Cardiovascular toxicity of local anesthetics is increased by hypoxia, acidosis, pregnancy, and hyperkalemia.
   e. Addition of EPI to a local anesthetic solution decreases absorption and also has sympathetic nervous system effects that tend to counter the circulatory effects of the local anesthetic.

D. **Treatment of systemic toxicity**
   1. The **best treatment of systemic toxicity** is prevention by meticulous attention to technique and recognition of intravascular injections with a preliminary test dose.
   2. **Oxygen must be administered at the first sign of systemic toxicity** because arterial hypoxemia and acidosis develop rapidly and further accentuate the toxicity of local anesthetics.
   3. **Seizure control** is provided by thiopental, succinylcholine (SCh), or diazepam. The optimal drug for treatment of seizures is controversial.

   a. Succinylcholine administered intravenously (0.2–0.5 mg·kg^{-1}) promptly stops peripheral muscular manifestations of seizures (decreases severity of metabolic acidosis) and facilitates ventilation of the lungs with oxygen. The disadvantage is the failure of SCh to suppress seizure activity in the CNS such that cerebral metabolic oxygen requirements remain elevated.

   b. Diazepam administered intravenously (0.1–0.3 mg·kg^{-1}) produces selective suppression of CNS seizure activity with minimal cardiovascular effects (in contrast to thiopental). The disadvantage of diazepam is a relatively slow onset (2–3 minutes) of seizure suppression.

4. Cardiovascular toxicity produced by local anesthetics is often resistant to treatment despite administration of high doses of EPI, atropine, and bretylium.

5. **Methemoglobinemia** reflects the metabolism of the aminoamide local anesthetic **prilocaine** to toludine, which is capable of producing detectable methemoglobinemia, especially when the total local anesthetic dose exceeds about 500 mg. **Methylene blue,** 1–5 mg·kg^{-1}, administered intravenously converts methemoglobin to reduced hemoglobin. Fetal blood is deficient in enzymes necessary to reduce methemoglobin, suggesting caution in the administration of prilocaine to parturients.

V. CLINICAL USES OF LOCAL ANESTHETICS

A. **Choice of local anesthetic** must take into consideration several factors (Table 16-6).

1. The concentration of local anesthetic selected is influenced by the diameter of the nerves to be blocked.

TABLE 16-6. Determinants of Choice of Local Anesthetic

Duration of surgery

Regional technique selected

Unique surgical needs (sensory blockade for obstetrics, motor blockade for orthopedics)

Skills of the anesthesiologist

Potential for systemic toxicity

Large-diameter nerves, as with epidural anesthesia, require higher concentrations than more peripheral nerves.

2. The quality of sensory and motor blockade produced by the various local anesthetics differs considerably. Intrathecal administration of tetracaine produces greater motor blockade than bupivacaine, whereas bupivacaine provides a longer duration of sensory analgesia. For brachial plexus block, mepivacaine produces greater motor and longer sensory blockade than lidocaine.

3. Bupivacaine and lidocaine can be used for all regional blocks and are currently the most widely used local anesthetics.

VI. ADJUVANTS AND COMBINATIONS

A. **Epinephrine** produces beneficial effects when added to local anesthetic solutions **(maximum dose, 200–250 μg)** (Table 16-7).

1. Epinephrine is less effective in prolonging the duration of action of bupivacaine than is tetracaine.

2. Epinephrine can decrease peak blood levels (lidocaine > bupivacaine), presumably by producing local vasoconstriction and decreasing the rate of local anesthetic systemic absorption.

3. Increased intensity of analgesia when EPI is added to local anesthetic solutions may result from a direct action of EPI (and other alpha agonists) on antinociceptive receptors in the spinal cord.

4. Vasoconstriction to reduce surgical bleeding is adequately produced by local infiltration of solutions containing EPI, 5 $\mu g \cdot ml^{-1}$ (1:200,000).

5. If the test dose contains 15 μg of EPI, intravascular injection can be detected by an increase in heart rate

---

TABLE 16-7. Effects of Epinephrine Added to the Local Anesthetic Solution

Prolongs duration of anesthesia
Reduces systemic absorption
Increases the intensity of blockade
Reduces surgical bleeding
Component of test dose to signal intravascular injection

TABLE 16-8. Manifestations of Systemic Epinephrine Absorption

Increased heart rate
Increased cardiac output
Decreased systemic vascular resistance

---

of at least 20%. This response is blunted in patients receiving beta antagonists.

6. **Use in obstetrics.** Alpha effects of EPI may decrease uterine artery blood flow and beta effects could slow labor, leading some to avoid inclusion of EPI in local anesthetic solutions administered to parturients.

7. **Systemic effects.** Absorbed EPI (except in subarachnoid placement, which is devoid of circulatory effects) produces predominantly beta effects, with little evidence of alpha effects at doses up to 400 µg (Table 16-8).

8. There are several situations in which the inclusion of EPI in local anesthetic solutions is not recommended (Table 16-9).

B. **Phenylephrine** (2–5 mg) in the local anesthetic solution injected into the subarachnoid space prolongs spinal anesthesia similarly to the use of EPI. Phenylephrine does not reliably reduce peak blood levels of local anesthetic when injected with local anesthetic solutions for blocks other than spinal block. Prominent alpha-mediated circulatory effects reflect systemic absorption

---

TABLE 16-9. Contraindications to the Inclusion of Epinephrine in Local Anesthetic Solutions

Unstable angina pectoris
Cardiac dysrhythmias
Uncontrolled hypertension
Uteroplacental insufficiency
Treatment with monoamine oxidase inhibitors or tricyclic antidepressants
Peripheral nerve blocks in areas that may lack collateral blood flow (penis, digits)
Intravenous regional anesthesia

of phenylephrine when placed at sites other than the subarachnoid space.

C. **Carbonated local anesthetics.** Despite a more rapid onset and intensity of blockade (diffusion of carbon dioxide into the nerve lowers intraneural pH, which promotes ion trapping), the use of these solutions remains controversial. Peak blood levels are higher, and a more rapid onset with epidural anesthesia may accentuate blood pressure decreases.

IV

MANAGEMENT OF ANESTHESIA

17

Epidural and
Spinal Anesthesia

Epidural and spinal anesthesia are the two most popular regional anesthetic procedures used for surgery, obstetrics, and postoperative analgesia (Covino BG, Lambert DH: Epidural and spinal anesthesia. In Barash PG, Cullen BF, Stoelting RK [eds]: Clinical Anesthesia, pp 809–840. Philadelphia, JB Lippincott, 1992) (see Table 16-1).

I. RATIONALE FOR THE USE OF EPIDURAL AND SPINAL ANESTHESIA

A. **Metabolic and endocrine alterations.** Most of the surgically induced endocrine and metabolic changes (increased plasma concentrations of catecholamines, cortisol, glucose, antidiuretic hormone, and growth hormone) are inhibited by an appropriate level of sensory blockade produced by regional anesthesia.

B. **Blood loss.** Reduced intraoperative blood loss (total hip replacement, transurethral resection of the prostate) compared with general anesthesia may reflect hypotension caused by sympathetic nervous system (SNS) blockade or redistribution of blood flow away from the operative site.

C. **Thromboembolic complications** are reduced by 50–60% when hip surgery or prostatectomy is performed under epidural anesthesia, presumably reflecting increased blood flow to the lower extremities. Mortality rates, however, are similar to those with general anesthesia.

D. **Cardiopulmonary complications**
   1. **Continuous epidural analgesia for postoperative pain relief** may ameliorate the usual postoperative deterioration of pulmonary function, as reflected by higher Pa_{O_2} values and fewer chest infections.

2. Patients who have cardiac disease and are undergoing major noncardiac surgery may develop fewer cardiovascular alterations during regional anesthesia (lower pulmonary capillary wedge pressure, fewer cardiac dysrhythmias, lower incidence of myocardial ischemia) than during general anesthesia.

3. No difference in the incidence of postoperative myocardial infarction or mortality has been documented with the use of regional versus general anesthesia.

II. ANATOMY

A. **Bony structures.** The spinal canal extends from the foramen magnum to the sacral hiatus (7 cervical, 12 thoracic, 5 lumbar vertebrae). The degree of angulation of the spinous processes influences the direction of a needle to be placed in the epidural or subarachnoid space. In the lumbar region, the spinal processes are almost horizontal, and the needle may be directed at right angles to the sagittal plane.

B. **Ligaments.** From the skin, a needle directed toward the subarachnoid space passes in sequence through several different structures (Table 17-1).

C. **The epidural space** is a potential space (completely filled with connective tissue, fatty tissue, and blood vessels) located **between the ligamentum flavum and the dura mater.** Solutions injected into the epidural space spread in all directions among the loose tissue structures that occupy this space.

1. **The subdural space** is a potential space (contains lymph) between the dura mater and the arachnoid mater.

2. **The subarachnoid space** is the space between the arachnoid mater and pia mater (closely attached to

---

TABLE 17-1. Structures Penetrated During Insertion of a Needle to Perform Spinal Anesthesia

Supraspinous ligament
Interspinous ligament
Ligamentum flavum (joins the laminae of the vertebrae)
Dura mater
Arachnoid mater

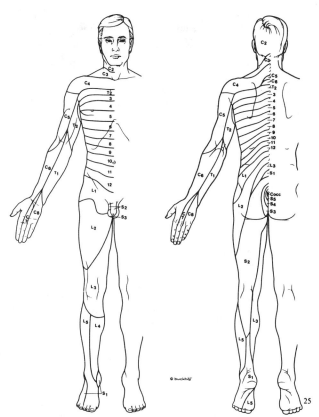

Figure 17-1. Dermatomes of the body.

the spinal cord and nerves), which contains cerebrospinal fluid (CSF) (Fig. 17-1).

III. PATIENT EVALUATION AND PREPARATION FOR EPIDURAL AND SPINAL ANESTHESIA

Patient evaluation and preparation for epidural and spinal anesthesia are similar to those scheduled for general anesthesia, with some special areas of emphasis (see Appendix F) (Table 17-2).

TABLE 17-2. Preparation Before Epidural and
Spinal Anesthesia

Physical examination of the back and history of back problems
Coagulation profile
Explanation of technique and perceived advantages
Description of the forms of sedation available
Tailor preoperative medication to level of anxiety and need for
  analgesia (anticholinergics are probably not necessary)

IV. CONTRAINDICATIONS FOR EPIDURAL AND SPINAL ANESTHESIA
(Table 17-3)

V. TECHNICAL ASPECTS

The most important landmarks for performance of lumbar epidural or spinal anesthesia are the **vertebral spinal processes (define the midline)** and the **iliac crests (a line drawn between the crests crosses L4),** which identify the spaces usually selected (L3–4 or L4–5) for insertion of the epidural or spinal needle (Fig. 17-2).

A. **Epidural anesthesia.** The epidural space is most easily entered in the lumbar region (the spinous processes are not angulated, and the space is wide) using a 17- or 18-gauge Tuohy needle. The curved Huber point of this needle decreases the possibility of accidental dural puncture and facilitates passage of a catheter. Patients remain sitting or are placed in the lateral position with the knees and head flexed to maximally open the intervertebral spaces. An intravenous infusion is initiated before performing the block, and the blood pressure, heart rate, and electrocardiogram are monitored.

1. The most common method to identify the epidural space is the **loss-of-resistance technique,** in which the dorsum of the anesthesiologist's noninjecting hand is placed on the patient's back (Fig. 17-3).

2. Loss of resistance to advancement of the plunger is noted as the needle passes through the ligamentum flavum to enter the epidural space.

3. **Catheter placement.** An important advantage of epidural anesthesia is the ability to insert a plastic catheter into the epidural space to permit repeated

**TABLE 17-3. Contraindications to Epidural and
Spinal Anesthesia**

Absolute Contraindications
  Patient refusal
  Infection at the puncture site
  Uncorrected hypovolemia
  Severe coagulation abnormalities
  Anatomic abnormalities

Relative Contraindications
  Bacteremia
  Pre-existing neurologic disorders (multiple sclerosis)
  Minidose heparin

    injections of local anesthetic and/or opioid solutions. The catheter is advanced only 2–3 cm into the epidural space to reduce the likelihood that it might exit through an intervertebral foramen, with resulting inadequate epidural anesthesia.

4. **Test dose.** A local anesthetic solution (3–4 ml containing 1:200,000 epinephrine [EPI]) injected through the epidural needle or catheter identifies **accidental intravascular injection** (increased heart rate and blood pressure due to EPI) or **unrecognized subarachnoid injection** (sensory blockade despite a low dose of local anesthetic). It is best to reinstitute epidural anesthesia at a different interspace if there is any evidence of an intravascular

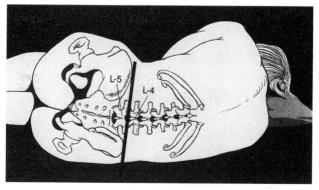

Figure 17-2. Anatomic landmarks for epidural or spinal block.

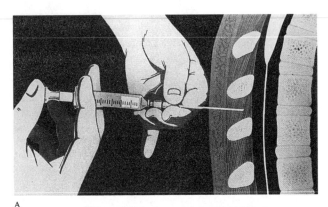

A

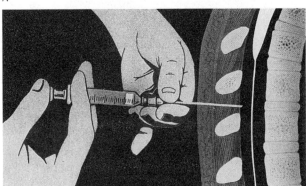

B

Figure 17-3. Hand position for identifying epidural space by the loss of resistance technique.

injection. Spinal anesthesia is an alternative if there is evidence of a subarachnoid injection.

5. The total dose of local anesthetic solution injected into the epidural space depends on the **physical status** of the patient and the **location of the surgical procedure.** The injection of local anesthetic solution is often slow (3- to 4-minute intervals) and incremental (3–5 ml), considering the large volumes required and rapid systemic absorption of drugs from the epidural space. The dermatomal

sensory level can be evaluated by pinprick or use of an alcohol swab.

B. **Spinal anesthesia** is induced with patients in the lateral or sitting position (proper curvature of the back is easier to obtain, but syncope is a risk).

1. **Midline approach.** A 22-gauge (patients >60 years of age) or 25- to 26-gauge needle (reduced incidence of postdural puncture headache) is inserted in the midline in the most easily palpable lumbar interspace below L2 (spinal cord ends at L1–2). The needle is inserted with the bevel parallel to the dural fibers and spinous processes and advanced at a slightly cephalad angle until it lodges in the interspinous ligament, after which it is no longer possible to change the direction of advancement. A distinct "pop" is often felt as the needle passes through the dura mater. If CSF is not obtained or if blood, paresthesia, or bone is encountered, the needle is withdrawn to subcutaneous tissue and redirected. When entrance into the subarachnoid space is confirmed by free flow of CSF, the dorsum of the anesthesiologist's noninjecting hand is placed on the patient's back and the hub of the needle grasped between the thumb and index finger. The syringe containing the local anesthetic solution is attached to the needle, a small amount of CSF is gently aspirated to again verify the placement, and the solution is injected.

2. **Paramedian or lateral approach.** The needle is inserted 1.5–2.0 cm lateral to the midline opposite the center of the selected interspace. This approach bypasses calcified supraspinous and interspinous ligaments in elderly patients.

3. **The Taylor approach** is entrance into the subarachnoid space at the L5–S1 interspace (the largest interspace in the vertebral column) with the needle directed cephalad and medial from a site 1 cm medial and 1 cm caudad to the posterior superior iliac spine.

4. **Continuous spinal anesthesia** is provided by a small (27–32 gauge) catheter threaded 2–3 cm into the lumbar subarachnoid space.

   a. To minimize the frequency of postdural puncture headache, the use of a 27-gauge needle and a 32-gauge catheter has been recommended for patients up to 50 years of age.

   b. Cauda equina syndrome, although rare, has followed continuous spinal anesthesia, perhaps reflecting maldistribution of the local anesthetic injected through the microcatheter.

VI. MECHANISM OF SPINAL AND EPIDURAL ANESTHESIA

A. **Spinal anesthesia.** The anatomy of the dorsal roots is such that small-diameter nerve fibers (preganglionic autonomic, dull pain, temperature, touch) are close to the surface, thereby shortening the distance for diffusion of local anesthesia and making it appear that these fibers are more susceptible to block than large-diameter fibers (motor, proprioception), which are situated in the core of the nerve bundle **("differential blockade")**.

B. **Epidural anesthesia.** Initial blockade occurs in the spinal roots, followed by some degree of spinal cord anesthesia as local anesthetic diffuses into the subarachnoid space. A delay in the onset or inadequate anesthesia at S1–2 when local anesthetic solutions are injected into the epidural space may reflect the large size of these spinal roots.

VII. PHYSIOLOGIC EFFECTS OF SPINAL AND EPIDURAL ANESTHESIA

A. **Spinal anesthesia**

1. **Sympathetic nervous system blockade** is unavoidable during spinal anesthesia, reflecting the fact that preganglionic SNS fibers originate in the spinal cord and travel with the spinal nerves. SNS fibers may be blocked to a greater extent than somatic sensory fibers because they are more peripherally located in the nerve roots than the sensory fibers. SNS blockade exceeds sensory blockade by two or more dermatomes.

2. **The cardiovascular system.** All the cardiovascular effects associated with spinal anesthesia are the direct result of preganglionic SNS blockade (Table 17-4).

3. **The respiratory system.** Intercostal muscle paralysis interferes with the ability to cough and clear secretions.

4. **The renal system.** Spinal anesthesia resulting in hypotension sufficient to reduce renal blood flow is accompanied by transient decreases in glomerular filtration rate and urinary output.

**TABLE 17-4. Cardiovascular Effects of
Spinal Anesthesia**

Bradycardia (blockade of cardioaccelerator fibers from T1–4
and decreased venous return)
Venodilation
Decreased blood pressure (due principally to reduced cardiac
output secondary to decreased venous return)

5. **The gastrointestinal system.** Hepatic blood flow is decreased in parallel with reductions in blood pressure. Blockade of sympathetic innervation (T5–L1) to the gastrointestinal tract leaves vagal tone intact and results in a contracted bowel. The etiology of nausea during spinal anesthesia is poorly understood (Table 17-5).

B. **Epidural anesthesia**
 1. **Hemodynamic effects.** SNS blockade sufficient to cause systemic hypotension is more gradual in onset than with spinal anesthesia and rarely occurs before sensory anesthesia is established. Changes in blood pressure, heart rate, and cardiac output during epidural anesthesia depend on multiple factors (Table 17-6).

**TABLE 17-5. Etiology and Treatment of Nausea During
Spinal Anesthesia**

Unopposed vagal activity and increased peristalsis (atropine,
0.4 mg iv)
Hypotension (ephedrine, 5–10 mg iv and oxygen)
Cerebral ischemia
Medications used for sedation (droperidol, 0.625 mg iv)

**TABLE 17-6. Determinants of Hemodynamic Responses
to Epidural Anesthesia**

Level of anesthesia (above T5)
Systemic absorption of local anesthetic
Inclusion of epinephrine (systemic beta$_1$ and beta$_2$ effects)
Intravascular fluid volume
Cardiovascular status of the patient

TABLE 17-7. Local Anesthetics Used for Spinal Anesthesia

Surgical Site	Drug	Concentration (%)	Usual Dose (mg)	Usual Volume (ml)	Usual Duration	
					No Epinephrine (h)	0.2 mg Epinephrine (h)
Above L1 (hyperbaric)	Bupivacaine	0.75	10–15	1.5–2.0	2	2
	Tetracaine	0.5	10–15	2–3	3	3
	Lidocaine	5.0	50–75	1.0–1.5	1	1
Below L1 (hypobaric)	Bupivacaine	0.5	15	3	3–4	4–6
	Tetracaine	0.5	15	3	3–4	4–6
	Lidocaine	2.0	60	3	1–2	2–4

2. **Effects on regional blood flow.** Increases in blood flow to the lower limbs are rarely associated with significant decreases in blood pressure because of compensatory vasoconstriction above the level of blockade. Decreases in cerebral blood flow, coronary blood flow, renal blood flow, and hepatic blood flow parallel reductions in blood pressure.

VIII. PHARMACOLOGIC CONSIDERATIONS

A. **Spinal anesthesia**
   1. **Selection of a specific local anesthetic.** Lidocaine, tetracaine, and bupivacaine are most often selected based on the site and duration of surgery and desired intensity of motor blockade. Hyperbaric solutions gravitate to the thoracic kyphosis in supine patients, ensuring an adequate level of spinal anesthesia for procedures above L1, whereas isobaric solutions tend to remain in the lower dermatomes, providing intense anesthesia of prolonged duration (Table 17-7).
      a. **Hyperbaric lidocaine** is useful for short duration surgical and obstetric procedures (30–90 minutes).
      b. **Hyperbaric tetracaine** is useful for abdominal surgical procedures of 2–4 hours' duration.
      c. **Isobaric bupivacaine** is particularly valuable for lower limb vascular and orthopedic procedures lasting 2–5 hours.
   2. **Factors that influence distribution of local anesthetics in the cerebrospinal fluid** (Table 17-8)
      a. Local anesthetic solutions are rendered hyperbaric by adding glucose to increase the density to >1.008.
      b. The high and low points in the spinal canal influence distribution of hyperbaric and hypo-

---

TABLE 17-8. Determinants of Local Anesthetic Distribution in Cerebrospinal Fluid

Baricity of the local anesthetic solution (hyperbaric, isobaric, hypobaric)

Shape of the spinal canal (when patient is supine, a high point at L3–4 and low point at T5–6)

Position of the patient (hyperbaric solutions gravitate to dependent areas and hypobaric solutions float upward)

baric solutions but not of isobaric solutions (Fig. 17-4).

3. **Vasoconstrictors.** EPI (200–250 µg) and phenylephrine (2–5 mg) are believed to prolong spinal anesthesia by localized vasoconstriction, although a direct antinociceptive effect may also be operative.

B. **Epidural anesthesia**

1. Local anesthetics used for epidural anesthesia are classified according to their onset and duration of action (Table 17-9).

    a. Bupivacaine 0.25% is useful for continuous epidural anesthesia during labor, producing analgesia with minimal motor blockade.

    b. Etidocaine provides rapid onset of analgesia and profound motor blockade that is considered useful for certain surgical but not for obstetric procedures.

    c. Tetracaine is rarely used for epidural block because of its slow onset of action.

2. The **quality of epidural anesthesia** is determined by several factors (Table 17-10).

    a. Cephalad spread occurs more easily than caudad spread following lumbar epidural injection, presumably reflecting the impact of negative intrathoracic pressure and narrowing of the epidural space at the lumbosacral junction (S1–2 is often slow to be blocked).

    b. Lumbar epidural administration of local anesthetic solutions usually requires the use of volumes of 15–25 ml (10–20 ml in a term parturient) to achieve sensory levels adequate for surgical anesthesia.

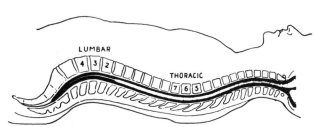

Figure 17-4. Shape of the spinal canal with the patient in the supine position.

TABLE 17-9. Local Anesthetics Used for Epidural Anesthesia

Anesthetic	Usual Concentration (%)	Usual Onset (min)	Usual Duration (h)	Clinical Use
2-Chloroprocaine	2–3	5–15	0.5–1.5	Obstetrics
Lidocaine	1–2	5–15	1–2	Obstetrics
				Surgery
Mepivacaine	1–2	5–15	1.0–2.5	Surgery
Bupivacaine	0.25–0.5	10–20	2–4	Obstetrics
	0.5–0.75	10–20	2–4	Surgery
Etidocaine	1.0–1.5	5–15	2–4	Surgery

TABLE 17-10. Determinants of the Quality of Epidural Anesthesia
Local anesthetic selected
Mass of drug injected (dose, volume, and concentration)
Addition of epinephrine (1:200,000) reduces systemic absorption, especially if lidocaine is used
Site but not speed of injection or patient position
Patients >40 years of age
Pregnancy (hormonal and/or mechanical factors)

IX. COMPLICATIONS OF SPINAL AND EPIDURAL ANESTHESIA

A. Spinal block

1. **Hypotension** reflects venodilation with decreased venous return and cardiac output, whereas declines in systemic vascular resistance are minimal. Adequate hydration (500 ml of crystalloid solution) before induction of spinal anesthesia and positioning to ensure adequate venous return (supine or modest 5–10 degrees head down) are often all that is necessary to prevent or treat the blood pressure manifestations of SNS blockade. A vasopressor that constricts veins in preference to arterioles (e.g., ephedrine, 5–10 mg iv) is occasionally necessary, especially in parturients to maintain placental perfusion.

2. **Postdural puncture headache** is believed to be caused by decreased CSF pressure resulting from leakage of CSF through the needle hole in the dura. The role of needle size (22 vs. 26 gauge) used to perform the block, especially in younger patients, is thus emphasized. A true postdural puncture headache has specific characteristics that distinguish it from a headache that is unrelated to the dural puncture (Table 17-11).

   a. Treatment of postdural puncture headache is symptomatic and specific (Table 17-12).

   b. **Low back pain and nuchal discomfort** are the most common complaints after an epidural blood patch. If two epidural blood patches are not effective, the diagnosis of postdural puncture headache is suspect.

3. **Extensive spread of spinal anesthesia** is suggested by several symptoms (Table 17-13).

TABLE 17-11. Characteristics of a Postdural Puncture Headache

Postural component (made worse by upright position)
Frontal or occipital
Tinnitus
Diplopia
Young females (especially parturients)
Use of a large-gauge needle

TABLE 17-12. Treatment of a Postdural Puncture Headache

Analgesics
Bed rest
Hydration
Epidural blood patch (aseptic placement of 10–20 ml of autologous blood, especially if headache persists >24 hours)
Caffeine infusion (?)

    a. The **phrenic nerves** are usually spared, and diaphragmatic breathing suffices. An exception may be parturients, in whom an enlarged uterus interferes with diaphragmatic excursions.

    b. **Treatment** is ventilation of the lungs with oxygen and support of blood pressure. Patients are placed in a head-down position to facilitate venous return. An attempt to limit the spread of local anesthetic solution in the CSF by placing patients in a head-up position is not warranted, as this position jeopardizes cerebral blood flow and contributes to medullary ischemia. Induc-

TABLE 17-13. Symptoms of an Accidental High Spinal Anesthesia

Agitation
Hypotension
Nausea
Absent intercostal muscle function
Inadequate air movement to generate an audible voice

tion of general anesthesia and intubation of the trachea may be necessary in some patients, especially if there is a risk of aspiration.

   c. Spread of local anesthetics to the cervical region usually produces short-lived effects because the concentration achieved is not great.

4. **Backache** is an infrequent problem. It most likely reflects ligament strain owing to profound skeletal muscle relaxation and surgical positioning.

5. **Major neurologic injury or infection** is extremely rare, especially since the introduction of disposable equipment.

B. **Epidural anesthesia**

1. **Toxicity due to local anesthetics.** Systemic absorption and potential toxicity produced by the relatively high doses of local anesthetics injected into the epidural space depend on several factors (Table 17-14).

2. **Local tissue toxicity.** There is a low potential for localized nerve damage, although accidental subarachnoid injection of high doses of local anesthetics (especially 2-chloroprocaine) may be of concern because the spinal cord and spinal roots lack a protective connective tissue sheath.

3. **Technique-related complications** (Table 17-15)

   a. Epidural anesthesia should not be attempted in patients who are fully anticoagulated or in whom a coagulopathy is present.

   b. Anticoagulation is not contraindicated after atraumatic placement of an epidural catheter. If an epidural blood vessel is punctured, at least 30–60 minutes should elapse before heparinization is performed.

   c. An epidural catheter must never be withdrawn backward through the epidural needle, as this could shear the catheter.

TABLE 17-14. Determinants of Systemic Toxicity Following Epidural Anesthesia

Site of injection (extravascular vs. accidental intravascular)

Total dose (not volume or concentration)

Vasoconstrictor (most useful with lidocaine)

Pharmacologic profile of local anesthetic (etidocaine blood levels lower than those of bupivacaine)

TABLE 17-15. Complications of Epidural Anesthesia

Hypotension (treat with hydration, position, ephedrine, phenylephrine, atropine)

Accidental subdural (delayed onset) or subarachnoid (signs of high block) injection

Dural puncture and postdural headache

Neural damage (epidural hematoma and anticoagulants)

Catheter complications (vascular or subarachnoid placement, shearing)

X. CAUDAL ANESTHESIA

Caudal anesthesia is produced by injection of local anesthetic through a needle introduced through the sacral hiatus into the sacral (epidural) canal. Compared with lumbar epidural anesthesia, approximately twice the dose is required because of the large volume of the sacral canal and free leakage of local anesthetic solution through the sacral foramina. Nearness to the rectum requires careful aseptic technique. Caudal anesthesia is a popular technique for providing anesthesia and postoperative analgesia in children; this reflects the ease of locating the sacral hiatus in children compared with in adults.

18

Peripheral Nerve Blockade

Regional anesthesia of the extremities and of the trunk may be a useful alternative to general anesthesia in selected patients (Mulroy MF: Peripheral nerve blockade. In Barash PG, Cullen BF, Stoelting RK [eds]: Clinical Anesthesia, pp 841–870. Philadelphia, JB Lippincott, 1992).

I. GENERAL PRINCIPLES

A. **Local anesthetic drug selection and doses** (see Table 16-1). Use low concentrations of local anesthetics, which permit injection of large volumes that are useful for peripheral nerve blocks. The addition of epinephrine (EPI) (1:200,000) to the local anesthetic solution is indicated to prolong the duration of anesthesia (exceptions are end-organ or intravenous regional blocks). The duration of blockade is also influenced by local blood flow.

B. **Nerve localization**
1. **Relationship of nerves to bones or arteries** improves the likelihood of technical success.
2. **Paresthesias** are considered the ultimate sign of nerve localization, but care must be taken to avoid intraneural injection **(cramping or aching during injection).** Even without intraneural injection, residual neuropathy of peripheral nerves appears more likely if paresthesias are elicited.
3. **Nerve stimulator.** A low-current electrical impulse (0.1–10.0 mA) delivered by a peripheral nerve stimulator and an insulated needle to a nerve produces stimulation of the motor fibers and thus identifies proximity to the nerve.

C. **Equipment**
1. Use of **disposable kits** is a matter of personal preference based on cost, quality of contents, and assurance of sterility.

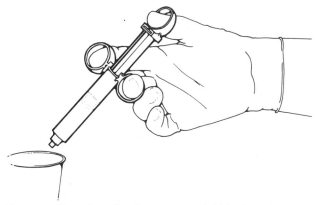

Figure 18-1. Three-ring syringe improves control of injection and ease of refilling.

2. **Needles** used for regional anesthesia have a shorter angulation to the bevel (to push the nerve away) and the addition of a small bead to the shaft about 6 mm from the hub, which prevents skin from retracting over the needle in the event that the shaft separates from the hub.

3. **Syringes** (10 ml is the best compromise between bulk and the need to inject large volumes) may include **control rings** to facilitate control of the injection and allow an operator to refill the syringe with one hand (Fig. 18-1).

4. **Organic iodine** preparations are useful for skin preparation.

D. **Complications** (Table 18-1)

II. PATIENT PREPARATION

A. **Patient selection.** Most operations can be performed with a regional anesthetic technique, but the decision

---

TABLE 18-1. Complications of Peripheral Nerve Block

Systemic toxicity

Peripheral neuropathy (intraneural injection vs. positioning injury)

Pain at injection site

Local hematoma

**TABLE 18-2. Contraindications to Peripheral
Nerve Blocks**

Patient refusal or objection to being "awake"
Local infection at block site
Coagulopathy
Pre-existing neuropathy

to select a peripheral nerve block may be influenced
by several factors (Table 18-2).
B. **Premedication and sedation** must be adjusted to the
required level of patient cooperation (report paresthesias), need for analgesia (fentanyl, 50–100 μg iv) and
subsequent amnesia (midazolam, 1–3 mg iv). Careful
titration of intravenous drugs at the time of performance of the block is the most effective way to adjust
the level of sedation. Benzodiazepines increase the
seizure threshold for local anesthetics.
C. **Monitoring** is the same as for patients undergoing
general anesthesia (see Appendix F), although it is
also important to maintain verbal contact as a means
of assessing a patient's mental status and of detecting
early signs of **local anesthetic (systemic) toxicity.**
D. **Discharge criteria.** It is acceptable to discharge a patient from the postanesthesia care unit in the presence
of residual numbness (analgesia) as long as blood
pressure is stable (no orthostatic hypotension) and
mental status is acceptable.

III. HEAD AND NECK

Regional anesthesia for the head and neck has limited application (Table 18-3).
A. **Cervical plexus blockade** is useful for operations on
the lateral (carotid endarterectomy) or anterior neck
(thyroidectomy). Complications of this block may be
serious (Table 18-4).
B. **Airway anesthesia** is useful to facilitate awake tracheal intubation or fiberoptic laryngoscopy, but caution must be exercised if loss of protective laryngeal
reflexes could place a patient at increased risk for aspiration.
1. **Topical anesthesia** is often provided with pledgets
or an atomizer using a solution of 4% lidocaine.
This higher concentration of lidocaine is required
to penetrate mucosal membranes. Premedication

with an **anticholinergic** to reduce secretions facilitates the onset of topical anesthesia.

  a. For effective **anesthesia of the posterior pharyngeal wall,** the tongue is first sprayed and the patient is encouraged to gargle and swallow the residual liquid in the mouth. The numb tongue is grasped with a gauze pad, and the patient is encouraged to take rapid deep breaths while the spray is applied on inspiration.

  b. For **nasal mucosal anesthesia,** a mixture of 3–4% lidocaine with 0.25–0.5% phenylephrine on cotton pledgets is an alternative to 4% cocaine and its unique vasoconstrictive properties.

2. **Superior laryngeal nerve blockade.** This nerve is a branch of the vagus that provides sensory fibers to the vocal cords, epiglottis, and arytenoids. The superior laryngeal nerve is blocked bilaterally as it penetrates the thyrohyoid membrane (Fig. 18-2).

3. **Tracheal anesthesia** is produced by rapid injection during inspiration of 4 ml of 4% lidocaine through

TABLE 18-4. Complications of Cervical Plexus Block

Phrenic nerve block (reason to avoid bilateral cervical plexus block)
Vertebral artery injection
Epidural injection
Subarachnoid injection
Recurrent laryngeal nerve block

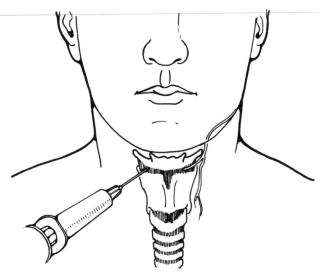

Figure 18-2. Superior laryngeal nerve block is performed through the thyrohyoid membrane.

a needle passed through the cricothyroid membrane into the trachea.

IV. UPPER EXTREMITY

Innervation of the upper extremity is from nerve roots derived from C5–T1. There are three anatomic locations where local anesthetic solutions are placed to block the brachial plexus (Table 18-5; Fig. 18-3).

A. Interscalene approach

1. The needle is inserted in the interscalene groove at the level of the cricoid cartilage and advanced perpendicular to the skin in all planes until the tubercle of C6 is contacted or a paresthesia is elicited, at which point 25–30 ml of 1% lidocaine or 0.25% bupivacaine is injected. Higher concentrations of local anesthetic are needed to produce more profound motor blockade.

2. Complications of the interscalene approach are related to the structures located in the vicinity of the tubercle (Table 18-6).

TABLE 18-5. Anatomic Approaches to Block of the Brachial Plexus

Interscalene groove near the transverse processes (blocks lower fibers of cervical plexus; therefore useful for shoulder surgery but may spare C8–T1 fibers, which innervate the ulnar border of the forearm)

Subclavian sheath at the first rib (most reliable for anesthesia of the forearm and hand)

Axillary sheath surrounding the artery in the axilla (technically easy but may not block the musculocutaneous nerve)

B. Supraclavicular approach
1. The needle is inserted in the interscalene groove 1 cm behind the midpoint of the clavicle and advanced caudad until the first rib is contacted or a paresthesia is elicited, at which point 25–40 ml of 1% lidocaine or 0.25% bupivacaine is injected. Higher

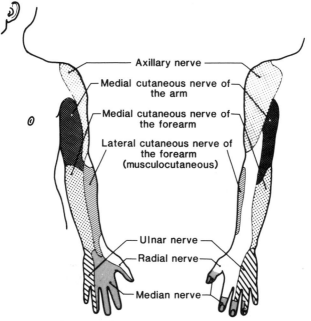

Figure 18-3. Sensory dermatomes of the arm.

TABLE 18-6. Complications of the Interscalene Approach to the Brachial Plexus

Pneumothorax (cough or chest pain while exploring for the nerve)

Spinal or epidural anesthesia

Vertebral artery injection

Diaphragm paralysis

Neuropathy of the C6 nerve root

Inadequate anesthesia in the ulnar distribution (use 30–40 ml)

---

concentrations of local anesthetic are needed to produce more profound motor blockade.

2. If a tourniquet is to be used, a ring of cutaneous anesthesia should be produced around the axilla to block sensory fibers from the chest wall.

3. **Pneumothorax** is the most serious complication of the supraclavicular approach.

C. **Axillary technique**

1. The axillary technique carries the least risk of pneumothorax, making it useful for outpatients. The nerves are anesthetized around the axillary artery. The median and musculocutaneous nerves lie above the artery, whereas the ulnar and radial nerves lie below and behind the vessel. Individual fascial septa may surround each nerve, necessitating separate injections into each compartment in contrast to other single-injection approaches (Fig. 18-4).

2. **Classic approach, seeking paresthesias.** The axillary artery is located as high as practical in the axilla as it courses in the groove between the coracobrachialis and triceps muscles (Fig. 18-5).

   a. The needle is advanced alongside the artery, ideally seeking paresthesias of the nerves serving the area of the proposed surgery (see Fig. 18-4). Injection of 15–20 ml of 1% lidocaine or 0.25% bupivacaine with each paresthesia or a single injection of 25–40 ml is carried out.

   b. Separate supplementary anesthesia of the **musculocutaneous nerve** is provided by injecting 5–10 ml of local anesthetic solution into the body of the coracobrachialis muscle.

3. **Alternate approach of multiple injections without paresthesias.** Local anesthetic solution is injected

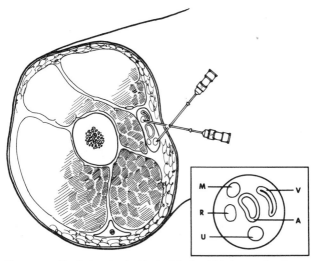

Figure 18-4. Needle location for block of the brachial plexus using the axillary technique.

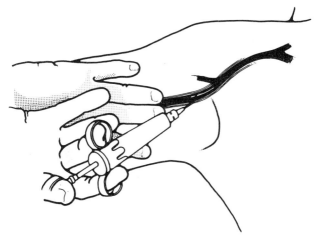

Figure 18-5. Hand position for block of the brachial plexus using the axillary technique.

on each side of the artery in multiple small increments.

4. **Transarterial approach.** The artery is deliberately entered, and the needle is advanced until aspiration confirms it has passed just posterior, at which point one half the local anesthetic solution is injected. The needle is then withdrawn until aspiration confirms it is just anterior to the artery, and the other half of the solution is injected.

5. **Complications** of the axillary technique are rare and include **neuropathy** (the reason some routinely avoid paresthesias), **hematoma** (small-gauge needles reduce the risk), and intravascular injection.

V. DISTAL UPPER EXTREMITY BLOCKADE

Nerves to the hand can be blocked at the elbow or wrist, where the muscles are thinned and prominent bony landmarks allow easier identification of the nerves. Blockade at the elbow does not produce greater anesthesia than blockade at the wrist, reflecting the extensive branching of the sensory nerves to the forearm, principally from the musculocutaneous nerve.

A. **Blockade at the elbow.** Seek paresthesias but carefully avoid intraneural injections (Table 18-7).

B. **Blockade at the wrist** is often preferred to more proximal approaches, as the nerves are associated with easily identified landmarks, and anesthesia is produced with or without paresthesia using 3 ml of local anesthetic solution (Fig. 18-6).

VI. INTRAVENOUS REGIONAL ANESTHESIA (BIER'S BLOCK)

Intravenous regional anesthesia (Bier's block) is produced by injection of **local anesthetic solution *without* EPI** (50 ml of 0.5% lidocaine or prilocaine or 0.25% bu-

---

TABLE 18-7. Block of Peripheral Nerves at the Elbow

Ulnar nerve (inject 1–4 ml of local anesthetic solution in the groove formed by the medial condyle of the humerus and the olecranon)

Median nerve (inject 5 ml of local anesthetic solution 1 cm medial to the brachial artery)

Radial nerve (inject local anesthetic solution in a fan-shaped pattern 2 cm lateral to the brachial artery)

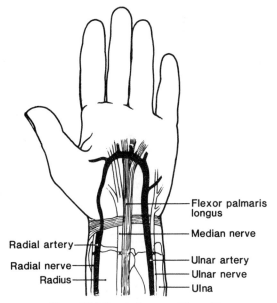

Figure 18-6. Terminal nerves at the wrist.

pivacaine) through a small-gauge intravenous catheter in
the dorsum of the hand. Injection is accomplished only
after exsangunation of the extremity and subsequent inflation of a tourniquet around the upper arm to 300 mm
Hg. Reinjection may be considered after 90 minutes. Systemic toxicity may occur if the tourniquet fails or is released prematurely (within 40 minutes after intravenous
injection).

VII. TRUNK

A. **Intercostal nerve blockade.** Anesthesia of the intercostal nerves provides both **motor and sensory anesthesia of the entire abdominal wall** from the xiphoid
process to the pubis **without sympathetic blockade.**
   1. When a patient is in the prone, lateral, or sitting
      position, the ribs are identified along the line of
      their most extreme posterior angulation (Fig. 18-7).
   2. The needle is **"walked off"** the lower border of the
      rib and advanced 4–6 mm while maintaining a 10-

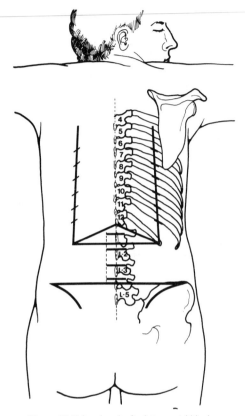

Figure 18-7. Landmarks for intercostal block.

degree cephalad angle, at which point 3–5 ml of
0.25–0.5% bupivacaine is injected after confirming
an extravascular location of the needle (Fig. 18-8).
3. **Complications** of intercostal nerve block are potentially serious (Table 18-8).
B. **Intrapleural anesthesia** is instituted by inserting an
epidural catheter 5–6 cm into the intrapleural space
(signaled by negative pressure that moves the plunger
of the attached glass syringe forward) at the level of
7th or 8th intercostal space.
1. Bupivacaine (20 ml of 0.5% with epinephrine) is
injected into the intrapleural space every 3–6

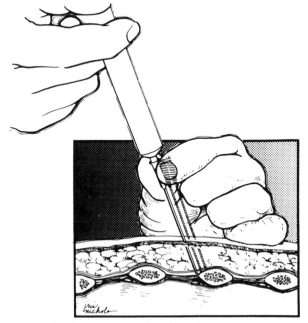

Figure 18-8. Hand and needle positions for intercostal block.

hours, or a constant infusion of 0.25% bupivacaine (0.125 ml·kg·h^{-1}) can be initiated.
2. The local anesthetic appears to diffuse through the parietal pleura onto the intercostal nerves.
3. Risks of this technique include systemic toxicity from absorption of the local anesthetic and pneumothorax.
   a. A major limitation is unilateral analgesia, which limits this technique to procedures such as cholecystectomy or nephrectomy.

TABLE 18-8. Complications of Intercostal Nerve Block

Pneumothorax
Intravascular injection
Systemic absorption (vascularity of the injection site is great)
Epidural or subarachnoid injection (most likely with an intrathoracic approach)

      b. Loss of local anesthetic solution to thoracotomy drainage makes this technique less reliable for thoracotomy pain.

C. Sympathetic blockade—stellate. This block provides selective sympathetic nervous system blockade of the upper extremity and head, which is especially useful in the **treatment of reflex sympathetic dystrophy.**

    1. The needle is inserted at the medial border of the sternocleidomastoid muscle, 1.5–2.0 cm caudad to the level of the cricoid cartilage (about 2 finger breadths above the clavicle) and advanced until it contacts bone (C7), at which point a test dose (2 ml) is injected followed by up to 8 ml of 1% lidocaine or 0.25% bupivacaine (Fig. 18-9).

      a. The sternocleidomastoid muscle and carotid sheath are retracted laterally. Paresthesia of the brachial plexus implies that the needle is too far lateral.

      b. Onset of ipsilateral sympathetic nervous system blockade is usually evident within 10 minutes (Table 18-9).

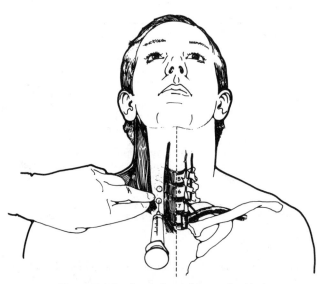

Figure 18-9. Landmarks for stallate ganglion block.

TABLE 18-9. **Signs of Sympathetic Nervous System Blockade Following Stellate Ganglion Block (Horner's Syndrome)**

Ptosis	Nasal congestion
Miosis	Vasodilation
Anhydrosis	Increased skin temperature

2. Potential complications of stellate ganglion block reflect the surrounding anatomy and detract from the use of neurolytic solutions (Table 18-10).

D. **Sympathetic blockade—celiac plexus.** This block provides relief of pain from malignancy of upper abdominal organs, especially the pancreas. The celiac plexus is a sympathetic ganglion that results from the merger of the greater and lesser splanchnic nerves at the level of L1 in the retroperitoneal space along the aorta.

1. The needle is advanced until it contacts the lateral border of L1 (the T12 spinous process partially overlies L1), at which point it is withdrawn and the angle steepened so it may be walked off the anterior border of L1 (Fig. 18-10).

a. **Radiographic verification** of needle location may be indicated, especially if neurolytic solutions are to be injected.

b. **A large volume** of local anesthetic (20–25 ml of 0.75% lidocaine or 0.25% bupivacaine) is needed to diffuse in the retroperitoneal space to reach the ganglia. The most reliable sign of **successful blockade** is **analgesia or hypotension** (prehydration with 1000 ml of crystalloid solution blunts this response).

TABLE 18-10. **Complications of Stellate Ganglion Block**

Pneumothorax
Intravascular injection (vertebral artery)
Block of cardioaccelerator fibers
Hoarseness from recurrent laryngeal nerve paralysis
Subarachnoid injection

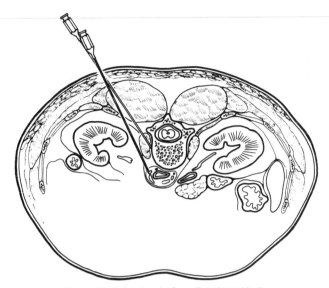

Figure 18-10. Landmarks for celiac plexus block.

2. Potential complications of celiac plexus block reflect the surrounding anatomy (Table 18-11).
3. **Chronic pain relief** with a neurolytic block lasts 2–6 months and may be repeated as necessary, although a trial diagnostic block with a local anesthetic is indicated before each use of neurolytic drugs.

TABLE 18-11. Complications of Celiac Plexus Block

Unrecognized subarachnoid injection (permanent paralysis if using a neurolytic solution)

Intravascular injection

Back pain if injecting neurolytic solution (treat with intravenous opioids)

Diaphragmatic irritation (shoulder pain)

Transiently increased peristalsis (reflects a shift in balance from sympathetic to parasympathetic nervous system innervation)

VIII. LOWER EXTREMITY

Nerves to the lower extremities are most easily blocked by spinal or epidural anesthesia. A peripheral nerve block may be indicated in the presence of sepsis, coagulopathy, or desire for selective anesthesia of the leg or foot. The nerves to the leg arise from the spinal roots of L2–S3, which form the lumbar plexus (lateral femoral cutaneous, femoral, and obturator nerves provide sensory and motor innervation to the upper leg) and the sciatic nerve (divides into the tibial and common peroneal nerves to supply the lower leg).

A. Sciatic nerve blockade, classic posterior approach. This block provides adequate anesthesia for the sole of the foot and lower leg. The needle is inserted at a point 5 cm caudad along the perpendicular line that bisects the line joining the posterior superior iliac spine and greater trochanter; it is advanced perpendicular to the skin in all planes until a **paresthesia is elicited,** at which point 25 ml of 1.5% lidocaine or 0.5% bupivacaine is injected (Fig. 18-11).

B. Ankle blockade. At least five nerves must be blocked to produce adequate anesthesia (Fig. 18-12).

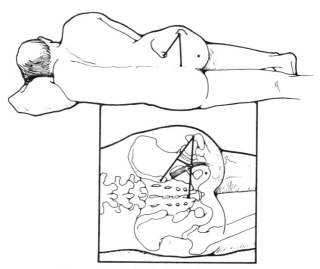

Figure 18-11. Landmarks for sciatic nerve block.

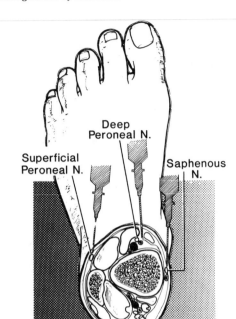

Figure 18-12. Landmarks for ankle block.

1. **Posterior tibial nerve.** The needle is introduced just behind the posterior tibial artery and advanced until a paresthesia to the sole of the foot is elicited, at which point 5 ml of local anesthetic solution is injected.

2. **Sural nerve.** The needle is advanced into the groove between the lateral malleolus and the calcaneus, where 5 ml of local anesthetic solution is injected.

3. **Saphenous nerve.** Infiltration of 5 ml of local anesthetic solution in the area where the saphenous

vein passes anterior to the medial malleolus blocks this nerve.

4. **Deep peroneal nerve.** This is the major nerve to the dorsum of the foot, and it is blocked by placement of 5 ml of local anesthetic solution just lateral to the anterior tibial artery.

5. **Superficial peroneal branches.** A subcutaneous ridge of anesthetic solution (5–10 ml) is placed between the anterior tibial artery and the lateral malleolus.

19

Neurophysiology and Neuroanesthesia

Knowledge of the neurophysiology of the brain is essential to the application of the principles of neuroanesthesia (Bendo AA, Kass IS, Hartung J, Cottrell JE: Neurophysiology and neuroanesthesia. In: Barash PG, Cullen BF, Stoelting RK [eds]: Clinical Anesthesia, pp 871–918. Philadelphia, JB Lippincott, 1992).

I. NEUROPHYSIOLOGY

A. **Membrane potentials.** Neurons have an electrical potential across their cell membranes (about -70 mV at rest) owing to different intracellular and extracellular ion concentrations. The conductance of ions across the cell membrane is *via* ion-specific **protein channels.** Neurons signal over long distances by propagating **action potentials,** which are brief and rapid depolarizations of the membrane.

B. **Synaptic transmission.** Neurons communicate *via* chemical synapses (an action potential evokes the presynaptic release of a neurotransmitter that combines with a postsynaptic receptor molecule to cause the opening of a channel or generation of second messengers).

1. If the neurotransmitter is **excitatory (glutamate),** the postsynaptic neuron is depolarized and, therefore, more likely to generate an action potential.

2. If the neurotransmitter is **inhibitory (gamma-aminobutyric acid, GABA),** the postsynaptic neuron is hyperpolarized and, therefore, less likely to generate an action potential.

C. **Brain metabolism.** The main substrate used for energy production (formation of adenosine triphosphate) in the brain is glucose; which requires oxygen (3.5 ml $100 \cdot g^{-1} \cdot min^{-1}$ in an adult and 5.2 ml $\cdot 100 \cdot g^{-1} \cdot min$ in a child) for its entrance into the glycolytic pathway. Pumping ions (sodium, potassium, calcium) across cell membranes is the largest energy requirement of the brain.

D. Cerebral blood flow (CBF). The brain receives about 15% of the cardiac output; yet it represents only 2% of total body weight, reflecting its high metabolic rate.

1. Regional CBF is coupled with metabolic rate, increasing dramatically when the cerebral metabolic rate for oxygen ($CMRO_2$) increases.

2. CBF parallels the $Paco_2$ (increasing the $Paco_2$ from 40 mm Hg to 80 mm Hg doubles the CBF, whereas decreasing the $Paco_2$ from 40 mm Hg to 20 mm Hg halves the CBF) (Fig. 19-1).

    a. Manipulating the CBF by acute changes in the $Paco_2$ or by drug-induced (thiopental) decreases in the $CMRO_2$ is an **important principle of neuroanesthesia.**

    b. The effects of increasing or decreasing the $Paco_2$ are transient, and CBF returns to normal in 6–8 hours even if the altered $Paco_2$ levels are maintained.

3. CBF is maintained at a constant rate **(autoregulated)** over a mean arterial pressure (MAP) from about 50–150 mm Hg, reflecting appropriate adjustments of the cerebral vascular resistance (Fig. 19-1).

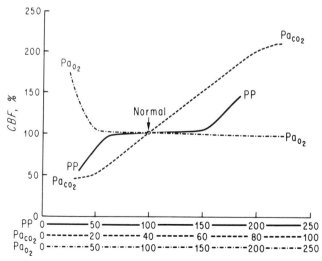

Figure 19-1. The effect of perfusion pressure (PP), $Paco_2$, and Pao_2 on CBF.

      a. This response takes 1–3 minutes to develop, such that an abrupt change in MAP over the autoregulation range is accompanied by a brief corresponding change in CBF.

      b. When MAP decreases below 50 mm Hg, the CBF is reduced and mild symptoms of cerebral ischemia may occur at a perfusion pressure of about 40 mm Hg.

      c. When MAP exceeds the autoregulated range, it may cause disruption of the blood-brain barrier and cerebral edema.

      d. Autoregulation can be abolished by trauma, hypoxia, and certain anesthetic and adjuvant anesthetic drugs.

      e. Systemic hypertension that persists for 1–2 months causes a shift of the autoregulation range to higher pressures, such that cerebral ischemia may occur at a MAP >50 mm Hg.

E. Cerebrospinal fluid is formed in the choroid plexus of the cerebral ventricles (0.3–0.4 ml·min^{-1}) and reabsorbed into the venous system of the brain *via* the arachnoid villi (volume of cerebrospinal fluid in the brain is 100–150 ml). Furosemide and acetazolamide may be used clinically to decrease the rate of cerebrospinal fluid formation.

F. Intracranial pressure (ICP) that is excessive (>15 mm Hg) reduces CBF (cerebral perfusion pressure is MAP minus ICP) and introduces the risk of brain herniation.

    1. Under normal circumstances, a small increase in intracranial volume does not greatly increase ICP because of the elasticity **(compliance)** of the components located in the cranium (Fig. 19-2).

    2. After a certain point, the capacity of the system to adjust to increased volume is exceeded, and even a small increase in volume (vasodilation, hematoma, tumor, or edema) increases ICP.

G. Pathophysiology. The brain is the most sensitive of all organs to ischemic damage, which may be **global** (cardiac arrest) or **focal** (localized stroke). Ischemic damage to neurons most likely reflects decreased energy production (blockage of oxidative phosphorylation), leading to decreased activity of adenosine triphosphate–dependent ion pumps and intracellular accumulation of sodium and calcium.

    1. Seizures greatly increase CMRo$_2$ and must be suppressed in conditions in which blood flow to the brain may be compromised.

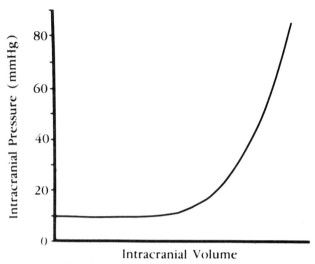

Figure 19-2. The effect of increasing intracranial volume on intracranial pressure.

    2. Brain trauma may produce irreversible neuronal damage, although much of the injury may be secondary and follow the initial insult (calcium influx, release of vasoconstrictive substances (see Section XII).

II. NEUROANESTHESIA

  A. Effects of Anesthetics and Other Adjunctive Drugs on Brain Physiology (Table 19-1).

    1. The importance of drug-induced increases in CBF is the possible corresponding increase in ICP.

    2. Isoflurane is often considered the preferred volatile anesthetic for neuroanesthesia because of its ability to greatly reduce CMR_{O_2}.

    3. Thiopental in doses sufficient to produce a flat electroencephalogram decreases CMR_{O_2} by 50%. The decrease in CMR_{O_2} results in constriction of the cerebral vasculature, leading to a decrease in CBF and ICP. A major problem with thiopental when used to lower ICP is decreased cerebral perfusion pressure.

TABLE 19-1. Effects of Drugs on Neurophysiology of the Brain

Drug	Cerebral Blood Flow	Cerebral Metabolic Oxygen Requirements	Direct Cerebral Vasodilation
Halothane	+ + +	−	Yes
Enflurane	+ +	−	Yes
Isoflurane	+ or NC	− −	Yes
Nitrous oxide with a volatile anesthetic	+	+	
Nitrous oxide with an injected anesthetic	NC	NC	
Thiopental	− − −	− − −	No
Etomidate	− − −	− − −	No
Propofol	− −	− −	No
Midazolam	− −	− −	No
Ketamine	+ +	+	Yes
Fentanyl	− or NC	− or NC	No

+ = increase; − = decrease; NC = no change.

260

TABLE 19-2. Techniques to Prevent Brain Damage

Hypothermia (even mild hypothermia, 32–34°C, present before an ischemic insult is protective)

Barbiturates (protective for focal ischemia but efficacy for global ischemia is controversial)

Channel blockers (nimodipine)

Free radical scavengers (corticosteroids, vitamin E)

---

    4. Methohexital is unique among the barbiturates in its ability to activate some seizure foci in patients with temporal lobe epilepsy.

    5. Etomidate is a direct cerebral vasoconstrictor even before $CMRO_2$ is suppressed.

    6. Ketamine can increase $CMRO_2$ and CBF and is therefore not commonly used in neuroanesthesia.

  B. Brain protection. Techniques to prevent brain damage are designed to maintain energy stores (adenosine triphosphate) by decreasing demand ($CMRO_2$) (Table 19-2).

III. MONITORING

  A. The electroencephalogram can be used to monitor cerebral function (early detection of cerebral ischemia) and localization of epileptic foci (Table 19-3).

TABLE 19-3. Electroencephalogram Frequency Changes

Delta rhythm (0–3 Hz)	Deep sleep
	Deep anesthesia
	Pathologic states (brain tumors, arterial hypoxemia, metabolic encephalopathy)
Theta rhythm (4–7 Hz)	Physiologic sleep and general anesthesia in adults
	Hyperventilation in awake children
Alpha rhythm (8–13 Hz)	Resting awake adult with eyes closed
Beta rhythm (>13 Hz)	Mental activity
	Light anesthesia

1. Anesthetic drugs and physiologic changes may alter electroencephalographic waveforms and interpretation (Table 19-4).
2. Efforts to use the electroencephalogram as a monitor of **depth of anesthesia** have been unreliable.
3. Verification of electrical silence *via* electroencephalogram is useful when determining the dose required to induce and maintain barbiturate coma.

B. **Computerized electroencephalographic processing** has facilitated intraoperative monitoring with the electroencephalograph. Control readings in awake pa-

---

TABLE 19-4. Electroencephalogram Changes Associated With Drugs and Physiologic Changes

Increased Frequency

Barbiturates (low doses)
Benzodiazepines (low doses)
Etomidate (low doses)
Nitrous oxide (30–70%)
Volatile anesthetics (<1 MAC)
Ketamine
Arterial hypoxemia (initially)
Hypercarbia (mild)
Seizures

Decreased Frequency/Increased Amplitude

Barbiturates (moderate doses)
Etomidate (moderate doses)
Opioids
Volatile anesthetics (>1 MAC)
Arterial hypoxemia (mild)
Hypocarbia (moderate to extreme)
Hypothermia

Decreased Frequency/Decreased Amplitude

Barbiturates (high doses)
Arterial hypoxemia (mild)
Hypercarbia (severe)
Hypothermia (<35°C)

Electrical Silence

Barbiturates (coma doses)
Etomidate (high doses)
Isoflurane (2 MAC)
Arterial hypoxemia (severe)
Hypothermia (<20°C)
Brain death

tients should be obtained prior to induction of general anesthesia. Bilateral data must be obtained to distinguish between anesthetic and systemic effects **(bilateral changes)** and surgical trauma or ischemia **(ipsilateral changes).**

C. **Evoked potentials** are used to monitor the functional integrity of ascending sensory pathways (sensory-evoked potentials) and descending motor pathways (motor-evoked potentials).

   1. **Sensory-evoked potentials** employed clinically are somatosensory, auditory, and visual.

      a. Compromise or injury of a neurologic pathway is manifested as an **increase in the latency and/or a decrease in the amplitude** of evoked potential waveforms (e.g., as with **sensory** pathway compromise during spinal column instrumentation).

      b. Anesthetics influence evoked potentials (Table 19-5). In general, volatile anesthetics cause a dose-dependent increase in latency and a decrease in amplitude (halothane less than enflurane).

   2. **Motor-evoked potentials** (detect **motor** pathway compromise) may obviate the need for an intraoperative wake-up test during scoliosis surgery and provide detection of intraoperative spinal cord dysfunction during aortic cross-clamping.

D. **Intracranial pressure monitoring** (see Chapter 7, Section V)

IV. Neuroradiology (Table 19-6)

A. These procedures require the patient's total immobility; this introduces the need for general anesthesia in uncooperative patients (see Chapter 38, Section III).

B. The need to avoid ferrous metal makes the management of anesthesia and intraoperative monitoring a challenge in the patient undergoing **magnetic resonance** imaging. Patients with artificial cardiac (demand) pacemakers or an intracranial clip (as is used to treat an intracranial aneurysm) should not undergo magnetic resonance imaging.

C. When general anesthesia is required for angiography, the angiogram quality may be enhanced by hyperventilation (hypocarbia slows CBF and improves clarity by constricting cerebral vessels).

D. **Adverse Reactions from Contrast Media**

   1. **Neurotoxic reactions** manifest as unconsciousness, seizures, and hemiplegia, presumably reflecting the hyperosmolality of the contrast medium.

TABLE 19-5. Effects of Intravenous and Inhaled Drugs on Sensory-Evoked Potentials

	Brain Stem Auditory-evoked Potentials		Cortical Somatosensory-Evoked Potentials		Visual-Evoked Potentials	
	Latency	Amplitude	Latency	Amplitude	Latency	Amplitude
Thiopental (4–6 mg·kg⁻¹)	NC	NC	NC	NC	?	?
Droperidol (0.1 mg·kg⁻¹)	?	?	I	D	?	?
Diazepam (0.1 mg·kg⁻¹)	NC	NC	I	D	?	?
Midazolam	?	?	NC	D	?	?
Fentanyl	NC	NC	I	D	?	?
Sufentanil	NC	NC	NC	D	?	?
Etomidate	NC	NC	I	I	?	?
Propofol (2–6 mg·kg⁻¹)	NC	NC	I	D	?	?
Enflurane	I	NC	I	I	I	D
Halothane	I	NC	I	D	I	NC
Isoflurane	I	NC	I	D	I	D
Nitrous oxide	NC	NC	NC	D	I	D

I = increase; D = decrease; NC = no change; ? = not studied.

2. **Allergic reactions** vary in manifestations from pruritus and skin rashes to wheezing and hypotension, most likely reflecting nonimmunologic release of histamine and other vasoactive mediators (see Table 38-5). **Prophylaxis** with a corticosteroid and an antihistamine is recommended for the patient with a history of allergy or specific reaction to contrast media (see Table 38-6).

V. ANESTHETIC MANAGEMENT OF NEUROSURGICAL PATIENTS

A. Neurosurgical procedures tend to be lengthy and require unusual positioning of the patient and the institution of special techniques such as hyperventilation, cerebral dehydration, and deliberate hypotension.

B. Except for neurosurgical emergencies (head trauma, impending herniation), most neurosurgical procedures can be delayed until after the treatment of medically unstable conditions.

C. **Preoperative evaluation** includes a complete neurologic examination with special attention to the patient's level of consciousness, the presence or absence of increased ICP, and the extent of focal neurologic deficits (Table 19-7).

D. Fluid and electrolyte abnormalities are common in patients with reduced levels of consciousness.

E. The location of the lesion (supratentorial or infratentorial compartment) determines its clinical representation and anesthetic management.

1. **Supratentorial disease** is usually associated with problems in the management of increased ICP.

2. **Infratentorial lesions** cause problems related to pressure effects on vital brain stem structures and

---

TABLE 19-6. Methods Used for Neuroradiology

Computed tomography (contrast enhancement is provided by intravenous injection of the dye)

Magnetic resonance imaging (provides excellent contrast between gray and white matter)

Angiography (used to delineate the vasculature of the brain or spinal cord)

Myelography

TABLE 19-7. Signs and Symptoms of Increased Intracranial Pressure

Headache

Nausea

Papilledema

Unilateral pupillary dilation

Oculomotor or abducens palsy

Depressed level of consciousness

Irregular breathing

Midline shift (0.5 cm) or encroachment of expanding brain on cerebral ventricles (computed tomography or magnetic resonance imaging)

---

increased ICP produced by obstructive hydrocephalus.

VI. SUPRATENTORIAL INTRACRANIAL TUMORS

A. Meningiomas, gliomas, and metastatic lesions eventually grow to the size at which compensatory mechanisms are exhausted, and additional increases in the size of the tumor (central area of hemorrhagic tissue, wider border of brain edema) manifest as progressive increases in ICP.

B. **Anesthetic Techniques and Drugs**

1. The goal is to maximize modalities that decrease intracranial volume (ICP) before the cranium is opened.

2. **Clinical Control of Intracranial Hypertension** (Table 19-8)

   a. **Severe fluid restriction** preoperatively can cause hypovolemia, resulting in hypotension with induction of anesthesia, unless intravascular fluid volume is restored with glucose-free isotonic crystalloid solutions (glucose-containing solutions may increase brain water content and exacerbate ischemic damage).

   b. Rapid brain dehydration and ICP reduction are often obtained by administration of an **osmotic diuretic** (mannitol, 0.25–1 g·kg^{-1} iv, works in 10–15 minutes and is effective for 2 hours) or a **loop diuretic** (furosemide, 0.5–1 mg·kg^{-1} iv, alone or 0.15–0.3 mg·kg^{-1} iv, in combination with mannitol). Furosemide may be the pre-

TABLE 19-8. Methods to Control Intracranial Pressure

Hyperventilation ($Paco_2$ 25–30 mm Hg)

Diuresis (mannitol as an osmotic diuretic; furosemide as a tubular diuretic)

Cerebral vasoconstriction (thiopental, lidocaine)

Cerebral spinal fluid drainage

Elevation of the head to 30 degrees (encourages venous return)

Blood pressure control

Fluid restriction

Corticosteroids (dexamethasone effective for localized cerebral edema surrounding tumors; requires 12–36 hours)

Surgical decompression (epidural hematoma)

ferred choice to decrease ICP in patients with impaired cardiac reserve.

c. **Corticosteroids** decrease edema around brain tumors, but neurologic improvement may precede a decrease in ICP, perhaps reflecting a restoration of the previously abnormal blood-brain barrier.

d. **Hyperventilation** of the lungs to maintain a $Paco_2$ of 25–30 mm Hg (every mm Hg decrease below 40 mm Hg decreases CBF about 4%) is the mainstay of acute and subacute management of increased ICP. Impaired responsiveness of the cerebrovasculature in areas of intracranial disease (ischemia, trauma, tumor, infection) interferes with the effectiveness of hyperventilation.

e. A head-down position or application of positive end-expiratory pressure may further increase ICP.

f. Pharmacologic agents (thiopental, etomidate, lidocaine) are potent cerebral vasoconstrictors that can acutely decrease ICP; or when administered prophylactically, they may attenuate any increase in ICP associated with a painful stimulus.

3. **Premedication** is not administered to lethargic patients.

4. **Monitoring** in addition to routine observations includes measurement of intra-arterial blood pressure, arterial blood gases, central venous pressure,

and urinary output. The need to monitor ICP for supratentorial operations is controversial.

5. **Muscle Relaxants**

   a. Succinylcholine and nondepolarizing muscle relaxants that evoke the release of histamine may accentuate coexisting intracranial hypertension or lower cerebral perfusion pressure.

   b. Atracurium and vecuronium have no effect on ICP or cerebral perfusion pressure in neurosurgical patients.

6. **Induction, Maintenance, and Emergence**

   a. A common induction sequence is thiopental (4–6 mg·kg^{-1} iv), followed by an opioid (fentanyl, 3–5 μg·kg^{-1} iv) and a muscle relaxant (vecuronium, 0.1 mg·kg^{-1} iv).

   b. Before laryngoscopy and intubation of the trachea, a surgical level of anesthesia is established so as to minimize any pain-induced increase in ICP.

   c. After induction of anesthesia, ventilation of the lungs is controlled mechanically and adjusted to maintain the Pa$_{CO_2}$ between 25 and 30 mm Hg.

   d. The most commonly administered maintenance anesthetics for patients with supratentorial tumors are nitrous oxide–opioids (most often fentanyl) and nitrous oxide–volatile drugs (most often isoflurane, $<1\%$).

   e. Reaction to the tracheal tube during emergence should be avoided (lidocaine, 1.5 mg·kg^{-1} iv, administered 90 seconds before suctioning and extubation of the trachea to minimize cough, straining, and hypertension). If the patient is not responsive, the endotracheal tube should remain in place.

   f. A brief neurologic examination is performed before and after extubation of the trachea.

VII. INFRATENTORIAL INTRACRANIAL TUMORS

A. Patients with infratentorial tumors (posterior fossa contains the medulla, pons, cerebellum, and lower cranial nerve nuclei) may exhibit depressed levels of consciousness secondary to increased ICP from obstructive hydrocephalus and/or exhibit signs of brain stem compression, with depressed ventilation and cranial nerve palsies.

B. **Special Anesthetic Considerations**

   1. **Surgical position.** Exploration of the posterior fossa has been traditionally performed with the pa-

tient in the sitting position because it provides excellent surgical exposure and facilitates venous and cerebrospinal fluid drainage. Other positions (lateral, prone) have been advocated because of the lower incidence of air embolism and greater cardiovascular stability.

2. **Monitoring** the electrocardiogram for alterations in heart rate and cardiac rhythm is important during posterior fossa exploration because surgical retraction or manipulation of the brain stem or cranial nerves can cause significant cardiac dysrhythmias or alterations in blood pressure. Alternatively, sensory-evoked potentials (brain stem auditory-evoked potentials during acoustic neuroma surgery; somatosensory-evoked potentials to monitor brain stem ischemia) have been used to monitor compromise of the brain stem or cranial nerves.

3. **Venous air embolism** may occur whenever the operative field is elevated 5 cm or more above the right atrial level (Tables 19-9 and 19-10).

4. **Anesthetic Management**
   a. When selecting an anesthetic technique for patients in the sitting position, conditions of particular concern are postural hypotension (minimized by adequate preoperative hydration, wrapping the legs, and flexing the patient's hips and knees at heart level) and the risk of venous air embolism (physiologic effect may be increased in the presence of nitrous oxide).

TABLE 19-9. Diagnosis of Venous Air Embolism

Precordial Doppler ultrasonic transducer (placed over right sternal border between the 3rd and 6th intercostal spaces; verify correct positioning by injection of 10 ml saline; most sensitive monitor detecting amounts of air as small as 0.25 ml)

Capnograph (air embolism reflected as decreased end-tidal CO_2; Doppler sounds without changes in end-tidal CO_2 are not hemodynamically significant)

Mass spectrometry (end-expired nitrogen reflects the volume of entrained air)

Transesophageal echocardiography (as sensitive as Doppler; can be used to determine presence of a probe patent foramen ovale)

Pulmonary artery catheter (increase in pressure correlates with the hemodynamic significance of the embolus)

TABLE 19-10. Treatment of Venous Air Embolism

Flood surgical field with saline and wax bone edges

Discontinue nitrous oxide

Compress neck veins

Aspirate air (maximum retrieval of air can be obtained from a multiorificed tip that is positioned at the junction of the superior vena cava and the right atrium)

Give vasopressors and volume infusion (treat hypotension)

Administer positive end-expiratory pressure (avoid in patients with a probe patent foramen ovale)

---

    b. Often a nitrous oxide-oxygen-opioid muscle relaxant anesthetic combined with controlled hyperventilation of the lungs is recommended for maximal cardiovascular stability and control of ICP.

  5. Postoperative Concerns (Table 19-11)

VIII. PITUITARY TUMORS

  A. Pituitary tumors can be categorized as **nonfunctioning** (chromophobe adenomas that enlarge and compress the normal gland) and **hypersecreting** (most often adenomas secreting prolactin or growth hormone).

  B. Special Anesthetic Consideration

    1. Preoperative evaluation of patients with pituitary tumors requires an assessment of endocrine function and associated medical disorders (systemic effects of excess cortisol; airway changes associated with acromegaly).

      a. Panhypopituitarism replacement therapy includes oral administration of corticosteroids and thyroxine and possibly intranasal instillation of synthetic vasopressin.

      b. All patients scheduled for pituitary surgery are given supplemental short-acting corticosteroid therapy perioperatively.

      c. The computed tomographic scan or magnetic resonance imaging scan and the neurologic examination are evaluated for signs of increased ICP.

    2. Surgical considerations. Trans-sphenoidal excision has been recommended for all pituitary tumors that do not have marked suprasellar extension.

TABLE 19-11. Postoperative Concerns Following Posterior Fossa Surgery

Central apnea

Impaired swallowing and pharyngeal sensation (at risk for aspiration)

Hypertension (requires prompt treatment to prevent brain edema and hematoma formation)

Cardiac dysrhythmias

Delayed awakening (brain stem compression)

3. **Anesthetic considerations** for patients undergoing pituitary surgery include measures to control ICP if a transcranial approach is used and right atrial catheterization for treatment of potential venous air embolism if a trans-sphenoidal procedure is planned.
   a. Visual evoked potential monitoring may be used to monitor compromise of blood supply to the optic nerves and chiasm.
   b. Cocaine and epinephrine used to prepare the nasal approach for trans-sphenoidal surgery may initially cause hypertension, tachycardia, cardiac dysrhythmias, and myocardial ischemia that necessitate treatment.
   c. Following trans-sphenoidal surgery, the patient awakens with nasal packing in place; this emphasizes the need for the patient to be fully awake before extubation of the trachea is performed.
4. **Postoperative concerns** include the need for continued corticosteroid supplementation and strict attention to fluid balance (diabetes insipidus may manifest in the first 12 hours postoperatively).

IX. INTRACRANIAL ANEURYSMS

A. The incidence of cerebral aneurysms in North America is estimated to be 1 in 50 persons, with the incidence of subarachnoid hemorrhage (SAH) being 1 in 8000 persons.

B. The most important complications of SAH are increased ICP, rebleeding, vasospasm (heralded by worsening headache, hypertension, and confusion), and hydrocephalus.

TABLE 19-12. Preoperative Evaluation of the Patient With a Subarachnoid Hemorrhage

Increased intracranial pressure

Hyponatremia (diabetes insipidus, syndrome of inappropriate antidiuretic hormone secretion)

Hypernatremia and hyperosmolarity

Hypertension

Cardiac dysrhythmias

ST segment depression or elevation on the electrocardiogram (subendocardial infarction is a possibility)

1. **Nimodipine** is a calcium antagonist that may prevent or reverse ischemic neurologic deficits produced by vasospasm.
2. **Hypervolemic hypertensive** therapy may be useful in reversing neurologic deficits caused by vasospasm.

C. **Special Anesthetic Considerations**
  1. **Preoperative Evaluation** (Table 19-12)
  2. **Anesthetic management** is designed to avoid aneurysm rupture (occurs intraoperatively in 20% of patients), maintain cerebral perfusion pressure, and provide optimal surgical access ("slack brain") (Table 19-13). The use of deliberate hypotension for cerebral aneurysm clip ligation is controversial.
  3. **Postoperative concerns** include hypertension leading to cerebral edema or hematoma (requires pharmacologic treatment) and vasospasm (maintain higher than normal intravascular fluid volume).

X. ARTERIOVENOUS MALFORMATIONS

A. Clinical features of an arteriovenous malformation (AVM) are SAH, focal epilepsy, and progressive focal neurologic sensory-motor deficits occurring in a child or young adult.
B. **Special Anesthetic Considerations**
  1. **Closed embolization of cerebral AVMs** may be performed with sedation (fentanyl-midazolam), which allows neurologic examinations during the procedure and permits immediate diagnosis of complications (stroke, hemorrhage).
  2. The anesthetic management of a patient with an AVM is similar to the management of patients for aneurysm surgery (see Section IX C).

TABLE 19-13. Management of Anesthesia for Treatment of Subarachnoid Hemorrhage Due to an Intracranial Aneurysm

Minimize hypertension associated with intubation of the trachea (establish surgical level of anesthesia, give short-acting opioid, brief duration of laryngoscopy, administer intravenous lidocaine and/or esmolol)

Mechanical control of ventilation to maintain $Paco_2$ at 25–30 mm Hg

Thiopental and fetanyl frequently used in conjunction with isoflurane to maintain anesthesia

Cerebrospinal fluid drainage and osmotic diuretics

Consider administration of thiopental or institution of deliberate hypotension during dissection of the aneurysm

Low-grade (32°C) hypothermia

Consider monitoring evoked potentials

Be prepared to treat sudden hemorrhage

Avoid reaction to tracheal tube at conclusion of surgery

---

    a. When the AVM is large, hypothermia and high-dose barbiturates may be recommended for brain protection.

    b. Deliberate hypotension may be instituted to decrease the size of the AVM.

    c. After removal of the AVM, breakthrough cerebral edema (blood flow diverted to vessels not accustomed to high flow), hemorrhage, or hypertension (beta antagonists are a useful treatment) may occur.

XI. DELIBERATE HYPOTENSION

    A. Mean arterial pressure can be safely decreased to 50 mm Hg in the patient with a normal healthy brain. In the patient with chronic hypertension, a guideline is to decrease the MAP no more than 50 mm Hg from the baseline pressure.

    B. Ventilation of the lungs during deliberate hypotension should be adjusted to maintain normocarbia.

    C. Commonly Used Drugs

        1. Sodium nitroprusside is the most commonly administered drug for production of deliberate hypotension because of its rapid onset and short duration of action. Side effects of sodium nitroprusside must be considered when the drug is administered (Table 19-14).

TABLE 19-14. Side Effects of Sodium Nitroprusside

Cyanide toxicity (most likely when >1 mg·kg⁻¹ in <2.5 hours
  or >0.5 mg·kg⁻¹·h⁻¹; treatment is thiosulfate)
Increased intracranial pressure
Inhibition of platelet aggregation
Increased pulmonary shunting (less likely in patients with
  chronic obstructive pulmonary disease)
Baroreceptor-mediated tachycardia (blunt with a beta
  antagonist)
Rebound hypertension

   2. **Nitroglycerin,** like sodium nitroprusside, may in-
       crease ICP but does not introduce the risk of cya-
       nide toxicity.
   3. **Volatile anesthetics** decrease MAP by combina-
       tions of myocardial depression (halothane) and pe-
       ripheral vasodilation (isoflurane). Relative to
       sodium nitroprusside, isoflurane blunts the stress
       response evoked by deliberate hypotension, and
       pulmonary shunting is not increased.

XII. HEAD INJURY

   A. Motor vehicle accidents are responsible for the major-
       ity of head injuries, and more than 50% of these pa-
       tients have multiple injuries resulting in significant
       blood loss, hypotension, and arterial hypoxemia.
   B. **Classification** of severe head injury is based on the
       Glasgow Coma Score (score <7 persisting for >6
       hours is severe head injury) (Table 19-15).
   C. Following head trauma, the primary injury results
       from the biomechanical effect of forces applied to the
       skull and brain (concussion, contusion, laceration,
       hematoma) and is **irreversible.** Secondary injury
       caused by arterial hypoxemia, anemia, hypotension,
       hypercarbia, or increased ICP is treatable.
       1. Nonoperative treatment of diffuse cerebral edema
           includes hyperventilation of the lungs, diuresis
           produced with mannitol and furosemide, barbitu-
           rates, and ICP monitoring.
       2. Depressed skull fractures and acute epidural, sub-
           dural, and intercerebral hematomas usually re-
           quire craniotomy.

TABLE 19-15. Glasgow Coma Score

Parameter	Response	Score
Eye opening	Spontaneously	4
	To command	3
	To pain	2
	No response	1
Motor response	Obeys verbal command	6
	Localizes pain	5
	Flexion withdrawal	4
	Decorticate rigidity	3
	Decerebrate rigidity	2
	No response	1
Verbal response	Oriented and converses	5
	Disoriented and converses	4
	Inappropriate words	3
	Incomprehensible words	2
	No response	1

D. Emergency Therapy
   1. Associated cervical spine injury must be considered before securing the head injury patient's airway.
   2. All head-injured patients are assumed to have full stomachs.
E. Anesthetic management is a continuation of the initial resuscitation efforts, including airway management, fluid and electrolyte balance, and ICP control (Table 19-16).
   1. A period of postoperative ventilation is often recommended because brain swelling is maximal 12–72 hours after injury.

TABLE 19-16. Preanesthetic Assessment of the Head-Injured Patient

Airway (cervical spine)
Breathing (ventilation and oxygenation)
Circulatory status
Associated injuries
Neurologic status (Glasgow Coma Score)
Pre-existing chronic illness
Circumstances of the injury (time of injury, duration of unconsciousness, associated alcohol or other drug use)

TABLE 19-17. Systemic Sequelae of Head Injury

Cardiopulmonary Problems
  Airway obstruction
  Arterial hypoxemia
  Shock
  Adult respiratory distress syndrome
  Neurogenic pulmonary edema
  Aspiration

Hematologic Problems
  Disseminated intravascular coagulation

Endocrine Problems
  Diabetes insipidus
  Syndrome of inappropriate antidiuretic hormone release

Gastrointestinal Problems
  Stress ulcers
  Hemorrhage

---

      2. Labetalol and esmolol may be used to treat hypertension, and supplemental barbiturates are given to sedate the patient.
   F. Systemic sequelae of head injury are diverse and can complicate its management (Table 19-17).

XIII. ELECTROCONVULSIVE THERAPY (see Chapter 38, Section V)

20

Anesthesia for Thoracic Surgery

Noncardiac thoracic surgical operations (on the lung, bronchus, mediastinum, thymus) may introduce unique physiologic, pharmacologic, and clinical considerations (Eisenkraft JB, Cohen E, Neustein SM: Anesthesia for thoracic surgery. In Barash PG, Cullen BF, Stoelting RK [eds]: Clinical Anesthesia, pp 943–988. Philadelphia, JB Lippincott, 1992).

I. PREOPERATIVE EVALUATION

Preoperative evaluation should focus on the extent and severity of pulmonary disease and cardiovascular involvement.

A. **History** (Table 20-1)

B. **Physical examination** (Table 20-2)

C. **Laboratory studies** (Table 20-3)

1. **A vital capacity** at least three times the **tidal volume** is necessary for an effective cough. A vital capacity <50% of predicted or <2 l is an indicator of increased risk.

2. **Mortality** after surgery increases when forced exhaled volume in 1 second **(FEV_1) is** <2 l.

3. The **ratio of FEV_1 to forced vital capacity** (FEV_1/FVC) is useful in differentiating restrictive (normal ratio as both are decreased) from obstructive (low ratio as FEV_1 is decreased) disease.

4. A 15% improvement in pulmonary function tests following **bronchodilator** therapy is an indication for continued preoperative therapy.

II. PREOPERATIVE PREPARATION

Several conditions predispose to postoperative complications, and their treatment preoperatively is associated with decreases in morbidity and mortality (Table 20-4).

TABLE 20-1. History Before Thoracic Surgery

Dyspnea (quantitate as to activity required to produce it; may warn of need for postoperative ventilation)

Cough (characteristics of sputum, culture)

Cigarette smoking

TABLE 20-2. Physical Examination Before Thoracic Surgery

Respiratory system
  Cyanosis
  Clubbing
  Breathing rate and pattern (distinguish between obstructive and restrictive disease)
  Breath sounds (wet sounds vs. wheezing)
Cardiovascular system (presence of pulmonary hypertension)

TABLE 20-3. Laboratory Studies Before Thoracic Surgery

Electrocardiogram (evidence of right ventricular hypertrophy)

Chest radiograph

Arterial blood gas determinations (blue bloaters vs. pink puffers)

Pulmonary function tests (evaluation for lung resectability)

TABLE 20-4. Factors That Predispose to Complications Following Thoracic Surgery

Smoking (carboxyhemoglobin declines in 48 hours; improvement of ciliary function and decrease in sputum production require 8–12 weeks)

Infection

Bronchial secretions

Wheezing

III. INTRAOPERATIVE MONITORING

Invasive monitoring and pulse oximetry have improved patient care (Table 20-5).

A. An arterial catheter is essential to provide continuous recordings of blood pressure, because surgical manip-

TABLE 20-5. Invasive Monitoring for Thoracic Surgery
Direct arterial catheterization (place in dependent arm for thoracotomy; right radial warns of innominate artery compression during mediastinoscopy)
Central venous pressure (acceptable in patients with good ventricular function)
Pulmonary artery catheter (during one-lung ventilation, accuracy of measurements may depend on position of the catheter)

     ulations or intravascular volume shifts can cause sudden changes in blood pressure.

B. Serial arterial blood gas determinations are necessary to confirm the adequacy of ventilation and oxygenation as suggested by capnography and pulse oximetry.

IV. PHYSIOLOGY OF THE LATERAL DECUBITUS POSITION (see Chapter 6)

In an open-chested, anesthetized, and paralyzed patient, the dependent lung is overperfused (gravity-dependent blood flow) and underventilated. Underventilation reflects minimal pressure of abdominal contents pressing against the upper diaphragm, making it easier for positive-pressure ventilation to distend the nondependent lung.

V. ONE-LUNG VENTILATION

A. Indications may be categorized as absolute and relative (Table 20-6).

B. **Methods of lung separation**

    1. **Double-lumen endobronchial tubes** are two catheters bonded together with one lumen long enough to reach a mainstem bronchus while the other ends in the trachea. Lung separation is achieved by inflation of the tracheal and bronchial cuff. The bronchial cuff on a right-sided tube is slotted to allow ventilation of the right upper lobe, because the right mainstem bronchus is too short to accommodate both the right lumen tip and cuff.

        a. A **Carlens** tube is a left-sided double-lumen tube with a carinal hook.

        b. A **White** tube is a right-sided Carlens tube.

        c. A **Robertshaw** tube is available as a left- or right-sided clear plastic disposable tube (No.

TABLE 20-6. Indications for One-Lung Ventilation

Absolute Indications

Prevent contamination of healthy lung (abscess, hemorrhage)

Control distribution of ventilation (bronchopleural fistula)

Relative Indications

Surgical exposure—high priority
Thoracic aneurysm
Pneumonectomy
Upper lobe lobectomy

Surgical exposure—low priority
Esophageal surgery
Middle and lower lobe lobectomy

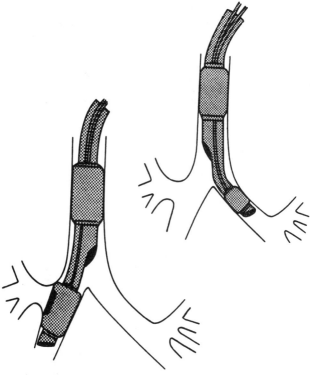

Figure 20-1. Schematic depiction of the proper placement of a right or left endobronchial tube.

**TABLE 20-7. Steps to Verify Proper Position of a
Double-Lumen Tube**

Inflate tracheal cuff and confirm bilateral and equal breath
sounds

Inflate bronchial cuff (rarely >2 ml of air) and confirm bilateral
and equal breath sounds (ensures that bronchial cuff is not
obstructing the contralateral hemithorax)

Selectively clamp each lumen and confirm one-lung
ventilation

Perform bronchoscopy using a pediatric fiberscope (nearly
one half of tubes thought to be properly positioned by
auscultation and examination were not confirmed by
bronchoscopy)

35–41 French) without a carinal hook. Lumina
are of sufficient size to facilitate suctioning and
offer low resistance to gas flow. The blue endobronchial cuff is easily recognized when fiberoptic bronchoscopy is used to confirm its
position.

2. **Positioning double-lumen tubes (Robertshaw)**
   a. Initial insertion of the tube is performed with
   the distal concave curvature facing anteriorly.
   After the tip of the tube is past the vocal cords,
   the stylet is removed and the tube is rotated
   90 degrees to direct the bronchial lumen appropriately toward the desired mainstem bronchus. Advancement of the tube is ended when
   moderate resistance to further passage is encountered, indicating that the tube tip has
   been firmly seated in the mainstem bronchus
   (Fig. 20-1).
   b. Once the tube is judged to be in the proper position, a sequence of steps (auscultation and
   physical examination) should be performed to
   check its location (Table 20-7).
   c. Confirmation of placement using a pediatric fiberscope is recommended (Table 20-8; Figs.20-
   2 and 20-3).

VI. MANAGEMENT OF ONE-LUNG VENTILATION

A. A goal of one-lung ventilation is to optimize arterial
oxygenation (Table 20-9).

**TABLE 20-8. Use of a Pediatric Fiberoptic
Bronchoscope to Verify Proper Placement
of a Double-Lumen Tube**

Left-sided Tube
   Tracheal lumen—carina visualized and upper surface of blue
      endobronchial cuff just below the carina
   Bronchial lumen—identify left upper lobe orifice

Right-sided Tube
   Tracheal lumen—carina visualized
   Bronchial lumen—identify right upper lobe orifice

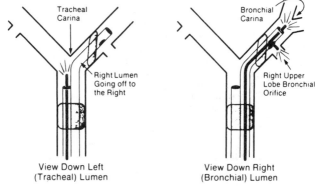

Figure 20-2. Use of a fiberscope to verify position of a double-lumen
tube.

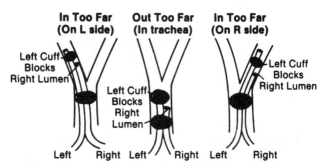

Figure 20-3. Examples of double-lumen tube malpositions.

**TABLE 20-9. Methods to Optimize Oxygenation
During One-Lung Ventilation**

Maximize delivered oxygen concentration (FIO_2 usually 1.0, but
this may contribute to absorption atelectasis)

Tidal volume to the dependent lung is 10–12 ml·kg^{-1}, and the
rate is adjusted to maintain $PaCO_2$ near 35 mm Hg

Positive end-expiratory pressure to the dependent lung (10 cm
H_2O increases functional residual capacity; consider when
PaO_2 is low)

Continuous positive airway pressure to the nondependent
lung (5–10 cm H_2O improves PaO_2 most reliably, distends
alveoli, and diverts blood flow to the dependent lung)

**B. Clinical approach to the management of one-lung
ventilation**
1. The position of the double-lumen tube should be
rechecked after the patient is placed in the lateral
decubitus position. Two-lung ventilation is maintained as long as possible.
2. After initiation of one-lung ventilation, PaO_2 can
continue to decrease for up to 45 minutes **(continuously monitor with pulse oximetry).**
a. If hypoxemia occurs during one-lung ventilation, it is important to verify proper tube position using a fiberscope.
b. If hypoxemia persists after verification of tube
position, consider addition of continuous positive airway pressure or positive end-expiratory
pressure.
c. Monitor airway pressure, as a sudden increase
may reflect tube dislocation.
d. Continuous auscultation by a stethoscope over
the dependent lung is useful.
3. Never hesitate to reinstitute two-lung ventilation
until a patient can be stabilized or the cause of a
patient's instability (hypoxemia, hypotension, cardiac dysrhythmias) is corrected.
C. Choice of anesthesia for thoracic surgery
1. Consider the likely presence of increased airway
reactivity (cigarette smoking, chronic bronchitis,
obstructive pulmonary disease) and the effect of
volatile anesthetics or ketamine on bronchomotor
tone.
2. Lidocaine, 1–2 mg·kg^{-1} iv, has been used before
airway manipulations to reduce the likelihood of
reflex bronchospasm.

3. An adequate depth of anesthesia before airway manipulation is the most important goal for managing patients with increased airway reactivity.

VII. HYPOXIC PULMONARY VASOCONSTRICTION

A. Hypoxic pulmonary vasoconstriction is a homeostatic mechanism that normally diverts blood flow away from hypoxic (atelectatic) regions of the lungs (local increases in pulmonary vascular resistance) and thereby optimizes oxygenation.

B. Inhibition of hypoxic pulmonary vasoconstriction during one-lung ventilation could accentuate arterial hypoxemia. Nevertheless, inhaled anesthetics do not seem to interfere with hypoxic pulmonary vasoconstriction.

VIII. ANESTHESIA FOR DIAGNOSTIC PROCEDURES

A. **Bronchoscopy** is most often performed with a fiberoptic bronchoscope that easily passes through a tracheal tube of 8.0–8.5 mm internal diameter.

B. **Mediastinoscopy.** Management of anesthesia includes several considerations (Table 20-10).

IX. ANESTHESIA FOR SPECIAL SITUATIONS

High-frequency jet ventilation techniques are often appropriate.

A. **Bronchopleural fistula and empyema** are more likely to occur after a pneumonectomy than after other types of lung resection. Management of anesthesia in such

---

TABLE 20-10. Anesthetic Considerations During Mediastinoscopy

Signs of Eaton-Lambert syndrome

Hemorrhage

Pneumothorax

Venous air embolism

Recurrent laryngeal nerve injury

Pressure on the innominate artery (manifests as reduced right radial pulse and necessitates repositioning of the mediastinoscope, especially in the presence of cerebrovascular disease)

patients includes several considerations (Table 20-11).

1. An alternative to tracheal intubation in awake patients is placement of a double-lumen tube under general anesthesia with a patient breathing spontaneously.

2. Rapid sequence induction of anesthesia plus a muscle relaxant, followed by placement of a single-lumen tracheal tube, may be acceptable if the air leak is small and an empyema is not present.

3. For a large bronchopleural fistula, high-frequency jet ventilation may be the nonsurgical treatment of choice.

B. **Lung cysts and bullae** usually represent an area of end-stage emphysematous destruction of the lungs associated with severe obstructive pulmonary disease and carbon dioxide retention.

1. Positive-pressure ventilation or nitrous oxide may cause bullae to expand or rupture (tension pneumothorax).

2. Ideally, a double-lumen tube is inserted with a patient breathing spontaneously while awake or during general anesthesia.

3. Gentle positive-pressure ventilation with rapid, small tidal volume and pressures not to exceed 10 cm H_2O may be used during the induction and maintenance of anesthesia, especially if the bullae have been shown to have no or only poor bronchial communication.

C. **Anesthesia for resection of the trachea** may be necessary to relieve stenosis that may follow tracheal intubation or tracheotomy (Table 20-12).

TABLE 20-11. Anesthetic Considerations in Management of a Patient with Bronchopleural Fistula

Drain empyema before induction of anesthesia

Awake tracheal intubation with a double-lumen tube (bronchial lumen directed to the side opposite the fistula; anticipate outpouring of pus from the tracheal lumen if an empyema is present)

Instituting controlled ventilation before placement of a double-lumen tube may result in hypoventilation because of a large air leak

Leave the chest drainage tube open to prevent tension pneumothorax

---

TABLE 20-12. Anesthetic Considerations for Tracheal Resection

Left radial artery cannulation (permits continuous monitoring of blood pressure during periods of innominate artery compression)

Corticosteroids to reduce tracheal edema

Deliver 100% oxygen to facilitate periods of apneic oxygenation

Consider placing a small anode (wire reinforced) tracheal tube above the stenosis, followed by distal placement of a sterile tracheal or bronchial tube after the trachea is exposed (other options include high-frequency jet ventilation or cardiopulmonary bypass)

Postoperatively, keep the head flexed and strive for early tracheal extubation

---

    D. Bronchopulmonary lavage is performed under general anesthesia using a double-lumen tube, most often for the treatment of cystic fibrosis.

X. MYASTHENIA GRAVIS

Myasthenia gravis is caused by a **decrease in the number of postsynaptic acetylcholine** receptors (circulating antibodies to the receptors), resulting in a decrease in the margin of safety of neuromuscular transmission (exercise-induced weakness).

    A. Medical therapy with anticholinesterases prolongs the action of acetylcholine. Anticholinesterase overdose causes a **cholinergic crisis** (treat with intravenous atropine), whereas underdose causes a **myasthenic crisis** (improves with edrophonium, 2–10 mg iv). Plasmapheresis reduces antibody titers, resulting in transient improvement (also causes a decrease in plasma cholinesterase).

    B. Thymectomy is considered the treatment of choice in most patients with myasthenia gravis. The gland is removed by a median sternotomy or transcervically using a technique similar to mediastinoscopy (lower incidence of postoperative ventilatory failure).

    C. Management of general anesthesia (Table 20-13)

    D. Nondepolarizing muscle relaxants. It is prudent to assume that even treated patients are sensitive and to greatly reduce the initial dose of muscle relaxant. One

---

TABLE 20-13. Anesthetic Considerations in Management of Thymectomy for Treatment of Myasthenia Gravis

Evaluate the adequacy of drug therapy (steroids, anticholinesterases)

Pulmonary function tests

Continue anticholinesterases preoperatively (controversial)

Modest preoperative medication (benzodiazepines, avoid opioids)

Induction of anesthesia with an intravenous drug followed by a volatile anesthetic (isoflurane <1%) to facilitate tracheal intubation

Anticipate the need for postoperative support of ventilation

Avoid drugs with skeletal muscle relaxing properties (antidysrhythmics, diuretics, aminoglycosides)

Sensitivity to nondepolarizing muscle relaxants

TABLE 20-14. Postoperative Considerations Following Thoracic Surgery

Atelectasis (rapid shallow breathing in response to pain; treatment is any maneuver that increases functional residual capacity)

Postoperative pain control (optimizes ventilation)
  Patient-controlled analgesia
  Intercostal nerve blocks (0.5% bupivacaine, 2–3 ml)
  Cryoanalgesia
  Neuraxial opioids (epidural or subarachnoid morphine diluted in saline, intrathecal dose about 1/10 epidural dose)

Low cardiac output syndrome (replace intravascular fluid volume; consider inotropes and/or vasodilators)

Cardiac dysrhythmias (supraventricular tachycardias; consider prophylactic digitalis if normokalemic)

Hemorrhage (re-explore if >200 ml·h^{-1})

Tension pneumothorax

Peripheral nerve injury (intercostal, brachial plexus, recurrent laryngeal)

---

approach is to titrate to effect using a peripheral nerve stimulator, beginning with doses of muscle relaxant that are 1/10–1/20 the usual dose.

1. Atracurium, because of its rapid elimination, is a useful drug. The intubating dose in patients with

myasthenia gravis is 0.1–0.2 mg·kg^{-1}, followed by a continuous infusion.

   2. Reversal with anticholinesterases has been safely accomplished but introduces the risk of a cholinergic crisis (titrate the anticholinesterase dose against response to peripheral nerve stimulation). Spontaneous recovery from a drug such as atracurium is an advantage if pharmacologic reversal of the muscle relaxant is deemed undesirable.

E. **Depolarizing relaxants.** Patients treated with anticholinesterases may be sensitive to succinylcholine, reflecting slowed metabolism of the muscle relaxant.

F. **Postoperative care.** Reduce opioid dose by one third, as anticholinesterases may increase the analgesic effect of these drugs.

XI. POSTOPERATIVE MANAGEMENT AND COMPLICATIONS (Table 20-14)

21

Anesthesia for Cardiac Surgery

Management of anesthesia for cardiac surgery requires a thorough understanding of normal and altered cardiac physiology; knowledge of the pharmacology of anesthetic, vasoactive, and cardioactive drugs; and familiarity with the physiologic derangements associated with cardiopulmonary bypass (CPB) and the surgical procedures themselves (Wray DL, Fine RH, Hughes CW, Thomas SJ: Anesthesia for cardiac surgery. In Barash PG, Cullen BF, Stoelting RK [eds]: Clinical Anesthesia, pp 1021–1057. Philadelphia, JB Lippincott, 1992).

I. CORONARY ARTERY DISEASE (CAD)

Prevention or treatment of myocardial ischemia before CPB in patients undergoing coronary artery bypass graft (CABG) surgery may reduce the incidence of perioperative myocardial infarction. Successful management of patients with CAD requires controlling the factors determining myocardial O_2 demand and optimizing O_2 supply to the heart (Table 21-1).

A. Coronary blood flow

1. The left ventricular subendocardium is most vulnerable to ischemia because myocardial O_2 requirements are great and perfusion is limited almost entirely to during diastole. The time available for diastole decreases with increasing heart rate, with the greatest percentage of reductions occurring at the lower heart rates.

2. A low ventricular filling pressure is ideal for improving perfusion (higher pressure gradient) and reducing myocardial O_2 requirements (decreased ventricular volume and wall tension).

3. It is not uncommon during an anesthetic for a patient to show signs of myocardial ischemia without any change in blood pressure, heart rate, or ventricular filling pressure.

TABLE 21-1. Myocardial Oxygen Balance

Demand	Supply
Wall tension	Coronary blood flow
Ventricular radius	(diastolic blood
Pressure generation	pressure)
Contractility	Diastolic time (heart rate)
Heart rate	Saturation
	Myocardial O_2 extraction

B. **Hemodynamic goals** of a successful anesthetic are to prevent myocardial ischemia by reducing myocardial O_2 requirements. Combinations of anesthetics, sedatives, muscle relaxants, and vasoactive drugs are selected to achieve this goal.

C. **Monitoring for ischemia** (Table 21-2). Myocardial ischemia reflects decreased O_2 delivery (hypotension, anemia, hypoxemia, coronary artery spasm) or increased myocardial O_2 requirements (hypertension, tachycardia, sympathetic nervous system stimulation).

D. **Selection of anesthetic.** Although there is no best anesthetic, the choice should depend primarily on the extent of pre-existing myocardial dysfunction and the pharmacologic properties of the drugs themselves. **Myocardial depression** and associated reductions in myocardial O_2 requirements are only harmful in a patient whose heart cannot be further depressed without precipitating congestive heart failure. All factors considered, there is **no evidence that the choice of anesthetic influences outcome** after CABG surgery.

   1. **Opioids** lack myocardial depressant effects and are useful in patients with severe myocardial dysfunction. In severely ill patients, opioids such as fentanyl (50–100 $\mu g \cdot kg^{-1}$) can be administered as the sole

TABLE 21-2. Monitoring for Myocardial Ischemia

Electrocardiogram (ST segment analysis of leads V_5 and II)

Heart rate and blood pressure

Pulmonary artery catheter (V waves reflect ischemia-induced papillary muscle dysfunction; probably not a sensitive indicator of myocardial ischemia.)

Two-dimensional transesophageal echocardiography (regional wall motion)

anesthetic. In patients with good left ventricular function, opioids may be inadequate to depress sympathetic nervous system activity, requiring the addition of volatile anesthetics or vasoactive drugs.

2. Inhalation anesthetics provide predictable dose-dependent responses, especially suppression of sympathetic nervous system responses. Disadvantages of volatile anesthetics include myocardial depression and lack of postoperative analgesia.

   a. Combinations of opioids and volatile anesthetics may produce the advantages of each with minimal undesirable effects.

   b. Isoflurane use in patients with CAD must consider the issue of **coronary steal** (appears to be clinically significant only in doses >1 **MAC** (see Chapter 14).

E. Treatment of ischemia. Selection of anesthetics or vasoactive drugs that enable the heart to return to the **slow, small, perfused state** is frequently required (Table 21-3) (see Chapter 11).

1. Nitroglycerin is the drug of choice for the treatment of coronary vasospasm. As a venodilator, this drug reduces venous return and decreases ventricular filling pressures and thus wall tension.

2. Phenylephrine increases myocardial O_2 requirements, but this increase is offset by improvements in O_2 delivery produced by the increased coronary perfusion pressure.

TABLE 21-3. Treatment of Intraoperative Ischemia

Event Associated With Ischemia	Treatment
Increased blood pressure and PCWP*	Increase anesthetic depth Nitroglycerin
Increased heart rate	Beta antagonist
Decreased blood pressure	Decrease anesthetic depth Phenylephrine
Decreased blood pressure and increased PCWP	Phenylephrine Nitroglycerin Inotrope
Normal hemodynamics	Nitroglycerin Calcium entry blocker

*PCWP = pulmonary capillary wedge pressure.

3. **Verapamil** is useful in the treatment of coronary vasospasm and supraventricular tachycardia. Simultaneous administration of phenylephrine may be necessary to counteract the peripheral vasodilation and hypotension that often accompany the use of verapamil.

II. VALVULAR HEART DISEASE

Valvular heart disease is characterized by pressure or volume overload of the atria or ventricles.

A. **Aortic stenosis**
   1. **Pathophysiology.** Chronic obstruction to left ventricular ejection results in concentric ventricular hypertrophy, which makes the heart susceptible to myocardial ischemia even in the absence of CAD. Because the ventricle is stiff, atrial contraction is critical for ventricular filling and stroke volume.
   2. **Anesthetic considerations.** Maintenance of adequate ventricular volume and sinus rhythm is crucial. Hypotension must be prevented and treated early if it develops in order to prevent the catastrophic cycle of hypotension-induced ischemia, subsequent ventricular dysfunction, and worsening hypotension. Bradycardia is a common cause of hypotension in patients with aortic stenosis.

B. **Hypertrophic cardiomyopathy** is a genetically determined disease characterized by development of a hypertrophic intraventricular septum, resulting in outflow obstruction. Outflow obstruction is increased by increases in myocardial contractility or heart rate or decreases in preload or afterload. Anesthetic management is based on maintenance of ventricular filling and controlled myocardial depression as produced by volatile anesthetics, especially halothane.

C. **Aortic regurgitation**
   1. **Pathophysiology.** Chronic volume overload of the left ventricle evokes eccentric hypertrophy but only minimal changes in filling pressures.
   2. **Anesthetic considerations.** Maintenance of adequate ventricular volume in the presence of mild vasodilation and increases in heart rate is most likely to optimize forward left ventricular stroke volume.

D. **Mitral stenosis**
   1. **Pathophysiology.** Increased left atrial pressure and volume overload are inevitable consequences of the narrowed mitral orifice. Persistent elevations in left atrial pressure are reflected back through the pul-

monary circulation, leading to right ventricular hypertrophy and perivascular edema in the lungs.

2. **Anesthetic considerations.** Avoiding tachycardia is crucial for preventing pulmonary hypertension as well as inadequate left ventricular filling with concomitant hypotension. Continued preoperative administration of digitalis and beta antagonists, selection of anesthetics with minimal propensity to increase heart rate, and achievement of an anesthetic depth sufficient to suppress sympathetic nervous system responses are recommended.

E. **Mitral regurgitation**

1. **Pathophysiology.** Chronic volume overload of the left atrium is the cardinal feature of mitral regurgitation.

2. **Anesthetic considerations.** Selection of anesthetics that promote vasodilation and increase the heart rate are useful.

III. CARDIOPULMONARY BYPASS

CPB incorporates a circuit to oxygenate venous blood and return it to a patient's arterial circulation (Table 21-4; Fig. 21-1).

TABLE 21-4. Components of Cardiopulmonary Bypass

Circuits (blood is drained from the right atrium and returned to the ascending aorta)

Oxygenators
  Bubble (time-dependent trauma to blood)
  Membrane (less damage to blood)

Pumps (generate pressure required to return perfusate to patient)
  Roller (nonpulsatile)
  Centrifugal
  Pulsatile

Heat exchanger (allows production of systemic hypothermia)

Prime (reduces hematocrit to <30%)

Anticoagulants (a common recommendation is to maintain activated coagulation time >400 seconds, although evidence to support this practice is not available)

Myocardial protection (hypothermia to 10–15°C and K^+ to ensure diastolic electrical arrest)

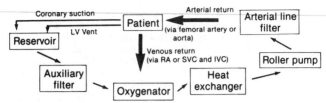

Figure 21-1. Diagram of a cardiopulmonary bypass circuit.

IV. PREOPERATIVE EVALUATION (CPB)

Data from the history, physical examination, and laboratory investigation are used to delineate the degree of left ventricular or right ventricular dysfunction (Table 21-5).

A. **Current drug therapy** is usually continued until the time of surgery, including digitalis preparations being administered for heart rate or rhythm control.

B. **Premedication** for cardiac surgery often combines an opioid (morphine, 0.1–0.2 mg·kg^{-1}) with scopolamine (0.006 mg·kg^{-1}) and/or a benzodiazepine (diazepam 0.05–0.1 mg·kg^{-1}, lorazepam 0.05–0.07 mg·kg^{-1}). Patients with valvular heart disease may be more susceptible to the ventilatory depressant effects of premedication than those with CAD scheduled for CABG operations.

C. **Monitoring** should emphasize those areas particularly relevant to cardiac surgery (Table 21-6) (see Chapter 7).

D. **Selection of anesthetic drugs.** There is no single best drug; the most critical factor governing anesthetic selection is the degree of ventricular dysfunction. The anticipated time to extubation of the trachea may influ-

---

TABLE 21-5. Data from Preoperative Evaluation

History of myocardial infarction

Signs of congestive heart failure

Evidence of myocardial ischemia or infarction on electrocardiogram

Chest radiograph

Left ventricular end-diastolic pressure >18 mm Hg

Ejection fraction <0.4

Cardiac index <2 l·min^{-1}·m^{-2}

Two-dimensional transesophageal echocardiography (wall motion abnormalities)

TABLE 21-6. Monitors for Cardiac Surgery Requiring Cardiopulmonary Bypass

Pulse oximeter (place as first monitor to detect unsuspected episodes of hypoxemia during catheter placement)

Electrocardiogram

Temperature (observe gradients during cooling and rewarming)

Intra-arterial blood pressure (radial artery blood pressure may be lower than central aortic pressure early after CPB)

Central venous pressure catheter (infusion of cardioselective drugs; assumed to reflect left-sided filling pressures in the absence of left ventricular dysfunction)

Pulmonary artery catheter (awake vs. asleep placement; distal migration occurs during CPB, so pull back a few centimeters before initiation of CPB)

Two-dimensional transesophageal echocardiography (role still evolving)

Central nervous system function (electroencephalogram, somatosensory-evoked potentials)

ence the choice of anesthetic. It is useful to be able to alter anesthetic depth in order to accommodate the varying intensity of surgical stimulus (intense with tracheal intubation, sternotomy, and manipulation of the aorta and minimal during hypothermic CPB).

1. **Potent inhalation anesthetics** are helpful as the primary anesthetic and as adjuvants to treat or prevent hypertension associated with high-dose opioid techniques. Volatile anesthetics can be administered during CPB through a vaporizer mounted on the pump.

2. **Opioids** lack negative inotropic effects and in high doses (fentanyl, 50–100 $\mu g \cdot kg^{-1}$; sufentanil, 10–20 $\mu g \cdot kg^{-1}$) may be used as the sole anesthetic. In patients with good left ventricular function, it is often necessary to include adjuvant drugs to provide amnesia (benzodiazepines) and control hypertension (volatile anesthetics, vasodilators). Excessive bradycardia may accompany the use of opioids, especially if nondepolarizing muscle relaxants without heart rate effects are administered (vecuronium or atracurium rather than pancuronium).

3. **Nitrous oxide** has limited usefulness because of its myocardial depressant effects in the presence of opioids and the ability to enhance the size of air

emboli, which may be present in coronary arteries after CABG operations.

   E. **Neuromuscular blocking drugs.** Doxacurium and pipecuronium may be useful in cardiac surgical patients because they do not produce significant heart rate and blood pressure effects.

V. INTRAOPERATIVE MANAGEMENT

Anticipation of needs specific to each stage of the procedure and ready availability of necessary equipment and drugs are essential (Table 21-7).

   A. **Induction and intubation.** The dose, speed of administration, and specific drugs selected depend primarily on a patient's cardiovascular reserve and desired cardiovascular profile. A brief duration of laryngoscopy is desirable, although intubation of the trachea may be a strong stimulus for coronary vasoconstriction regardless of the anesthetic selected and even in the absence of hemodynamic changes.

   B. The **preincision** period between intubation of the trachea and skin incision is one of minimal stimulation. Therefore, blood pressure may need to be supported.

   C. **Incision for CPB** is characterized by periods of intense surgical stimulation, which often require alteration in the depth of anesthesia or administration of a vasodilator to blunt responses (hypertension, tachycardia) that may predispose to myocardial ischemia.

   D. **CPB** is initiated after confirmation of adequate heparin effect.

      1. There is no consensus about the optimal mean arterial pressure during CPB, although flows of 50–60 ml·kg^{-1} usually produce perfusion pressures of 50–60 mm Hg. The effect of decreased viscosity (acute hemodilution) and loss of pulsatile flow may initially cause the perfusion pressure to decrease below 40 mm Hg. Phenylephrine may be administered to increase perfusion pressure if it is deemed important to maintenance of organ blood flow.

      2. Once full CPB is established, there is no need to continue ventilation of the lungs. There is no consensus about care of the lungs (positive end-expiratory pressure vs. zero airway pressure, O_2 vs. room air) during CPB.

      3. Anesthetic requirements are reduced during hypothermic CPB, an effect that may offset the dilutional effect of CPB on plasma concentrations of injected drugs.

TABLE 21-7. Use of the Mnemonic LAMPS to Guide Management

Before Cardiopulmonary Bypass

Laboratory	Activated coagulation time, hematocrit
Anesthesia	Adequate depth, nitrous oxide off, paralysis
Monitor	Blood pressure, central venous pressure, pulmonary capillary wedge pressure
Patient	Cannulas in place and patient's facial appearance (suffusion, unilateral blanching)
Support	Usually unnecessary

During Cardiopulmonary Bypass

Laboratory	Activated coagulation time, hematocrit, arterial blood gases, K^+
Anesthesia	What to do with lungs?
Monitor	Blood pressure (check cannulas, flows, transducers), central venous pressure, pulmonary capillary wedge pressure, electrocardiogram (flat line if cardioplegia), urine output, temperature
Patient	Conduct of operation, cyanosis, movement or breathing
Support	Control blood pressure (phenylephrine, vasodilator, anesthetic)

Before Separation from Cardiopulmonary Bypass

Laboratory	Arterial blood gases, hematocrit, K^+
Anesthesia	Ventilation initiated, vaporizers off, alarms on
Monitor	Transducers zeroed and calibrated, electrocardiogram, temperature
Patient	Look at the heart (contractility, rhythm, size), hemostasis
Support	As necessary (inotrope, vasodilator)

---

    4. Continued skeletal muscle paralysis is desirable to prevent increases in O_2 requirements owing to skeletal muscle activity.

  E. Central nervous system protection. Neurologic injury after CPB is most likely the result of emboli. Nevertheless, hypoperfusion due to hypotension can be a contributing cause.

F. **Monitoring and management during cardiopulmonary bypass.** It is important to continuously observe the surgical field and cannulas to permit early detection of mechanical causes of hypotension or hypertension during CPB.

1. Addition of carbon dioxide to the oxygenator gas mixture based on Pa_{CO_2} values corrected for temperature is not recommended.

2. Maintenance of urine output with diuretics is a common practice during CPB. Nevertheless, the likelihood of postoperative renal failure is determined by aggravation of pre-existing renal dysfunction or persistent low cardiac output following CPB.

G. **Rewarming** is begun when the surgical repair is nearly complete, remembering that patients may regain awareness as the anesthetic effects of hypothermia dissipate.

H. **Discontinuation of cardiopulmonary bypass** is considered when rewarming is adequate. Inadequate cardiac output must prompt a search for explanations (kinked grafts, air in coronary grafts, coronary artery spasm, global ischemia from inadequate myocardial protection) and consideration of pharmacologic support (inotropes, vasodilators) (Table 21-8).

I. An **intra-aortic balloon pump** is a mechanical assist device (25-cm balloon on a 90-cm stiff vascular catheter) that uses the principle of synchronized counterpulsation to enhance left ventricular stroke volume. The balloon deflates immediately before systole to reduce afterload and myocardial O_2 requirements. Subsequently, the balloon inflates during diastole to provide diastolic augmentation that increases coronary blood flow. It is crucial to control heart rate and to suppress cardiac dysrhythmias to ensure proper balloon timing. As cardiac function improves, the assist ratio is gradually weaned from every beat to every other beat (finally to 1:8) and then removed.

J. **Postcardiopulmonary bypass.** Heparin is partially reversed with protamine administered intravenously while the arterial cannula remains in place for continued transfusion of pump contents.

1. Adequate reversal of anticoagulation with protamine is verified by measurement of the activated coagulation time.

a. Protamine administration may be accompanied by side effects (Table 21-9).

b. Whether protamine should be administered through the right atrium, left atrium, aorta, or a peripheral vein remains controversial.

TABLE 21-8. Diagnosis and Therapy of Cardiovascular Dysfunction Following Cardiopulmonary Bypass

Blood Pressure	Filling Pressures	Cardiac Output	Diagnosis	Treatment
↑	↑	↑	Hypervolemia	Remove volume, vasodilation
↑	↑	↓	Vasoconstriction Decreased contractility	Vasodilation Possible inotrope
↑	↓	↑	Hyperdynamic	Anesthetic, beta antagonist(?)
↑	↓	↓	Vasoconstriction	Vasodilation, administer volume
↓	↑	↑	Vasodilated Hypervolemia	Wait Vasoconstriction
↓	↑	↓	Left ventricular dysfunction	Inotrope Vasodilate Mechanical assist
↓↓	↓↓	↑↓	Vasodilated Hypovolemia	Vasoconstriction Administer volume

---

TABLE 21-9. Side Effects of Protamine

Hypotension (less likely when administered over 5 minutes)
Allergic reaction (more likely in patients receiving protamine-containing insulin preparations—NPH, PZI
Pulmonary hypertension (mediated by release of thromboxane and C5a anaphylatoxin)

---

2. **Postcardiopulmonary bypass bleeding,** despite adequate reversal of heparin, is not uncommon and most often reflects inadequate surgical hemostasis or platelet dysfunction.
3. Closure of the chest is occasionally associated with transient decreases in blood pressure. If hypotension persists despite volume replacement, the chest must be reopened to rule out cardiac tamponade or kinking of a graft.
4. **Bring-back** of the patient for postoperative re-exploration is necessary in 4–10% of cases, usually in the first 24 hours (Table 21-10).

TABLE 21-10. Reasons for Postoperative Re-exploration

Persistent bleeding
Excessive blood loss
Cardiac tamponade
Unexplained low cardiac output

TABLE 21-11. Manifestations of Cardiac Tamponade

Hypotension
Equalization of diastolic filling pressures (when the pericardium is no longer intact, loculated areas of clot may compress only one chamber, causing isolated increases in filling pressures)
Fixed stroke volume (cardiac output and blood pressure become dependent on heart rate)
Peripheral vasoconstriction (maintain venous return)
Tachycardia
Potential for concurrent myocardial ischemia

      a. The possibility of **cardiac tamponade** must always be included in the differential diagnosis of unexplained low cardiac output (Table 21-11).

      b. Ketamine is useful for induction and maintenance of anesthesia in patients with cardiac tamponade, as the goal is to avoid vasodilation or cardiac depression.

VI. CONGENITAL HEART DISEASE

    A. Classification of congenital heart disease is based on the direction of blood flow through the shunt or obstruction to blood flow (Table 21-12).

    B. **Systemic and pulmonary vascular resistance.** It is important to understand each patient's cardiac anatomy and pattern of blood flow in order to predict effects of drug-induced changes in systemic vascular resistance (SVR) and pulmonary vascular resistance (PVR) on the magnitude of shunt flow and arterial oxygenation. For example, increases in SVR (ketamine, phenylephrine)

TABLE 21-12. Classification of Congenital Heart Defects

Left-to-Right Shunt (Increased Pulmonary Blood Flow)
   Atrial septal defect
   Ventricular septal defect
   Patent ductus arteriosus

Right-to-Left Shunt (Decreased Pulmonary Blood Flow)
   Tetralogy of Fallot
   Pulmonary atresia
   Ebstein's anomaly

Mixing of Systemic and Pulmonary Circulations
   Truncus arteriosus
   Transposition of the great arteries
   Total anomalous pulmonary venous drainage

Obstructive Lesions
   Aortic stenosis
   Pulmonary stenosis
   Coarctation of the aorta

increase pulmonary blood flow and improve oxygenation in patients with a right-to-left shunt.

C. **Preoperative evaluation** should determine the presence or absence of congestive heart failure and cyanosis. Polycythemia occurs in response to chronic arterial hypoxemia. When the hematocrit exceeds 60%, a child is at risk for cerebral infarction or coagulation abnormalities.

D. **Cardiac catheterization** is the traditional means of assessing the physiologic consequences of congenital cardiac lesions. Nevertheless, echocardiography also provides an assessment of blood flow patterns, cardiac anatomy, and shunt flow (direction and magnitude).

   1. A step-up in oxygen saturation from the superior vena cava to the right atrium or right ventricle is indicative of left-to-right shunting. Desaturation of left ventricular or aortic blood suggests right-to-left shunting of venous blood into the systemic circulation.

   2. Oxygen saturations are used to calculate the intrapulmonary to systemic blood flow ratio ($\dot{Q}p/\dot{Q}s$) and flows using the Fick equation.

E. Premedication is useful to reduce struggling and crying in infants and children, which may increase the magnitude of right-to-left shunt (Table 21-13).

F. **Preparation for anesthesia** is based on the recognition that arterial hypoxemia and hypotension can occur quickly. Care must be taken to eliminate all air from intravenous lines, as systemic embolization can occur in the presence of a right-to-left shunt. Cardioactive drugs must be immediately available (Table 21-14).

G. **Anesthetic selection** must consider depressant effects on the heart and impact on SVR and PVR. Regardless of age, **all pediatric patients require anesthesia.**

TABLE 21-13. Premedication for Hemodynamically Stable Children Over 6 Months of Age

Scopolamine	$10–20 \ \mu g \cdot kg^{-1}$	im
Atropine	$10–20 \ \mu g \cdot kg^{-1}$	im
Diazepam	$0.4 \ mg \cdot kg^{-1}$	im
Midazolam	$0.08 \ mg \cdot kg^{-1}$	im
Pentobarbital	$2–4 \ mg \cdot kg^{-1}$	im/oral
Morphine	$0.05–0.15 \ mg \cdot kg^{-1}$	im
Meperidine	$1–2 \ mg \cdot kg^{-1}$	im

TABLE 21-14. Cardioactive Drugs for Intravenous Administration to Patients with Congenital Heart Disease

Atropine	10–20 $\mu g \cdot kg^{-1}$
Calcium chloride	10 mg·kg^{-1}
Lidocaine	1 mg·kg^{-1}
	0.02–0.05 mg·kg^{-1}·min^{-1}
Propranolol	10–20 $\mu g \cdot kg^{-1}$
Verapamil	125–250 $\mu g \cdot kg^{-1}$
Digoxin	20–40 $\mu g \cdot kg^{-1}$
Nitroprusside	0.5–10.0 $\mu g \cdot kg^{-1} \cdot min^{-1}$
Prostaglandin E$_1$	0.1 $\mu g \cdot kg^{-1} \cdot min^{-1}$
Isoproterenol	0.1–0.5 $\mu g \cdot kg^{-1} \cdot min^{-1}$
Epinephrine	0.1–1.0 $\mu g \cdot kg^{-1} \cdot min^{-1}$
Dopamine	1–20 $\mu g \cdot kg^{-1} \cdot min^{-1}$
Dobutamine	1–10 $\mu g \cdot kg^{-1} \cdot min^{-1}$
Norepinephrine	0.1–0.5 $\mu g \cdot kg^{-1} \cdot min^{-1}$

H. **Induction of anesthesia** may include awake tracheal intubation in neonates, whereas older children may be managed with an inhalation or intravenous induction. Combative children may benefit from intramuscular ketamine, 5–10 mg·kg^{-1}.

 1. Theoretically, speed of anesthetic induction can be altered by the presence of shunts. For example, a right-to-left shunt slows equilibration with inhaled anesthetics, especially poorly soluble drugs such as nitrous oxide. Conversely, intravenous drugs reach the brain more quickly in the presence of a right-to-left shunt.

 2. A left-to-right shunt dilutes the plasma concentration of intravenous drugs, whereas the effect on the rate of inhalation induction is minimal if the cardiac output is maintained.

I. **Maintenance of anesthesia** is based on a patient's hemodynamic status and plans for the postoperative course. High-dose opioid techniques (fentanyl, 25–50 $\mu g \cdot kg^{-1}$ or sufentanil, 5–15 $\mu g \cdot kg^{-1}$) provide cardiovascular stability but prohibit early tracheal extubation. Volatile anesthetics with or without opioids are useful in children with better cardiovascular function, remembering that the immature myocardium and vascular system are very sensitive to the depressant effects of these drugs.

J. **Cardiopulmonary bypass** in infants requires a high flow rate (150–175 ml·kg⁻¹·min⁻¹), and the presence of an intracardiac shunt may make it difficult to maintain perfusion pressure.

K. **Deep hypothermic circulatory arrest** (10–15°C) is used in infants weighing less than 10 kg and requiring repair of complex congenital lesions. Most consider 60 minutes as the upper limit of safe continuous arrest.

L. **Timing of extubation.** Repair of simple congenital lesions (atrial septal defect, patent ductus arteriosus, coarctation) may be followed by early tracheal extubation. Repair of more complex lesions is often followed by postoperative mechanical support of ventilation.

22

Anesthesia for Vascular Surgery

Cardiac dysfunction is the most common cause of morbidity following vascular surgery (Roizen MF, Ellis JE: Anesthesia for vascular surgery. In Barash PG, Cullen BF, Stoelting RK [eds]: Clinical Anesthesia, pp 1059–1094. Philadelphia, JB Lippincott, 1992).

I. CAUSES OF MORBIDITY AFTER OPERATIONS FOR CEREBROVASCULAR INSUFFICIENCY

Morbidity and mortality following carotid endarterectomy vary directly with the preoperative neurologic and cardiac status of patients, especially if they are of advanced age. Patients with symptomatic carotid artery disease are at greater risk for stroke following coronary artery bypass graft operations.

II. CAUSES OF MORBIDITY AFTER OPERATIONS FOR VISCERAL ISCHEMIA, THORACOABDOMINAL ANEURYSMS, AND AORTIC RECONSTRUCTION FOR ANEURYSM OR ATHEROSCLEROTIC DISEASE

A. Occlusive vascular disease is often associated with smoking (chronic obstructive pulmonary disease), hypertension, and diabetes mellitus.

B. Improved survival makes patients with abdominal aortic aneurysms <6 cm in diameter candidates for reconstructive surgery.

C. Better perioperative fluid management has reduced the incidence of acute renal failure in this patient population.

D. **Spinal cord ischemia** may occur in 1–11% of operations involving repair of the distal descending thoracic aorta. Somatosensory-evoked potentials may be useful in detecting cord ischemia before it becomes irreversible. Low pressures in other areas of the body, such as those that accompany application of a high aortic occluding clamp, may result in diversion (steal) of spinal cord blood flow to low-pressure areas.

III. SURGERY FOR CEREBROVASCULAR INSUFFICIENCY

A. **Surgical considerations** (Table 22-1)

B. **Anesthetic goals and monitoring techniques.** For minimal morbidity, the anesthetic goals are to protect the heart and brain from ischemia.

1. **Myocardial ischemia.** A calibrated ECG (diagnostic mode) using lead V_5 is usually selected, although the sensitivity of this lead for detecting ischemic changes is questionable. The incidence of myocardial ischemia and death from myocardial mechanisms after carotid endarterectomy performed during regional anesthesia is similar to that following general anesthesia.

2. **Cerebral ischemia**

   a. **Repeated neurologic evaluation of conscious patients** is cited as the principal reason for choosing regional anesthesia.

   b. Several techniques are available for evaluation of neurologic function during general anesthesia (Table 22-2).

C. **Anesthesia for surgery for cerebrovascular insufficiency.** General anesthesia is most often selected (Table 22-3).

1. Patients who are deeply anesthetized and whose systemic vascular resistance is maintained with an infusion of phenylephrine have more than twice the

---

TABLE 22-1. Surgical Considerations in Performance of a Carotid Endarterectomy

Isolate the diseased portion of the internal carotid artery

Heparin followed by test occlusion (monitor electroencephalogram, somatosensory-evoked potentials, stump pressure)

Insert shunt (controversial)

Awaken patient promptly to permit evaluation of neurologic status

---

TABLE 22-2. Evaluation of Neurologic Function During General Anesthesia

---

Electroencephalogram (complex and may not be useful in predicting or preventing new neurologic deficits)

Somatosensory-evoked potentials (value unproved)

Regional cerebral blood flow (too complex for routine use)

Carotid stump pressure (maintain >60 mm Hg during anesthesia with a volatile drug; higher value recommended if an opioid-based anesthetic is used)

TABLE 22-3. Considerations in the Management of Anesthesia for Carotid Endarterectomy

---

Establish a normal range of blood pressure and heart rate as guidelines for acceptable intraoperative values

Preoperative interview to allay anxiety (avoid drugs that could delay postoperative awakening)

Normal saline for intravenous fluids (glucose and associated hyperglycemia may increase neurologic damage after global ischemia)

Place an arterial catheter

Thiopental—succinylcholine acceptable

Controlled ventilation of the lungs ($Paco_2$ 35–40 mm Hg)

Maintenance with minimal doses of volatile anesthetic (muscle relaxant optional)

Limit maintenance fluids to 10 ml·kg^{-1} (excess fluids may contribute to postoperative hypertension)

Ask the surgeon to infiltrate the carotid bifurcation with 1% lidocaine to prevent carotid sinus reflex responses

---

TABLE 22-4. Possible Postoperative Complications Following Carotid Endarterectomy

---

Hypertension (treat with nitroprusside, hydralazine, esmolol, labetalol)

Hypotension (attributed to hypersensitivity of the carotid sinus; often associated with myocardial ischemia)

Vocal cord paresis

Hematoma (stridor; may require urgent opening of the suture line)

New neurologic dysfunction (most often embolic; may necessitate immediate re-exploration)

Carotid sinus denervation

incidence of myocardial ischemia than do patients whose blood pressure is maintained by light anesthesia and endogenous vasoconstrictors.

2. There are several possible problems in the early postoperative period (Table 22-4).

IV. SURGERY FOR VISCERAL ISCHEMIA, THORACOABDOMINAL AORTIC ANEURYSMS, AND INFRARENAL AORTIC RECONSTRUCTION

A. **Cardiac and renal function are principal concerns** during these operations, with patients known to have preoperative renal insufficiency being at greatest risk of developing renal failure. It is important to minimize the duration of ischemia to viscera, especially to the renal circulation (infrarenal vs. suprarenal clamping of the aorta). During operative manipulation and clamping, great care must be taken that material is not dislodged into the renal arteries. Heparin is commonly administered to reduce the risk of thromboembolic complications, especially if there is a need for clamping the aorta.

B. **Anesthetic goals in surgery for aortic and visceral artery reconstruction.** The goal is to reduce myocardial oxygen requirements and at the same time maintain adequate perfusion to all other organs.

1. **Pathophysiologic events** that accompany cross-clamping of the aorta must be considered.

   a. In the absence of collateral circulation, aortic occlusion increases systemic vascular resistance in proportion to the level of occlusion.

   b. Myocardial performance and circulatory variables often remain within an acceptable range after the aorta is occluded at infrarenal levels. Nevertheless, cross-clamping the aorta may require deepening of anesthesia or use of vasodilating drugs.

   c. Despite the negligible cardiovascular effects of temporarily applying an infrarenal aortic occlusion clamp, hypotension (systolic blood pressure often decreases about 40 mm Hg) still may occur on restoration of flow through the aorta.

   d. Hypotension with release of the occlusion clamp most likely reflects reactive hyperemia in the freshly revascularized area, emphasizing the importance of volume expansion before removal of the clamp. In this regard, blood loss is replaced milliliter for milliliter during occlusion, and filling pressures are allowed to increase as much as possible without producing myocardial ischemia. If hypotension persists, it may be necessary for the surgeon to reapply the aortic occlusion clamp.

   2. **Monitoring** is designed to reflect preservation of central nervous system, myocardial, pulmonary, and renal function as well as intravascular volume (Table 22-5).

   3. **Infusion of mannitol** (0.2–1.5 $g \cdot kg^{-1}$) is sometimes recommended when renal ischemia is considered likely or in the presence of a ruptured aneurysm. Maintenance of an adequate intravascular volume and myocardial function is the most important concept in preventing renal insufficiency.

C. **Anesthetic agents and techniques for aortic reconstruction.** The quality and attentiveness of the anesthesiologist are more important than the choice of anesthetic.

   1. Isoflurane seems less likely than halothane to produce hepatic hypoxia when there is occlusion of the aorta at the supraceliac level.

   2. Selection of epidural anesthesia must consider the administration of heparin and the theoretical risk of an epidural hematoma. Skeletal muscle relaxation is an advantage of this technique. Postoperative analgesia can also be provided through the lumbar epidural catheter previously inserted for operative anesthesia. Outcome may be better in those patients receiving optimal analgesia with neuraxial opioids.

D. **Anesthesia for aortic reconstruction** (Table 22-6)

E. **Anesthesia for emergency aortic reconstruction.** When rupture of an abdominal aneurysm is known or sus-

---

TABLE 22-5. Monitoring of Organ Function

Intra-arterial catheter

Urine output

Pulmonary artery catheter

Electrocardiogram

Two-dimensional transesophageal echocardiography (limited use at present)

Electroencephalogram or somatosensory-evoked potentials (limited usefulness)

TABLE 22-6. Considerations in the Management of Anesthesia for Aortic Reconstruction

Prehydration to maintain normal hydration status before induction of anesthesia

Establish normal range of blood pressure and heart rate with a goal to maintain at ±20% of these values

Before cross-clamping of the aorta, maintain intravascular fluid volume and body temperature

Anticipate blood pressure decline with removal of cross-clamp and optimize blood volume

Provide postoperative analgesia (neuraxial opioids)

---

pected, rapid control of the proximal portion of the aorta is probably more important than optimizing a patient's preoperative condition.

V. SURGERY FOR PERIPHERAL VASCULAR INSUFFICIENCY

A. Obstruction most often is in the aortoiliac segment (aortofemoral bypass) or distal to the inguinal ligament (femoropopliteal bypass).

B. Operative arteriography is commonly used for evaluation of the adequacy of the surgical repair.

C. Major blood loss or hemodynamic changes are not usually encountered, but the procedures tend to be prolonged.

D. Anesthetic goals and management include avoidance of intraoperative overhydration, which may lead to congestive heart failure, especially as sympathectomy wanes during epidural anesthesia.

1. Dye administered for angiography may contribute to fluid shifts.

2. When surgery is an emergency, the choice of anesthetic technique may be influenced by the need for anticoagulation.

3. Hyperkalemia and acidosis owing to ischemic extremities may be present, and myoglobin can be released into the circulation.

23

Anesthesia and the Eye

Anesthesia for ophthalmic surgery presents unique anesthetic challenges and requirements (Table 23-1) (McGoldrick KE: Anesthesia and the eye. In Barash PG, Cullen BF, Stoelting RK [eds]: Clinical Anesthesia, pp 1095–1112. Philadelphia, JB Lippincott, 1992).

I. MAINTENANCE OF INTRAOCULAR PRESSURE (IOP)

IOP normally varies between 10 and 25 mm Hg but becomes atmospheric when the globe has been entered. Any sudden rise in IOP when the globe is open may lead to prolapse of the iris and lens, extrusion of vitreous, and loss of vision.

II. EFFECTS OF ANESTHESIA AND ADJUVANT DRUGS ON INTRAOCULAR PRESSURE
(Table 23-2)

A. Intravenous injection of succinylcholine (SCh) transiently increases IOP about 8 mm Hg, with return to baseline in 5–7 minutes. This effect of SCh on IOP may be a reason to avoid administration of this drug to patients with an open eye injury or recent ocular incisions.

B. Pretreatment with a nondepolarizing muscle relaxant as a means to prevent SCh-induced increases in IOP has not always been shown to be effective.

C. Etomidate-induced myoclonus may be hazardous in the setting of an open globe.

III. OCULOCARDIAC REFLEX

Oculocardiac reflex manifests as bradycardia and occasionally as cardiac dysrhythmias, elicited by pressure on

TABLE 23-1. Requirements for Ophthalmic Surgery

Akinesia
Profound analgesia
Minimal bleeding
Avoidance of the oculocardiac reflex
Control of intraocular pressure
Awareness of drug interactions
Smooth emergence with no vomiting or coughing

the globe and by traction on the extraocular muscles, especially the medial rectus. Monitoring the electrocardiogram is essential for early recognition of this reflex. Prevention and treatment are with intravenous atropine. During pediatric strabismus surgery, atropine (20 $\mu g \cdot kg^{-1}$ iv) is often recommended before beginning surgery. Atropine administered intramuscularly for preoperative medication is not effective for preventing this reflex.

IV. ANESTHETIC RAMIFICATIONS OF OPHTHALMIC DRUGS

Topical ophthalmic drugs may produce undesirable systemic effects or have deleterious anesthetic implications.
  A. Echothiophate is a long-acting anticholinesterase miotic that decreases IOP and prolongs the effect of SCh.

TABLE 23-2. Events That Alter Intraocular Pressure

Decreased	Increased
Volatile anesthetics	Increased venous pressure owing to cough or vomiting
Injected anesthetics (? ketamine)	Direct laryngoscopy
Hyperventilation	Succinylcholine
Hypothermia	Arterial hypoxemia
Mannitol	Hypoventilation
Glycerin	
Nondepolarizing muscle relaxants	
Timolol	

B. **Cyclopentolate** is a mydriatic that may produce central nervous system toxicity.

C. **Phenylephrine** is a mydriatic that may produce cardiovascular effects.

D. **Acetazolamide,** when administered chronically to lower IOP, may be associated with renal loss of bicarbonate and potassium ions.

E. **Timolol** lowers IOP, but systemic absorption may result in cardiac depression and increased airway resistance.

F. **Sulfur hexafluoride (SF6)** is injected into the vitreous to mechanically facilitate retinal reattachment. Nitrous oxide (N_2O) (blood:gas solubility 0.47) should be avoided for 10 days following intravitreous injection of SF6 (blood:gas solubility 0.004).

V. PREOPERATIVE EVALUATION

Patients with eye lesions are often at the extremes of age. Elderly patients may have age-related organ dysfunction unrelated to ocular disease necessitating surgery. Diabetes mellitus is the most common metabolic disease that is associated with ocular manifestations.

VI. SELECTION OF ANESTHESIA

Most ophthalmic procedures may be performed in adults under either local or general anesthesia. Available data have failed to demonstrate a significant difference in complications between local and general anesthesia for cataract surgery (Table 23-3).

A. **Akinesia** of the globe is provided by retrobulbar block, deep general anesthesia, or skeletal muscle paralysis. Patient comfort is improved by administration of methohexital, 10–30 mg iv, before performance of the retrobulbar block. Retrobulbar block may be associated with significant complications, emphasizing

---

TABLE 23-3. Factors That Influence Choice of Anesthesia

Nature and duration of procedure
Coagulation status
Patient's ability to communicate and cooperate
Personal preference of the anesthesiologist

TABLE 23-4. Complications of Retrobulbar Block

Stimulation of the oculocardiac reflex arc
Retrobulbar hemorrhage
Puncture of the posterior globe, resulting in retinal
detachment and vitreous hemorrhage
Central retinal artery occlusion
Penetration of the optic nerve
Accidental brain stem anesthesia
Accidental intraocular injection

that local anesthesia does not necessarily involve less physiologic trespass than general anesthesia (Table 23-4).

B. **Opioids** are avoided in view of their presumed emetic potential. In this regard, prophylactic administration of antiemetics (droperidol, 2.5–7.5 $\mu g \cdot kg^{-1}$) is a consideration.

C. If general anesthesia is elected, extubation of the trachea should be accomplished before there is a tendency for the patient to cough. Administration of lidocaine (1.5–2.0 $mg \cdot kg^{-1}$ iv) before extubation of the trachea may be helpful in attenuating the cough reflex.

VII. ANESTHETIC MANAGEMENT OF SPECIFIC SITUATIONS

A. **Open eye–full stomach.** Anesthesiologists must weigh the risk of aspiration against the risk of blindness in an injured eye that could result from elevated IOP and extrusion of ocular contents.

1. Consider preoperative administration of H_2 antagonists or metoclopramide or both.

2. **Induction of anesthesia** is often with thiopental (4 $mg \cdot kg^{-1}$) plus a high dose of a nondepolarizing muscle relaxant such as pancuronium, atracurium, or vecuronium. A dose of muscle relaxant equivalent to three times that necessary to depress twitch 95% (3 × ED_{95}) is often recommended. An advantage of a nondepolarizing muscle relaxant is unchanged or decreased IOP in contrast to transient increases produced by SCh. This advantage may be offset by delayed onset and prolonged duration of action for what otherwise may be a short opera-

TABLE 23-5. Considerations for Strabismus Surgery

Oculocardiac reflex
Increased incidence of malignant hyperthermia
Interference by succinylcholine in interpretation of forced duction test
Increased incidence of postoperative nausea and vomiting

tion. Although the method is controversial, there are no published reports of loss of intraocular contents from a nondepolarizing muscle relaxant pretreatment-barbiturate-SCh induction sequence when used in this setting.

3. Regardless of the muscle relaxant selected, any premature attempt at intubation of the trachea produces coughing, straining, and a dramatic rise in IOP, emphasizing the need to confirm the onset of drug effect with a peripheral nerve stimulator.

4. Intubation of the trachea in the awake patient is not acceptable because a patient's reaction elevates IOP.

B. **Strabismus surgery** is the most common pediatric ocular operation and is often performed on an outpatient basis. Unique concerns may be associated with this operation (Table 23-5).

C. **Intraocular surgery** (glaucoma drainage surgery, open eye vitrectomy, corneal transplants, cataract extraction). Unique concerns and requirements are associated with these operations (Table 23-6).

1. Epinephrine 1:200,000 may be infused into the anterior chamber to produce mydriasis. Systemic absorption and resulting cardiac dysrhythmias in the presence of volatile anesthetics have not been documented to be a problem.

2. Nondepolarizing muscle relaxants administered to provide akinesia can be safely reversed even in patients with glaucoma because the combination of

TABLE 23-6. Considerations for Intraocular Surgery

Control of intraocular pressure
Continue miotics in glaucoma patients
Need for complete akinesia
Provide an antiemetic effect

anticholinesterase and anticholinergic drugs, in conventional doses, has minimal effects on pupil size and IOP.

D. Retinal detachment surgery

1. Internal tamponade of the retinal break may be accomplished by injecting the expandable gas SF6 into the vitreous. Owing to blood:gas partition coefficient differences, the concomitant administration of N_2O may enhance the internal tamponade effect of SF6 intraoperatively, resulting in elevations in IOP and interference with retinal circulation (see Section IV F). For this reason, N_2O probably should be discontinued for at least 15 minutes before injection of SF6 and likewise N_2O probably should not be administered for 10 days after the injection.

2. Reduction of IOP is often provided by intravenous administration of acetazolamide or mannitol.

3. Akinesia is not critical, and inhalation anesthetics need not be accompanied intraoperatively by nondepolarizing muscle relaxants.

VIII. CORNEAL ABRASION

Corneal abrasion is the most common ocular complication following general anesthesia. Patients complain of pain and a foreign body sensation that is exacerbated by blinking. An ophthalmology consultation is appropriate, and treatment is prophylactic topical application of antibiotic ointment and patching the injured eye. Healing usually occurs within 24–48 hours.

24

Anesthesia for Ear, Nose, and Throat Surgery

A common feature of many otorhinolaryngology procedures is the need for the anesthesiologist and the surgeon to share the patient's airway (Feinstein R, Owens WD: Anesthesia for Ear, Nose, and Throat Surgery. In Barash PG, Cullen BF, Stoelting RK [eds]: Clinical Anesthesia, pp 1113–1124. Philadelphia, JB Lippincott, 1992). In some patients, edema, infection, or tumor may compromise the airway preoperatively.

I. LARYNGOSCOPY AND MICROLARYNGOSCOPY

   A. Many patients presenting for endoscopic procedures have disease that is compromising the airway.
   B. An antisialagogue is useful to minimize oral secretions and provide optimal surgical working conditions.
   C. Immobility during general anesthesia is often provided by muscle relaxants.
   D. Intubation of the trachea with a small internal diameter endotracheal tube (5–6 mm internal diameter) permits adequate ventilation of the lungs and still provides the surgeon with acceptable visualization. If the endotracheal tube interferes with the surgeon's view, an alternate method of ventilating the lungs (Carden's tube, high-frequency jet ventilation) may be selected. Location and position of the tracheal tube must be frequently evaluated because movement of the head may cause the tube to move.

II. LASER LARYNGOSCOPY

   A. Advantages of lasers include extreme precision, almost no blood loss (because the heat generated produces immediate coagulation), and minimal tissue edema.
   B. The primary anesthetic consideration in laser surgery is avoidance of damage to viable tissue in the patient or among operating room personnel. **The eyes are most vul-**

nerable to injury and must be protected. Patient immobility produced by muscle relaxants is important so as
to be able to direct the laser beam precisely.

C. The most serious danger during any laser surgery is **fire**;
this consideration is especially important in laser surgery in the airway. Polyvinylchloride is highly flamma-
ble, and tracheal tubes made of this material should not
be used. Nitrous oxide (N_2O) supports combustion but
does offer protection as a diluent to reduce delivered
concentrations of oxygen. Helium may be a useful diluent to replace N_2O and permit maintenance of inhaled
oxygen concentrations at the lowest acceptable level
(ideally <40%).

1. Tracheal tube cuffs may be filled with water or saline
to enable them to absorb more energy before becom-
ing hot or disrupted. Furthermore, if the cuff is penetrated by the laser beam, the escaping liquid helps
extinguish any fire.

2. Airway fire is treated by turning off the oxygen, removing the flaming endotracheal tube from the airway, and extinguishing the fire with sterile water or
saline (Table 24-1).

III. ADENOTONSILLECTOMY

A. Airway obstruction is likely to be present in patients
with **obstructive sleep apnea.** Visualization of the glottis
by direct laryngoscopy so as to intubate the trachea may
be difficult in these patients. Consider awake tracheal
intubation.

B. An antisialagogue is useful to minimize oral secretions
and provide optimal surgical working conditions.

C. Once the trachea is intubated, the surgeon places a
mouth gag, and the position and patency of the tube are

TABLE 24-1. Procedure for Extinguishing Airway Fires

Disconnect the breathing circuit from the endotracheal tube

Remove the endotracheal tube and any remaining smoldering
components in the patient's airway

Re-establish the airway and ventilate the lungs with air until
you are certain that nothing is left burning in the throat;
then switch to 100% oxygen

Examine the patient's airway to determine the extent of
damage and treat accordingly

Save the tube for later examination

again confirmed. Anesthesia is maintained with or without muscle relaxants.

D. Blood loss during tonsillectomy averages 4 ml·kg^{-1} but is often underestimated because of an undetermined amount of blood that drains into the stomach.

E. The most frequent complication of tonsillectomy is postoperative bleeding (90% occurs in the first 9 hours), with resultant hypovolemia and airway obstruction. Intubation of the trachea while the patient is awake may be considered if reoperation is required to control bleeding. Alternatively, ketamine (1–2 mg·kg^{-1} iv) or an inhalation induction may be chosen. The most important goal is to restore and maintain intravascular fluid volume (rehydration with lactated Ringer's solution, 15–20 ml·kg^{-1}) before induction of anesthesia. The stomach should be emptied by means of an orogastric tube after placement of the tracheal tube.

IV. CANCER OF THE HEAD AND NECK

A. Patients are often elderly and have a history of cigarette smoking and alcohol abuse with associated chronic obstructive pulmonary disease, hypertension, coronary artery disease, and liver disease. Unless airway obstruction is imminent, surgery should be delayed until a patient's medical condition can be optimized.

B. If airway obstruction is present, an anesthesiologist should consider intubation of the trachea in the awake patient with the aid of a flexible fiberscope or should recommend a tracheostomy using local anesthesia.

C. Blood loss is difficult to estimate because much of it is hidden from view. Controlled hypotension may be considered in an attempt to reduce blood loss. Use of controlled hypotension is limited by the presence of associated atherosclerosis, especially coronary artery disease.

D. No specific anesthetic technique or drug combination has been shown to be superior to any other. Use of muscle relaxants may be limited by a surgeon's need to evaluate intactness of nerves (facial nerve) during neck dissection or parotid surgery.

E. If the procedure involves a neck dissection, manipulation of the carotid sinus can result in cardiac dysrhythmias and wide fluctuations in blood pressure. Infiltration of the surrounding tissues with lidocaine is the recommended treatment.

F. Neck veins that are open during neck dissection can be a source of venous air embolism.

G. If a tracheostomy is not performed as part of the operation, an anesthesiologist must decide whether the surgical procedure produced sufficient edema or distortion to compromise the airway. If there is any doubt, the patient's trachea should remain intubated in the immediate postoperative period.

V. SURGICAL PROCEDURES INVOLVING THE EAR

A. The majority of procedures done on the ear involve the middle ear in otherwise young and healthy patients with hearing loss. Nausea and dizziness are common postoperative problems, emphasizing the possible value of avoiding opioids in the preoperative medication and anesthetic management as well as considering the administration of prophylactic antiemetics.

B. Use of N_2O is controversial because this gas can enter the closed space represented by the middle ear more rapidly than air can leave. As a result, middle ear pressures may increase during administration of N_2O, only to become negative when the gas is discontinued. Discontinuation of N_2O at least 5 minutes before placement of a tympanic membrane graft prevents subsequent dislodgment of the graft or drug-induced increases in middle ear pressure.

C. A bloodless operative field is important for microsurgical procedures in the ear. Controlled hypotension or local infiltration of the surgical site with epinephrine-containing solutions may be a consideration.

D. Identification and preservation of the facial nerve are always given consideration in surgical procedures on the ear. For this reason, intense drug-induced skeletal muscle paralysis that would prevent a surgeon from eliciting a facial nerve response with direct electrical nerve stimulation is avoided.

E. Volatile anesthetics can produce an adequate level of anesthesia and obviate the need for muscle relaxants and N_2O. In addition, the incidence of nausea and vomiting may be less with a volatile anesthetic in the absence of N_2O or opioids.

VI. TRACHEOSTOMY

Tracheostomy is best performed electively in the operating room with a translaryngeal tracheal tube in place to facilitate ventilation of the lungs and permit an unhurried surgical procedure.

25

Anesthesia and the Renal System

The kidneys receive 20–25% of the cardiac output. About 10% of the renal blood flow (RBF) (1250 ml·min^{-1}) is filtered, producing a glomerular filtration rate (GFR) of 125 ml·min^{-1} (180 l·day^{-1}), which contrasts strikingly with the urine production of about 1–2 ml·min^{-1} (Prough DS, Foreman AS: Anesthesia and the renal system. In Barash PG, Cullen BF, Stoelting RK [eds]: Clinical Anesthesia, pp 1125–1155. Philadelphia, JB Lippincott, 1992).

I. PHYSIOLOGY OF URINE FORMATION

A. Filtration, reabsorption, and secretion are the three major functions of the kidneys.

B. **Neurohumoral regulation of the renal function**

1. The major physiologic influences determining the reabsorption of filtered Na$^+$ and water are the hormonal factors (Table 25-1).

2. The physiologic stress of trauma and surgery is associated with reduced urinary excretion of Na$^+$ and water, which reflects changes in intravascular and extracellular fluid volume as well as neuroendocrine effects.

II. RENAL PHARMACOLOGY

A. **Comparative renal pharmacology of inhaled and injected anesthetics.** Virtually all anesthetic drugs and techniques are associated with **decreases in RBF, GFR, and urinary output,** reflecting multiple mechanisms (Table 25-2).

1. Significant amounts of **fluoride ion** are released from enflurane but not from halothane or isoflurane. Clinically, this may manifest as decreases in urine concentrating ability, as the renal tubules are unresponsive to antidiuretic hormone (ADH), especially

TABLE 25-1. Hormonal Factors Responsible for Na⁺ and Water Reabsorption

Aldosterone (most important regulator of Na^+ reabsorption)
Antidiuretic hormone (reabsorption of water at collecting ducts)
Atrial natriuretic factor
Prostaglandins

TABLE 25-2. Mechanisms for Anesthetic-Induced Changes in Renal Function

Decreases in cardiac output (myocardial contractility, venous return, blood volume)
Altered autonomic nervous sytem function
Neuroendocrine changes
Mechanical ventilation (positive end-expiratory pressure)

when serum fluoride concentrations exceed 50 $\mu M \cdot l^{-1}$ **(high-output renal failure).**

2. Pre-existing intravascular fluid volume and the amount of intravenous fluid influence the renal response to anesthesia.

B. **Pharmacology of diuretics** (Table 25-3)

III. CHRONIC RENAL FAILURE

A. **Clinical characteristics.** Until <40% of normal functioning nephrons remain, there are no signs, symptoms, or laboratory abnormalities suggestive of renal failure. The **uremic syndrome** occurs with loss of >95% of functioning nephrons and requires dialysis for continued survival (Table 25-4).

1. Complications of renal failure are multiple (Table 25-5).

TABLE 25-3. Pharmacology of Diuretics

Osmotic diuretics (mannitol, 0.25–1.5 $g \cdot kg^{-1}$ iv, to reduce brain size or protect the kidneys during abdominal aneurysm surgery; hypovolemia can occur)
Loop diuretics (furosemide)
Aldosterone antagonists (spironolactone, K^+ sparing)

TABLE 25-4. Stages of Chronic Renal Failure

	Glomerular Filtration Rate (ml·min^{-1})	Signs and Symptoms	Laboratory Abnormalities
Normal	125	None	None
Decreased renal reserve	50–80	None	None
Renal insufficiency	12–50	Nocturia	Increased blood urea nitrogen and serum creatinine levels
Uremia	<12	Uremic syndrome	See Table 28–5

TABLE 25-5. Complications of Renal Failure

Fluid overload (congestive heart failure, hypertension)

Hyperkalemia

Metabolic acidosis

Platelet dysfunction

Neurologic complications (central, peripheral, and autonomic nervous systems)

Pericarditis

Anemia (erythropoietin deficiency and shortened erythrocyte survival time)

Nausea and vomiting

Sepsis

Hepatitis

    a. Most of the fluid and electrolyte, pH, neurologic, and platelet abnormalities improve with dialysis.

    b. Anemia (hemoglobin 5–7 $g \cdot dl^{-1}$) is well tolerated (transfusions not needed) because tissue blood flow increases secondary to decreased blood viscosity and increased cardiac output. A further aid to tissue oxygenation is a **shift of the oxyhemoglobin dissociation curve to the right** owing to acidosis and increased concentrations of 2,3-diphosphoglycerate.

TABLE 25-6. Indications for Dialysis

Intravascular fluid volume overload

Azotemia

Hyperkalemia

Acid-base disturbances

TABLE 25-7. Complications of Dialysis

Central nervous system disturbances (seizures, dementia)

Hypotension

Arterial hypoxemia

Skeletal muscle cramping

Nutritional depletion

B. **Dialytic treatment.** Many such patients require surgery for maintenance of vascular access (hemodialysis). Indications for acute dialytic therapy in acute renal failure are well defined (Table 25-6).

C. Physiologic effects and **complications of dialysis** and ultrafiltration (Table 25-7).

IV. ANESTHETIC MANAGEMENT OF PATIENTS WITH CHRONIC RENAL FAILURE

A. **Preoperative evaluation** (Table 25-8)

B. **Intraoperative management**
   1. **Monitoring.** An electrocardiogram may provide early detection of hyperkalemia. Pulse oximetry is especially useful because of the increased risk of tissue hypoxia in the presence of anemia if the oxygen saturation decreases.
   2. Dialysis can be repeated in the immediate postoperative period if intraoperative fluid requirements increase intravascular fluid volume to a postoperative level that is unsatisfactory.

C. **Selection of anesthetic agents**
   1. **Intravenous agents.** Reduced protein binding (especially thiopental) and uremia-induced alterations in the blood-brain barrier may result in the need for lower induction doses of intravenous drugs. Accumulation of morphine glucuronides may account for the prolonged depression of ventilation observed in some patients with renal failure. This complication should be less likely with low doses of fentanyl.

TABLE 25-8. Preoperative Evaluation of Patients with Renal Failure

---

Renal function tests (insensitive and influenced by hydration, nutrition, age, skeletal muscle mass)

    Blood urea nitrogen, 8–20 mg·dl^{-1}

    Creatinine, 0.5–1.2 mg·dl^{-1}

    Creatinine clearance, 120 ml·min^{-1}

Adequacy of dialysis (pH, electrolytes, blood pressure)

Hemoglobin concentration

Neurologic dysfunction (influences choice of regional anesthesia)

Consider delayed gastric emptying time

Reduce doses of sedative premedicant drugs

TABLE 25-9. Advantages of Volatile Anesthetics in Patients with Renal Failure
Lack of dependence on renal function for clearance
Permit delivery of maximal oxygen concentrations
Decrease muscle relaxant dose requirements

2. **Inhalation anesthetics.** Compared with intravenous drugs, the potent volatile anesthetics may have some advantages in patients with renal failure (Table 25-9).
3. **Neuromuscular blocking agents** (see Chapter 15)
   a. Atracurium and to a lesser extent vecuronium are preferable to long-acting nondepolarizing muscle relaxant drugs because of their minimal to absent dependence on renal clearance.
   b. Succinylcholine-induced K^+ release is not altered by renal failure, but in the presence of pre-existing hyperkalemia the additional drug-induced increase in serum K^+ (about 0.5 $mEq \cdot l^{-1}$) could produce cardiac dysrhythmias.
   c. Recurarization is unlikely because elimination of anticholinesterases is also dependent on renal function.

V. ACUTE RENAL FAILURE

Perioperative acute renal failure accounts for one half of all patients requiring acute dialysis and is associated with a mortality in excess of 50% (see Chapter 25).
A. **Pathophysiology.** Oliguric states (urine output < 30 $ml \cdot h^{-1}$) are defined as prerenal, renal (acute tubular necrosis), and postrenal (obstructive) (Table 25-10).
   1. Prerenal refers to oliguria produced by hemodynamic effects (**most often hypovolemia and/or decreased cardiac output** with associated decreases in RBF) that may progress to acute renal failure. Acute renal failure is especially likely in the presence of sepsis, burns, or in elderly patients undergoing high-risk surgery such as cardiopulmonary bypass or resection of an abdominal aneurysm.
   2. The early phase of acute renal failure is often amenable to prompt therapeutic interventions, whereas

TABLE 25-10. Differential Diagnosis of
             Causes of Oliguria

	Prerenal	Renal
Urine osmolarity	>500 mOsm·l^{-1}	<350 mOsm·l^{-1}
Urine/plasma osmolality	>1.3	<1.1
Urine Na$^+$	<20 mEq·l^{-1}	>40 mEq·l^{-1}
Urine/plasma urea	>8	<3

delayed improvement in RBF may not reverse acute renal failure.

B. **Comparison of oliguric and nonoliguric acute renal failure.** Nonoliguric renal failure is somewhat easier to manage clinically because it requires less scrupulous control of fluid and electrolyte intake. Chemical conversion of oliguric to nonoliguric acute renal failure does not improve outcome.

C. **Therapeutic conflicts in the management of acute oliguria**
   1. **Kidney/lung therapeutic conflicts.** Aggressive expansion of intravascular fluid volume in the management of prerenal oliguria may put patients at risk for the development of pulmonary edema, which is easier to treat than acute renal failure.

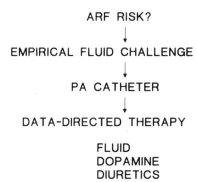

Figure 25-1. Algorithm for management of acute renal failure (ARF). PA = pulmonary artery.

2. **Kidney/heart therapeutic conflicts.** Aggressive volume expansion may increase left ventricular end-diastolic pressure, which limits subendocardial perfusion. Vasodilators may improve cardiac function in these patients.

D. **Suggested management.** No specific therapy guidelines routinely produce the least compromise to the kidneys, lungs, and heart (Fig. 25-1).

26

Anesthesia for Genitourinary Surgery

An increasing elderly population and important technological advances such as shock wave lithotripsy are changing traditional concepts of genitourinary surgery (Liu W-S, Wong KC: Anesthesia for genitourinary surgery. In Barash PG, Cullen BF, Stoelting RK [eds]: Clinical Anesthesia, pp 1157–1168. Philadelphia, JB Lippincott, 1992).

I. REGIONAL ANESTHESIA IN GENITOURINARY PROCEDURES

A. With the exception of operations on the kidney, most urologic operations are on the lower abdomen and thus are easily performed under regional anesthetic techniques.

B. Deep vein thrombosis of the legs occurs more often in patients undergoing urologic surgery, but the incidence may be less in patients receiving lumbar epidural anesthesia (greater blood flow) than in those receiving general anesthesia.

C. It is commonly believed that regional anesthesia causes a higher incidence of postoperative urinary retention than does general anesthesia, presumably reflecting delayed recovery of autonomic and somatic nerve functions.

II. POSITIONS IN GENITOURINARY PROCEDURES

Positions in genitourinary procedures are often anatomically unusual (lithotomy, lateral position with kidney rest elevated) and physiologically disturbing (water bath) (see Chapter 6).

III. ANESTHESIA FOR URETHRAL, BLADDER, AND URETERAL PROCEDURES

A. **Urethral procedures.** Penile block is useful for operations on the distal urethra. Internal urethrotomies require good sacral anesthesia. Urethroplasties require the exaggerated lithotomy position, and general anesthesia is often selected.

B. **Bladder procedures.** Cystoscopy is usually performed as an outpatient procedure under general or regional (T9 sensory level needed) anesthesia. Repeated cystoscopies are often necessary in patients with spinal cord injury, introducing the risk of autonomic hyperreflexia, especially if the level of cord transection is above T5. To reduce the risk of autonomic hyper-reflexia, spinal or epidural anesthesia is often selected.

IV. ANESTHESIA FOR OPERATIONS ON THE EXTERNAL GENITALIA

A. Deep general anesthesia is needed, as the genital and perineal areas are highly innervated.

B. Neural blockade (caudal, subarachnoid, penile) suppresses operative responses and provides much needed postoperative analgesia. Testicular surgery requires a T10 sensory level. Caudal anesthesia (bupivacaine, 1.25–1.5 mg·kg^{-1}) using a 20-gauge needle provides excellent analgesia in children following hypospadias repair, orchiopexy, and circumcision. Penile anesthesia is also useful in children and adults.

V. ANESTHESIA FOR PROSTATIC SURGERY

Patients are usually elderly and often have coexisting cardiopulmonary disease.

A. **Open prostatectomy.** Choice of regional or general anesthesia is influenced by a patient's mental status, associated cardiopulmonary diseases, and the surgical position. For example, the perineal approach necessitates an exaggerated lithotomy position, which favors general anesthesia.

B. **Transurethral resection of the prostate** is performed through a resectoscope and consists of excising the hypertrophied lateral and median lobes of the prostate gland with an electrically energized wire loop. Bleeding is controlled with a coagulating current. Continuous irrigating fluid (nonelectrolyte solutions consisting of sorbitol, mannitol, or glycine) is used to distend the bladder and to wash away blood and dissected prostatic tissue. The amount of irrigating fluid absorbed depends on the hydrostatic pressure driving fluid into prostatic veins and the duration of resection ($10-30$ ml·min^{-1}; limit resection time to 60 minutes).

1. **Transurethral resection of the prostate syndrome.** Headache, confusion, and hypertension reflect intravascular absorption of irrigating solution (Table 26–1).

2. **Blood loss during transurethral resection of the prostate** is difficult to estimate but averages about 15 ml·g^{-1} of prostatic tissue resected.

3. **Hypothermia during transurethral resection of the prostate** reflects intravascular absorption of cold fluid, which rapidly lowers core body temperature.

4. **Bacteremia** manifests as sudden cardiovascular collapse after transurethral resection of the prostate.

5. **Perforation of the bladder** in conscious patients may result in upper abdominal pain or referred pain from the diaphragm to the shoulder. Subdiaphragmatic irritation from intraperitoneal irrigating fluid may induce hiccups and dyspnea. Catheter drainage is often sufficient treatment for bladder perforation.

6. **Choice of anesthetic techniques**
   a. Spinal anesthesia (5% lidocaine, 0.5% tetracaine) provides a predictable block (at T10 sensory level) in awake patients who can give early warning of fluid overload or bladder perforation.
   b. Epidural anesthesia may miss sacral segments.
   c. General anesthesia allows support of ventilation and is indicated for uncooperative patients.
   d. Monitoring central venous pressure provides early evidence of fluid overload, which is best treated with saline-containing solutions and diuretics.
   e. Only modest discomfort is associated with this operation; therefore postoperative analgesia is usually not a problem.

TABLE 26-1. Complications of Transurethral Resection

Hypervolemia
Dilutional hyponatremia
Decreased serum osmolarity
Ammonia toxicity (limited to glycine)
Blindness (limited to glycine)

VI. ANESTHESIA FOR OTHER UROLOGIC PROCEDURES

A. **Percutaneous ultrasonic lithotripsy.** Normal saline is recommended for irrigation to avoid acute hyponatremia caused by fluid absorption. General, epidural, and local anesthesia have been successfully used.

27

Anesthesia and Obesity and Gastrointestinal Disorders

Obesity and gastrointestinal disorders are characterized by pathophysiologic changes that often impact on the management of anesthesia (Buckley PP: Anesthesia and obesity and gastrointestinal disorders. In Barash PG, Cullen BF, Stoelting RK [eds]: Clinical Anesthesia, pp 1169–1183. Philadelphia, JB Lippincott, 1992).

I. OBESITY

A. Obesity is frequently defined in terms of the **body mass index,** which is calculated as body weight (kilograms) divided by height squared (meters) (Table 27-1).

B. Patients with **android obesity** have fat distributed in the truncal (abdominal) region. Patients with **gynecoid obesity** have fat in the thighs and buttocks and are less prone to the respiratory or cardiovascular complications of obesity.

C. **Pathophysiology**

1. **Airway management** can be particularly difficult when anesthetizing obese patients. **Anatomic factors** that may interfere with mask ventilation and endotracheal intubation are listed in Table 27-2.

2. Obese patients have an increased incidence of hiatal hernia, increased intra-abdominal pressure, and increased gastric fluid volume and acidity. Thus, they are at increased risk for gastric aspiration and **pneumonitis.**

3. **Respiration.** Obesity can affect **ventilation** through both metabolic and mechanical means (Table 27-3; Fig. 27-1).

TABLE 27-1. Body Mass Index* As a Reflection of Obesity

Normal 24
Obesity >28
Morbid obesity >35

*Weight (kilograms) divided by height squared (meters).

TABLE 27-2. Anatomic Features of the Upper Airway in Obese Patients

Short and thick neck
Redundant pharyngeal and palatal soft tissue
Anterior larynx
Large tongue

---

4. **The Pickwickian syndrome** is associated with severe obesity and respiratory compromise. Manifestations can include those listed in Table 27-4.
5. **Circulation.** Because of an increased tissue mass and increased oxygen consumption, considerable stress is placed on an obese patient's cardiovascular system (Table 27-5; Fig. 27-2).

D. **Pharmacokinetics**

1. The behavior of many drugs may be altered in obese patients. The large volume of fat has limited blood supply and does not play a significant role in the **acute** phase of drug distribution and elimination. However, drug doses should be carefully tailored when administered on a mg·kg^{-1} basis.

TABLE 27-3. Effects of Obesity on Ventilation

Increased oxygen consumption
Increased carbon dioxide production
Increased minute ventilation
Increased work of breathing
Decreased chest wall compliance
Decreased lung volumes
Hypoxemia

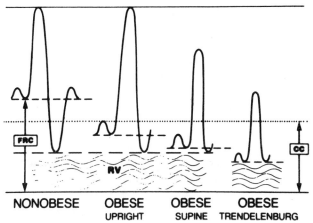

Figure 27-1. The effects of change in position on lung volumes in nonobese and obese patients. FRC = functional residual capacity; RV = residual volume; cc = closing capacity.

TABLE 27-4. Manifestations of the Pickwickian Syndrome
Hypercarbia
Hypoxemia
Polycythemia
Sleep apnea
Pulmonary hypertension
Congestive heart failure
Predisposition to upper airway obstruction

TABLE 27-5. Effects of Obesity on Circulation
Increased cardiac output
Increased blood volume
Systemic hypertension
Pulmonary hypertension
Cardiac ventricular hypertrophy

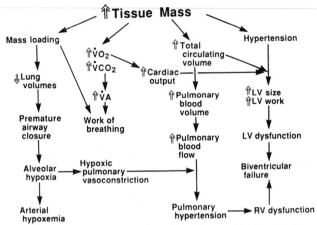

Figure 27-2. Cardiovascular and ventilation abnormalities in morbidly obese patients. LV = left ventricle; RV = right ventricle.

2. Theoretically, **lipid-soluble** anesthetics, such as fentanyl, thiopental, benzodiazepines, and volatile anesthetics, would be expected to have longer elimination half-times ($T_{1/2\beta}$) and decreased clearance when given to obese patients. Clinically, this does not appear to be the case. The central nervous system response of obese patients to an induction dose of **thiopental** does not differ from that of lean patients. **Hydrophilic** drugs, such as muscle relaxants, have similar volumes of distribution, $T_{1/2\beta}$, and clearance in obese and lean patients.

E. **Preoperative preparation of obese patients**
   1. Several factors must be taken into consideration when planning an anesthetic for obese patients (Table 27-6).
   2. Obese patients may benefit from **premedication** with H_2 antagonists, metoclopramide, and/or antacids to decrease the volume and acidity of gastric contents. Anticholinergic drugs may be indicated if awake or fiberoptic intubation of the trachea is planned. Sedatives, hypnotics, and opioids should be used with extreme caution, particularly if a patient may have the sleep apnea syndrome.

F. **Intraoperative management**
   1. **Monitoring** of obese patients is extremely important. A blood pressure cuff is acceptable if the anesthetic

TABLE 27-6. Problems Associated With Obesity

Problem	Signs/Symptoms	Tests
Airway obstruction	Sleep disturbances Snoring	Physical examination Review previous anesthetic history
Cardiovascular disease	Dyspnea Orthopnea Angina	Blood pressure Electrocardiogram Chest radiograph Two-dimensional transesophageal echocardiography
Respiratory disease	Cyanosis Dyspnea	Arterial blood gases Pulmonary function tests Chest radiograph
Gastrointestinal disease	Heartburn Reflux	History Upper gastrointestinal radiographs
Metabolic disease	Diabetes mellitus Fatty liver infiltration	Blood glucose Liver function tests

is to be short and the operation minor. Oscillometric devices work well on the forearm or calf if a cuff cannot easily be placed on the upper arm. An **arterial catheter** is frequently desirable because obese patients are susceptible to large blood pressure fluctuations and **arterial blood gas** determinations are often needed. **Central venous** or **pulmonary artery pressure** monitoring is indicated if a patient has evidence of impaired cardiac function. **End-tidal carbon dioxide** measurement and **pulse oximetry** are advisable, because obese patients are prone to hypoxia and hypoventilation. Because obese patients need full muscle function to breathe postoperatively, muscle relaxation should be continuously assessed with a peripheral **nerve stimulator.**

2. **Airway management** can be exceedingly difficult. Except for very short procedures, endotracheal intubation should be performed whenever general anesthesia is administered (Table 27-7).

  a. **Awake tracheal intubation** is a safe and conservative approach for massively obese patients, for those with small mouths or short necks, for patients with sleep apnea, and for patients with

---

TABLE 27-7. Reasons to Intubate the Trachea of Obese Patients

May be difficult to maintain a patent upper airway with only a mask and oral airway
High risk for aspiration of gastric contents
Controlled ventilation is usually indicated

---

compromised pulmonary or cardiovascular function. Alternatively, the ease of tracheal intubation can be assessed using a laryngoscope and topical anesthesia in awake patients. If the pharynx is spacious and the epiglottis or vocal cords can be seen, it may be safe to induce general anesthesia before intubation of the trachea. Because of the propensity of obese patients to have gastric regurgitation, induction with a **rapid-sequence** technique with cricoid pressure should be considered.

b. **Denitrogenation** of the lungs by breathing 100% oxygen before induction of anesthesia is recommended because obese patients have decreased lung volumes and increased oxygen consumption, which can cause desaturation to occur rapidly during apnea.

3. **Regional anesthesia** may be difficult to administer because of body fat and indistinct landmarks. The use of a peripheral nerve stimulator and insulated needles may facilitate performance of brachial plexus and peripheral **nerve blocks. Spinal anesthesia** is useful for lower abdominal and extremity surgery, but the dose of local anesthetics must be reduced by 20–25% below that used for lean patients. Having patients sit up makes location of the midline and insertion of the spinal needle easier. **Epidural anesthesia** may be safely administered to obese patients, but the dose of local anesthetic should also be reduced. If the level of anesthesia is high, it is often advisable to supplement epidural anesthesia with "light" general anesthesia delivered through an endotracheal tube. Epidural anesthesia has the added benefit that the catheter can be used to provide postoperative opioid analgesia. Despite the use of regional anesthesia, obese patients must be monitored as intensely as if general anesthesia were used, and anesthe-

siologists must be fully prepared to convert to general anesthesia if the need arises.

4. **General anesthesia** may be accomplished using various anesthetic agents. The dose of **thiopental** must be tailored to a patient's needs and not arbitrarily administered on a $mg \cdot kg^{-1}$ basis. The usefulness of nitrous oxide is limited because obese patients frequently have a large pulmonary shunt and usually require a minimum fractional inspired oxygen (FIO_2) of 0.5. Obese patients metabolize volatile anesthetics to a greater extent than do lean patients. **Halothane** is probably not a wise choice for routine use, because obese patients metabolize the drug by the potentially hepatotoxic reductive pathway. The metabolism of **methoxyflurane** and **enflurane** is also increased in obese patients, placing them at possible risk for fluoride-induced renal toxicity. **Isoflurane** appears to be a logical volatile anesthetic for use with obese patients. The supposition that obese patients absorb large quantities of fat-soluble anesthetic gases into their tissues and that recovery from anesthesia is prolonged has been disproved.

   a. Great care should be exercised when administering **opioids** to obese patients, because these patients are predisposed to hypoxia and hypoventilation in the postoperative period. If opioids are necessary, the use of temporary mechanical ventilation of the lungs in the recovery period should be considered.

   b. General anesthesia worsens an obese patient's already compromised ventilatory status by further decreasing functional residual capacity, disrupting ventilation-to-perfusion relationships, and predisposing a patient to the development of increasing venous admixture. **Controlled ventilation** with an $FIO_2 > 0.5$ is recommended. Assessment of oxygenation by pulse oximetry or re-

---

TABLE 27-8. Postoperative Care of Obese Patients

Supplemental oxygen
Monitor with pulse oximetry
Recovery in semisitting position
Early ambulation
Regional techniques for pain control

peated arterial blood gas determinations or both are indicated.

    c. It is best to wait until patients are awake and their normal muscle function has returned before extubating the trachea.

  5. Postoperative care of obese patients should include the measures listed in Table 27-8.

II. GASTROINTESTINAL DISORDERS

  A. Esophagus

    1. The major barrier to gastroesophageal reflux is the **lower esophageal sphincter.** The tendency for reflux to occur is a function of sphincter tone and the pressure gradient between the stomach and the esophagus. Conditions associated with decreased lower esophageal tone are listed in Table 27-9.

    2. Many drugs may alter lower esophageal tone (Table 27-10).

  B. The **stomach.** Gastric secretions are produced at a rate of 2000 ml·day^{-1}, usually with a pH of 1–3.5. Multiple factors can influence the rate of gastric emptying (Table 27-11).

    1. Having a patient consume nothing by mouth for the customary 4–6 hours preoperatively does not guar-

---

TABLE 27-9. Conditions Associated With Decreased Lower Esophageal Sphincter Tone

Obesity

Pregnancy

Hiatal hernia

History of gastroesophageal reflux

TABLE 27-10. Drugs That Alter Lower Esophageal Sphincter Tone

Increase	Decrease
Metoclopramide	Atropine
Neostigmine	Glycopyrrolate
Edrophonium	Opioids
Succinylcholine	Volatile anesthetics
	Thiopental

TABLE 27-11. **Factors That Influence the Rate of Gastric Emptying**

Cause	Increase	Decrease
Physiologic	Gastric distention Neurosis	Food Acid Pregnancy
Pathologic	Thyrotoxicosis	Anxiety Pain Shock Diabetes Angina
Pharmacologic	Metoclopramide Neostigmine Nicotine (smoking)	Opioids Alcohol Anticholinergics Tricyclic antidepressants

antee an empty stomach, particularly if a patient is anxious or is in pain.

2. Recent studies suggest that oral intake of small volumes of clear liquids may actually facilitate gastric emptying.

C. **The small intestine** is presented with 5–6 l of fluid per day, of which 80–90% is absorbed. Motility is **increased** by stimulation of the parasympathetic nervous system. Sympathetic nervous system stimulation, bowel manipulation during surgery, and distention of the intestine **decrease** motility.

D. **The colon** functions primarily to absorb fluid and is under control of the parasympathetic nervous system.

E. **Splanchnic blood flow** can be influenced by a number of factors (Table 27-12).

TABLE 27-12. **Factors That Influence Splanchnic Blood Flow**

Increase	Decrease
Beta stimulation	Alpha stimulation
Parasympathetic nervous system stimulation	Sympathectomy
Morphine	Hemorrhage
Hypercarbia	Hypocapnia
High spinal or epidural anesthesia	Neostigmine

TABLE 27-13. **Causes of Dehydration in Patients With Gastrointestinal Disorders**

Decreased fluid intake
Vomiting
Diarrhea
Paralytic ileus
Intestinal inflammation and edema

F. **Fluid and electrolyte balance** is important because patients with gastrointestinal disease are usually dehydrated (Table 27-13).
   1. Vomiting is typically associated with hypochloremic, hypokalemic alkalosis, whereas diarrhea may be associated with hypokalemic acidosis.
   2. When patients have a gastrointestinal disorder, preoperative assessment of **electrolytes** is essential. **Fluid resuscitation** with a balanced salt solution and K^+ usually corrects the imbalance. Patients with malnutrition or a malabsorption syndrome should receive parenteral nutrition.

III. ANESTHETIC MANAGEMENT

A. Many patients with gastrointestinal disorders, including decreased lower esophageal sphincter tone, gastroesophageal reflux, hiatal hernia, bowel obstruction, and abdominal distention, are at risk for **aspiration** of gastric contents into the lungs. When they are anesthetized, aspiration can result from active vomiting or passive regurgitation, most commonly during induction of anesthesia, when the airway is unprotected. Aspiration of solid material causes airway obstruction. Large volumes of fluid produce a syndrome similar to what occurs during drowning. If the material aspirated has a pH < 3, pneumonitis may result. Acid aspiration has also resulted in cardiovascular collapse and death. **Prevention** of aspiration of gastric contents and the acid aspiration syndrome can be facilitated by certain measures (Table 27-14).
B. Nitrous oxide has a solubility in blood that is 30 times that of nitrogen; thus, it enters gas-containing body cavities at a faster rate than the nitrogen in those cavities is removed by the circulation. Nitrous oxide entering distended bowel may interfere with surgical exposure, decrease the blood supply to the intestines, and make

TABLE 27-14. Approaches to Reduce the Risk of Aspiration

Nasogastric suction to reduce gastric volume
Facilitation of gastric emptying with metoclopramide
Increase gastric fluid pH with H_2 antagonists and/or nonparticulate antacids
Tracheal intubation in awake patients
Rapid-sequence induction of general anesthesia with application of cricoid pressure

closure of the abdomen difficult. If nitrous oxide is desired as a part of the anesthetic technique, the concentration should not exceed 50% and its use should be limited to short periods, such as during induction of and emergence from anesthesia. The amount of nitrous oxide that enters the bowel is a function of several factors (Table 27-15).

C. **Anticholinesterase drugs,** such as neostigmine, increase bowel peristalsis. Although it has not been proved, administration of these drugs theoretically may stress a recently created bowel anastomosis.

IV. SPECIFIC GASTROINTESTINAL DISORDERS

A. **Small bowel obstruction** usually is manifested as vomiting with subsequent dehydration and electrolyte abnormalities. Decompression of the stomach with a nasogastric tube, fluid resuscitation, and K^+ therapy are indicated preoperatively. Induction of general anesthesia should be accompanied by measures to protect against aspiration.

B. **Large bowel obstruction** takes longer to develop than small bowel obstruction and may result in massive abdominal distention, feculent vomiting, dehydration,

TABLE 27-15. Determinants of Nitrous Oxide Entry into the Gastrointestinal Tract

Amount of pre-existing gas in the bowel
Inspired concentration of nitrous oxide (50% is usually acceptable)
Duration of administration (equilibration takes about 100 minutes)

and electrolyte abnormalities. Gastric decompression, fluid resuscitation, and correction of electrolyte imbalance are indicated preoperatively. Measures to reduce the risk of gastric aspiration should be followed when proceeding with general anesthesia. Muscle relaxation and control of ventilation are indicated if abdominal distention is severe.

C. **Esophageal perforation** may result from ingestion of a foreign body or a corrosive fluid, a tumor, or a complication of endoscopy. If it is not detected early, patients may be severely dehydrated, in shock, and have sepsis. Ventilation and circulation may be impaired as a result of pneumomediastinum, pneumothorax, or a pleural effusion. Because of their inability to swallow, patients may have copious oral secretions. The usual operation is esophagoscopy and a thoracotomy. **Anesthetic considerations** should include those listed in Table 27-16.

D. **Intestinal perforation** results in ileus, abdominal distention, dehydration, and sepsis. **Anesthetic considerations** are described in Table 27-16.

E. **Pancreatitis** may necessitate an exploratory laparotomy. Alcoholism is a frequent cause, so patients must be evaluated for malnutrition, abnormal liver function, and early signs of alcohol withdrawal. Pancreatitis may be associated with dehydration, hypocalcemia, hyperglycemia, and adult respiratory distress syndrome.

F. **Crohn's disease,** or regional enteritis, is manifested by chronic illness, dehydration, malnutrition, anemia, bowel obstruction, and electrolyte imbalance. Patients may be receiving steroid therapy or immunosuppressants.

TABLE 27-16. Anesthetic Considerations in the Presence of Esophageal or Intestinal Perforation

Assessment of the airway (lye ingestion may cause laryngeal edema)

Preoperative correction of fluid and electrolyte disturbances

Consider the need for preoperative blood transfusion

Invasive cardiovascular monitoring

Presence of a full stomach

Anticipate exaggerated cardiovascular depressant effects of anesthetics, especially if a patient has sepsis

Do not instrument the esophagus

TABLE 27-17. **Adverse Responses That May Occur in Patients with Carcinoid Syndrome**

Dehydration	Bronchospasm
Hypotension	Cardiac failure
Hypertension	

G. **Ulcerative colitis** can result in chronic debilitation, anemia, dehydration, malnutrition, and electrolyte abnormalities. Many patients may also have coexisting arthritis, iritis, and hepatitis. Surgery may be required for bowel perforation, bowel obstruction, and hemorrhage. Patients with **toxic megacolon** are septic, critically ill, and may be in shock. Steroid therapy may be instituted. Critically ill patients may require steroid supplementation.

H. **The carcinoid syndrome** results when a carcinoid tumor in the gastrointestinal tract metastasizes to the liver. Hormones secreted by these tumors, such as **serotonin, kinins,** and **histamine,** are usually deactivated by the liver. The classic presentation of the syndrome is not always evident but may include **cutaneous flushing, hypotension, tachycardia, hypertension, diarrhea,** and **bronchospasm.** Rarely, patients may develop **cardiomyopathy.** The exact presentation depends on the predominant hormone being secreted. Taking a careful **history** is important in order to determine which symptoms patients are experiencing. **Anesthetic management** of these patients varies, depending on the nature of their disease and its complications (Tables 27-17 and 27-18).

TABLE 27-18. **Treatment of Adverse Responses Due to Carcinoid Tumors**

Fluid resuscitation
H_1 and H_2 antagonists
Steroids
Ketanserin (serotonin antagonist)
Bronchodilation with volatile anesthetics
Avoidance of drugs associated with histamine release
Use of direct-acting vasopressors
Use of vasodilators

28

Anesthesia and
the Liver

Management of anesthesia for patients with liver disease requires an understanding of the pathophysiology of liver disease (Gelman S: Anesthesia and the liver. In Barash PG, Cullen BF, Stoelting RK [eds]: Clinical Anesthesia, pp 1185–1214. Philadelphia, JB Lippincott, 1992).

I. INCIDENCE OF POSTOPERATIVE HEPATIC COMPLICATIONS

A. Patients who are scheduled for elective surgical procedures may have **unknown hepatic disease** or may be in the **prodromal phase of viral hepatitis.** Most patients who demonstrate postoperative hepatic dysfunction manifest only a transient increase in liver enzymes and/or bilirubin.

B. Severe hepatic necrosis following surgery and anesthesia is most often due to causes other than the anesthetic (Table 28-1).

C. The presence of ascites or prolonged prothrombin time is associated with a high postoperative mortality rate.

II. ANATOMY AND PHYSIOLOGY OF THE LIVER AND BILIARY TRACT

The liver is the largest gland in the body, receiving 25% of the cardiac output by way of the hepatic artery and portal vein. The hepatic artery provides 25% of the total hepatic blood flow (HBF) and 45–50% of the hepatic oxygen supply. Portal vein pressure (7–10 mm Hg) is determined by resistance to flow through the liver. The sympathetic nervous system, by way of alpha receptors, influences resistance to blood flow through the liver and modulates the reservoir function of this organ. For example, during hemorrhage, the liver may infuse an additional 500 ml of blood into the systemic circulation. Anesthetics may interfere

---

TABLE 28-1. Causes of Postoperative Hepatic Necrosis

Hepatocyte oxygen deprivation (hypotension, hypoxemia, drug-induced decreases in hepatic blood flow)
Sepsis
Viral infection
Congestive heart failure
Pre-existing hepatic disease
Concomitant drug therapy
Volatile anesthetic

---

with this compensatory response and lead to decompensation if blood is not promptly replaced.

A. **Metabolic functions of the liver** (Table 28-2)

B. **Pharmacokinetics and pharmacodynamics.** The response to drugs in patients with liver disease is unpredictable because of changes in HBF, hepatic clearance, and receptor responsiveness. Doses of drugs such as morphine or diazepam often need to be reduced in patients with hepatic cirrhosis. Conversely, these patients manifest reduced responses to catecholamines, presumably owing to increased plasma glucagon concentrations. Glucagon reduces the response of vascular smooth muscle to catecholamines.

III. PATHOPHYSIOLOGY OF LIVER DISEASE

A. **Parenchymal disease (viral hepatitis, cirrhosis).** The function of every organ and system is altered in patients with advanced parenchymal hepatic disease.

TABLE 28-2. Functions of the Liver

Stores glycogen
Gluconeogenesis
Maintains blood glucose concentration
Deamination of amino acids
Beta oxidation of fatty acids
Excretes bile salts
Synthesizes plasma proteins
Metabolizes endogenous and exogenous compounds
Phagocytizes bacteria
Excretes bilirubin

---

1. **Cardiovascular function** in cirrhosis is characterized by a **hyperdynamic circulation** and the presence of **arteriovenous fistulas** in many sites, including the splanchnic organs and lungs (Table
   28-3).
   a. Glucagon and other vasodilating substances may
      be responsible for the hyperdynamic circulation
      and development of arteriovenous fistulas.
   b. Total HBF is typically reduced in patients with
      cirrhosis, but hepatic oxygen supply is often
      maintained by hepatic artery blood flow.
   c. **Vasopressin** is administered to control bleeding
      from esophageal varices in patients with portal
      hypertension. The beneficial effect of this drug
      is related to vasoconstriction in the preportal
      area, with a subsequent decrease in portal blood
      flow and portal pressure.
2. **Respiratory function and pulmonary circulation.**
   Patients with cirrhosis commonly demonstrate
   varying degrees of arterial hypoxemia as a result of
   intrapulmonary shunting and mechanical effects of
   ascites.
3. **Blood and coagulation** in cirrhosis (Table 28-4)
4. **Encephalopathy** is presumed to reflect insufficient
   hepatic elimination of nitrogenous compounds (especially ammonia). Gastrointestinal bleeding, infection, or an overdose of diuretics is often responsible for an increase in the blood concentration of
   nitrogenous compounds.
5. **Renal function** in patients with liver disease. Renal
   dysfunction characterized by decreased urinary excretion of Na^+ results in increased extracellular
   fluid volume manifesting as ascites and edema. Na^+

**TABLE 28-3. Circulatory Changes in Patients with
Hepatic Cirrhosis**

Increased cardiac output
Decreased systemic vascular resistance
Increased blood volume
Unchanged blood pressure and heart rate
Decreased portal vein blood flow
Maintained or decreased hepatic artery blood flow
Maintained or decreased renal blood flow
Possible cardiomyopathy

> **TABLE 28-4. Characteristic Changes in the Hematopoietic System in Patients with Cirrhosis**
>
> Anemia (increased plasma volume, malnutrition, gastrointestinal bleeding, hemolysis)
> Thrombocytopenia (hypersplenism, alcohol-induced depression of bone marrow)
> Prolonged prothrombin time and partial thromboplastin time (Factors II, VII, IX, and X)
> Decreased albumin production

retention in patients with hepatic cirrhosis may reflect a compensatory response to a decrease in the effective blood volume. Diuretics are often used to increase urine output and decrease ascites.

  a. Hepatorenal syndrome may develop in patients with portal hypertension and ascites. Urine from patients with hepatorenal syndrome resembles that from patients with hypovolemia (urine Na^+ < 10 mEq·l^{-1}), as may follow vigorous diuretic therapy or gastrointestinal bleeding.

  b. Acute tubular necrosis (urine Na^+ > 30 mEq·l^{-1}) is more likely to occur in patients with obstructive jaundice.

  6. Ischemic hepatitis is characterized by dramatic increases in liver transaminase enzymes in patients with circulatory or pulmonary dysfunction. If cardiopulmonary function is normalized, ischemic hepatitis usually resolves spontaneously.

B. Cholestasis (obstructive jaundice) is a reduction in the hepatic secretion of bile owing to dysfunction of hepatocytes or extrahepatic biliary obstruction that requires surgical intervention. Bilirubin accumulates in the blood and may produce toxic effects on enzyme systems involved in cellular respiration, heme biosynthesis, and lipid, amino acid, and protein metabolism.

  1. Cardiovascular function in patients with biliary obstruction mimics (but to a lesser extent) the pattern observed in patients with hepatic cirrhosis (see Table 28-3). Decreased tolerance to blood loss in patients with biliary obstruction may reflect reduced responsiveness to catecholamines.

  2. Blood coagulation abnormalities in the presence of biliary obstruction initially reflect deficiency of vitamin K–dependent coagulation factors. Chronic biliary obstruction may subsequently result in decreased hepatic synthesis of coagulation factors owing to hepatocyte dysfunction.

3. **Renal function** is not altered by moderate elevations in plasma bilirubin concentrations.

IV. BLOOD TESTS FOR PATIENTS WITH LIVER DISEASE

Blood tests help distinguish between **prehepatic** (bilirubin overload), **intrahepatic** (parenchymal), and **posthepatic** (cholestasis) liver disease (Table 28-5).

V. ANESTHESIA, SURGERY, AND LIVER FUNCTION

Perioperative hepatic dysfunction may result from the direct toxic effect of an anesthetic on hepatocytes or from the indirect effect of decreased oxygen and blood supply to the liver.

A. **Halothane** is the anesthetic most studied regarding possible hepatotoxocity, with severe hepatic dysfunction occurring in approximately 1 of 6000 to 1 of 20,000 halothane administrations. It is difficult to differentiate halothane-associated hepatic dysfunction from viral hepatitis, which develops in the postoperative period. It is estimated that approximately 1 of every 1000 to 10,000 anesthetized patients may have unrecognized viral hepatitis before anesthesia and surgery and subsequently may develop signs of hepatitis postoperatively.

1. In the absence of previous hepatic dysfunction related to halothane, there is no contraindication to the use of this anesthetic in the presence of known liver disease. In this situation, postoperative outcome is determined by the degree of preoperative liver dysfunction and the extent of the surgical procedure.

2. Halothane decreases hepatic oxygen supply to a greater extent than isoflurane or enflurane.

3. Halothane decreases the intrinsic clearance of diazepam, propranolol, and lidocaine.

B. **Enflurane** is associated with such a low incidence of hepatic dysfunction that it is doubtful that a cause-and-effect relationship exists. In contrast to halothane administration, repeated administrations of enflurane do not increase the incidence of liver function test abnormalities.

TABLE 28-5. Liver Function Tests and Differential Diagnosis of Hepatic Dysfunction

	Bilirubin Overload (Hemolysis)	Hepatocellular Dysfunction	Cholestasis
Bilirubin	Unconjugated	Conjugated	Conjugated
Aminotransferases	Normal	Increased	Normal to increased
Alkaline phosphatase	Normal	Normal	Increased
Prothrombin time	Normal	Prolonged	Normal to prolonged
Serum proteins	Normal	Decreased	Normal to increased

TABLE 28-6. Delayed Elimination in the Presence of Hepatic Cirrhosis	
Midazolam	Morphine (?)
Fentanyl	Thiopental
Alfentanil	

C. **Isoflurane** is associated with an estimated incidence of postoperative hepatic dysfunction of 0.00032%, which is less than the incidence of viral hepatitis.

D. **Nitrous oxide.** Currently there is no convincing evidence that N_2O causes hepatotoxicity.

E. **Intravenous anesthetics** seem to cause only minimal alterations in routinely measured liver function tests.

1. **Opioids** can induce spasm of the sphincter of Oddi, with a subsequent increase in intrabiliary pressure (morphine and fentanyl more than meperidine and pentazocine) as well as severe abdominal pain. This spasm may suggest common duct obstruction on intraoperative cholangiography. Although some anesthesiologists avoid opioids for this reason, it is important to recognize that only about 3% of patients receiving these drugs experience sphincter spasm.

2. **Pharmacokinetics.** Severe hepatic disease delays the elimination of some injected drugs (Table 28-6).

VI. EFFECTS OF SURGICAL STRESS ON LIVER FUNCTION

Upper abdominal operations, independent of the anesthetic technique, result in decreased HBF, most likely as a result of traction on the viscera and release of vasoconstricting substances. Peripheral operations are accompanied by a relatively small reduction in HBF. The dose-related and drug-specific decrease in HBF produced by volatile anesthetics is additive to that produced by surgical stimulation.

VII. ANESTHESIA FOR PATIENTS WITH LIVER DISEASE

A. **Preoperative evaluation** of patients with liver disease includes a history, physical examination, analysis of laboratory tests, and institution of appropriate therapy (Table 28-7).

TABLE 28-7. Preoperative Evaluation of Patients with Liver Disease

History
    Jaundice
    Blood transfusions
    Gastrointestinal bleeding
    Prior anesthetics
    Exercise tolerance

Physical Examination
    Hepatosplenomegaly
    Arteriovenous fistulas (spider nevi)
    Ascites
    Cardiomyopathy
    Encephalopathy

Laboratory Tests
    Liver function tests
    Platelets
    Prothrombin time
    Partial thromboplastin time
    Renal function
    Electrolytes
    Glucose
    Arterial blood gases

Treatment
    Normalize coagulation (vitamin K)
    Hydration (albumin?)
    Diuresis (furosemide and/or mannitol, dopamine)

  B. Premedication must consider the decreased ability of the liver to metabolize drugs. Sedatives should be omitted or the dose decreased. Patients with advanced liver disease may be at risk for pulmonary aspiration because of hiatal hernia, ascites, or decreased gastric motility.

  C. Monitoring may include invasive measurement of blood pressure and cardiac filling pressures. Urine output should always be monitored in patients who have advanced liver disease and are undergoing surgery lasting more than 1–2 hours.

  D. Induction of anesthesia must consider the risk of pulmonary aspiration and the need to titrate injected anesthetics and muscle relaxants to effect (succinylcholine and decreased cholinesterase activity, pancuronium and increased volume of distribution).

E. **Maintenance of anesthesia** must consider the concept of hepatic oxygen delivery and demand. A decrease in HBF and oxygen delivery may be caused by several mechanisms (Table 28-8).

1. Regional anesthesia is useful in patients with advanced liver disease, assuming that coagulation status is acceptable.

2. When general anesthesia is selected, administration of modest doses of isoflurane (limit decrease in blood pressure to about 20% of awake values) with or without N_2O or fentanyl is often recommended.

3. Selection of nondepolarizing muscle relaxants should consider clearance mechanisms for these drugs. In this regard, atracurium has a theoretical advantage because its metabolism is not dependent on liver function. Vecuronium in doses <0.15 $mg \cdot kg^{-1}$ is acceptable in patients with liver disease.

4. Renal function must be maintained by administering a proper fluid load (fluid selection influenced by serum Na^+ concentration) and maintaining diuresis (furosemide or mannitol). A low dose of dopamine ($2-4$ $\mu g \cdot kg^{-1} \cdot min^{-1}$) may be beneficial because of a drug-induced improvement in renal blood flow and antialdosterone effect. Fluid replacement is optimally guided by measuring cardiac filling pressures.

5. **Opioid-induced spasm of the sphincter of Oddi** is infrequent (incidence <3%) and is attenuated by volatile anesthetics. Drugs that are effective in the treatment of sphincter spasm include atropine, naloxone, nitroglycerin, and glucagon.

F. **Postoperative hepatic dysfunction** usually resolves without treatment, but it is important to optimize car-

---

TABLE 28-8. Causes of Decreased Hepatic Oxygen Delivery

Arterial hypoxemia
Anemia
Hypotension
Hypovolemia
Decreased cardiac output
Surgical manipulation near the liver
Vasoconstrictive substances
Drug-induced (halothane > isoflurane)

TABLE 28-9. Causes of Postoperative Jaundice

Bilirubin Overload (Hemolysis)

Blood transfusion (500 ml of whole blood results in 250 mg of bilirubin)

Hematoma resorption

Hemolytic anemia (prosthetic heart valve, sickle cell disease, glucose-6-phosphate deficiency)

Hepatocellular Injury

Viral hepatitis

Exacerbation of pre-existing liver disease (stress response to surgery)

Hepatic ischemia

Drug-induced (volatile anesthetics, antibiotics)

Cholestasis

Intrahepatic (infection, drug-induced)

Extrahepatic (bile duct injury, pancreatic, gallstones)

diopulmonary function and treat infection. Postoperative jaundice can be attributable to one of three causes or any combination of three causes (Table 28-5; Table 28-9).

1. The most common cause of postoperative hepatic dysfunction is probably intraoperative hepatic oxygen deprivation.

2. **Benign postoperative intrahepatic cholestasis** mimics biliary obstruction and typically occurs after major surgery associated with hypotension or hypoxemia and multiple blood transfusions.

29

Anesthesia for Orthopaedic Surgery

Advances in technology have increased the need for anesthesiologists to understand the complicated apparatus and procedures of today's orthopaedic surgeon (Smith TC: Anesthesia and orthopaedic surgery. In Barash PG, Cullen BF, Stoelting RK [eds]: Clinical Anesthesia, pp 1215–1235. Philadelphia, JB Lippincott, 1992).

I. PREOPERATIVE CONSIDERATIONS

A. Unique considerations may accompany the needs of patients undergoing orthopedic surgery (Table 29-1).

B. The presence of **arthritis** introduces several concerns.

1. **Difficult tracheal intubation** may necessitate a flexible fiberoptic laryngoscope to expose the glottic opening. **Hoarseness** may indicate cricoarytenoid joint dysfunction and associated glottic narrowing. Instability of C1 or C2 (computed tomography examination) may interfere with positioning during direct laryngoscopy.

2. **Drugs** used to treat arthritis may interfere with coagulation (aspirin) or adrenal gland responses to stress (steroids). It may be necessary to consider steroid supplementation while recognizing that chronic steroid-induced skin changes may make venipuncture difficult.

II. INTRAOPERATIVE MANAGEMENT

A. **Choice of anesthetic technique** depends on interplay of patient and surgical factors, but anesthesia for orthopaedic surgery often lends itself to regional anesthesia. There is evidence that hip operations are associated with fewer short-term complications (reduced blood loss and a lower incidence of thromboembolism) when performed under spinal or epidural anesthesia. Provi-

---

TABLE 29-1. Likely Characteristics of Patients Undergoing Orthopaedic Surgery

Extremes of age

Acutely traumatized (open fractures require intervention within 6 hours to reduce risk of infection)

Arthritis (neck and temporomandibular joint immobility, glottic narrowing)

---

sion of **postoperative analgesia** is often a logical extension of regional anesthesia.

B. **Positioning** (see Chapter 6). The need to facilitate operative exposure of bones and joints (lateral position for hip replacement) dictates positioning for surgery. Pain may necessitate institution of anesthesia before positioning is accomplished.

C. **Prevention of blood loss**

1. **Tourniquets**

   a. The limb should be elevated for about 1 minute and tightly wrapped with an Esmarch bandage before inflating the cuff.

   b. Suggested tourniquet inflation pressures are 50 mm Hg and 100 mm Hg above a patient's systolic blood pressure for the arm and leg, respectively.

   c. Duration of safe tourniquet inflation time is unknown, but recommendations range from 30 minutes to 4 hours. Reperfusion between 1- and 2-hour inflations is not universally recommended, as some believe it supplies more substrate for free radical production without prolonging safe inflation time.

   d. Damage to underlying vessels, nerves, and skeletal muscles is a function of both pressure and duration of inflation. Damage is usually completely reversible for inflations of 1–2 hours.

   e. Transient metabolic acidosis, washout of K^+, and elevation of $Paco_2$ may follow deflation of the tourniquet.

   f. When a tourniquet is used with regional anesthesia, patients may complain of dull aching pain after about 45 minutes, even though analgesia appears to be adequate. During general anesthesia, increases in blood pressure and heart rate may reflect a similar phenomenon. Treatment in awake patients (assuming tourniquet deflation is not possible) is intravenous sedation and in extreme situations induction of general anesthesia.

   2. Deliberate hypotension is most often considered for scoliosis and hip surgery. Combinations of volatile anesthetics and peripheral vasodilators may be used to reduce blood pressure (epidural anesthesia may also reduce blood loss).

D. Replacement of blood. Despite efforts to reduce bleeding, some orthopedic procedures are associated with major blood loss, necessitating consideration of steps to reduce requirements for homologous transfusion (Table 29-2).

E. Intraoperative radiography. Use of a lead apron, maximizing the distance from the axial beam (doubling the distance from the source reduces the dose fourfold), and turning away at the moment of exposure are important to minimize thyroid and lens radiation dosage. Intraoperative fluoroscopy and arthroscopy may require darkness in the operating room.

F. Control of infection

   1. Postoperative infections in orthopaedic surgery delay healing or destroy the operative repair. An implanted device or prosthesis that becomes infected may have to be removed. Sources of infection are multiple (Table 29-3).

   2. Laminar flow ventilation removes airborne particles by virtue of filters and increases in air movement at the operative site. For example, laminar flow provides up to 500 air exchanges per hour as opposed to 12–15 exchanges in ordinary operating rooms. Noise generated by the laminar flow equipment may limit or obscure some of the auditory clues relied on by an anesthesiologist. Increased air flow at the op-

---

TABLE 29-2. Steps to Reduce Requirements for Homologous Transfusion

Donation of 2–3 units of blood in the 1–2 weeks before surgery

Removal of 1–2 units of blood immediately before surgery (replace with colloid or crystalloid solution) for reinfusion at end of procedure

Reinfuse blood recovered from the operative field (marrow fat and bone chips may limit)

Hemodilution (oxygen transport maximal at a hematocrit of 30%)

TABLE 29-3. Sources of Infection
Patient's skin
Oropharyngeal bacteria
Cross-infection from other patients
Bacteria on dust and lint particles
Airborne bacteria (originate from head and neck of operating room personnel)

erative site promotes drying of the operative field and leads to reductions in body temperature.

G. **Autonomic hyper-reflexia**
   1. Sudden massive sympathetic nervous system discharge with severe hypertension results from reflex stimulation of sympathetic nervous system neurons below the level of the cord lesion (most common if level T5 or above).
   2. Patients with spinal cord injuries may require orthopaedic interventions necessitating general or regional anesthesia to avoid autonomic hyper-reflexia.

III. POSTOPERATIVE CONSIDERATIONS

A. **Positioning and immobilization.** General anesthesia should be maintained until the desired immobilization is ensured by a cast, splint, or dressing. To minimize postoperative edema and circulatory embarrassment, it is often desirable to keep the operative site elevated.

B. **Relief of pain** that is likely to be intense is best managed by immobilization and optimal use of opioids (especially neuraxial) or local anesthetics (continuous epidural infusions).

C. **Embolic phenomena**
   1. **Fat embolism** is suspected in patients who have long bone fractures (mobilization of marrow fat from the bone cavity) and who develop tachypnea, tachycardia, decreased end-tidal carbon dioxide pressure, and arterial hypoxemia.
   2. **Thromboembolism.** Venous thrombosis and pulmonary embolism are common complications following orthopaedic surgery. Pulmonary emboli most often originate in the iliofemoral segment or the deep veins of the calf.
      a. Risk of postoperative thromboembolism is increased by several factors that are likely to be

TABLE 29-4. Risk Factors for Thromboembolism

Advanced age
Immobilization
History of previous embolism
Congestive heart failure
Estrogen therapy
Gram-negative sepsis
Carcinoma
Trauma

present in patients undergoing orthopaedic surgery (Table 29-4).
   b. Measures to reduce the incidence of thromboembolism are often used (Table 29-5).

IV. SPECIAL CONSIDERATIONS FOR SPECIFIC PROCEDURES

   A. Hip fractures occur most often in elderly patients, usually those with cardiopulmonary disease.
   1. Careful assessment of blood volume (central venous pressure, urine output, orthostatic hypotension) is important, as dehydration may mask hemoglobin changes due to hematoma formation (up to 1 l of blood sequestered) at the fracture site.
   2. Choice of anesthetic technique for urgent hip fractures remains controversial. There is no difference in mortality after 1 month in patients receiving general versus those receiving regional anesthesia. It is likely that age, physical status, and type of fracture are most important in determining survival. Delayed gastric emptying associated with trauma, pain, opioids, and age is an obvious consideration in

TABLE 29-5. Measures to Minimize Thromboembolism

Early ambulation
Anticoagulation (minidose heparin initiated before surgery
   and may have implications for regional anesthesia)
Dextran infusion
Aspirin
Regional anesthesia

choice of anesthesia. **Hypobaric spinal anesthesia** may be induced in the lateral position, eliminating the need for further surgical positioning.

B. Hip joint replacement

   1. There is no evidence that a specific anesthetic technique is preferable, although blood loss and thromboembolism may be less with regional anesthesia.

   2. Methylmethacrylate cement is used as a space-filling mortar to transmit compression loads from bone to prosthesis and to provide a tight fit and fixation for the prosthesis. Placement of the cement may result in hypotension within 30–60 seconds of cement insertion or up to 10 minutes after the prosthesis is inserted. Blood pressure usually recovers spontaneously but in some instances may require treatment with ephedrine, 10–15 mg iv. Multiple mechanisms are likely to be responsible for methylmethacrylate-induced hypotension (Table 29-6).

C. Procedures on the extremities

   1. Operations on the upper limb (see Chapter 18 for description of regional anesthetic procedures).

   2. Closed reduction of fractures or dislocations are often short-duration procedures that require analgesia and skeletal muscle relaxation (intravenous regional anesthesia, brachial plexus anesthesia, general anesthesia plus succinylcholine).

   3. Operations on the shoulder. General anesthesia is often selected, although a regional procedure is acceptable.

   4. Operations on the knee. Arthroscopy may be performed with regional anesthesia or local field blockade plus intra-articular local anesthetic.

   5. Amputations. Diabetes mellitus is often an associated disease when amputation is necessitated by insufficient blood supply. Spinal anesthesia is useful for lower extremity surgery, with a hypnotic dose of a barbiturate administered intravenously just before

---

TABLE 29-6. Mechanisms of Hypotension

Vasodilation (importance of pre-existing blood volume)

Emboli forced into the circulation (may result in arterial hypoxemia)

Release of vasoactive materials

Production of methacrylate acid

TABLE 29-7. Considerations in Spinal Fusion

Controlled hypotension (often includes nitroprusside)
Monitoring spinal cord function
  Intraoperative awakening
  Somatosensory-evoked potentials (opioid infusion is least
    likely to interfere with interpretation)
Increased risk of malignant hyperthermia

---

sawing of the bone is begun. It is particularly important to document any pre-existing neuropathy in a patient's medical record, especially when a regional anesthetic is selected.

6. **Joint manipulation and examination.** Adhesions may be broken under nitrous oxide–thiopental anesthesia plus succinylcholine, 0.5 mg·kg^{-1} (tracheal intubation is not mandatory).

D. **Replantation of limbs and digits.** Microsurgical anastomosis of vessels and nerves requires many hours, often necessitating continuous regional anesthetic techniques and a team of anesthesiologists to ensure optimal vigilance.

E. **Operations on the spine**

1. **Spinal fusion** is most often performed for treatment of scoliosis. There are unique anesthetic considerations in these patients (Table 29-7).

2. **Herniated intervertebral disk**

a. Microlaminectomy and diskectomy are performed with the patient in the prone position, most often using general anesthesia and partial skeletal muscle paralysis to facilitate surgical exposure. Complete paralysis is often avoided because it interferes with skeletal muscle responses to nerve root stimulation.

b. Dark blood in the surgical field may be due to venous stasis and not to hypoxia.

c. **Chymopapain** lyses mucopolysaccharides to decrease the size of the herniated disk, but a significant incidence of life-threatening allergic reactions detracts from the use of this approach.

30

Anesthesia and
the Endocrine System

An understanding of the pathophysiology of endocrine function is important in the management of anesthesia for patients with disorders of hormone-producing glands (Graf G, Rosenbaum S: Anesthesia and the endocrine system. In Barash PG, Cullen BF, Stoelting RK [eds]: Clinical Anesthesia, pp 1237–1265. Philadelphia, JB Lippincott, 1992).

I. THYROID GLAND

A. Thyroid metabolism and function

1. Thyroxine (T_4) and triiodothyronine (T_3) are the major regulators of cellular metabolic activity. The thyroid gland is solely responsible for the daily secretion of T_4 (80–100 $\mu g \cdot day^{-1}$, elimination half-time [$T_{1/2\beta}$] 6–7 days). About 80% of T_3 is produced by extrathyroidal deiodination of T_4 ($T_{1/2\beta}$ 24–30 hours). Thyroid hormone synthesis consists of four stages (Fig. 30-1).

2. Most of the excess effects of thyroid hormones **(hyperadrenergic state)** are mediated by T_3 (Table 30-1).

B. Tests of thyroid function (Table 30-2)

C. Hyperthyroidism

1. **Treatment and anesthetic considerations** (Table 30-3).

   a. A combination of propranolol (in doses titrated to effect) plus potassium iodide is frequently used preoperatively to render patients "euthyroid." Esmolol may be administered as a continuous intravenous infusion to maintain heart rate at <90 beats·min^{-1} both preoperatively and intraoperatively.

   b. The goal of intraoperative management is achievement of a depth of anesthesia (often with isoflurane) that prevents an exaggerated sympathetic nervous system response to surgical stim-

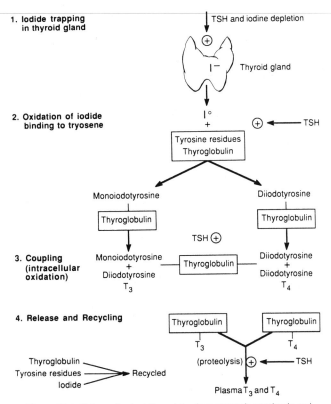

Figure 30-1. Schematic depiction of the four stages in synthesis and release of thyroid. TSH = thyroid-stimulating hormone.

TABLE 30-1. Effects of Triidothyronine on Receptor Concentrations

Increased number of beta receptors
Decreased number of cardiac cholinergic receptors

TABLE 30-2. Tests of Thyroid Function

	Thyroxine	T$_3$ Resin Uptake	Triiodothyronine	Thyroid-Stimulating Hormone
Hyperthyroidism	Elevated	Elevated	Elevated	Normal or low
Primary hypothyroidism	Low	Low	Low or normal	Elevated
Secondary hypothyroidism	Low	Low	Low	Low
Pregnancy	Elevated	Low	Normal	Normal

TABLE 30-3. Preparation of Hyperthyroid Patients

Propylthiouracil (inhibits synthesis and decreases peripheral conversion of thyroxine to triiodothyronine)

Inorganic iodide (inhibits release)

Beta-adrenergic antagonists (rapidly reverse tachycardia and anxiety)

ulation. Drugs that activate the sympathetic nervous system (ketamine) or increase the heart rate (pancuronium) should be avoided.

   c. If a regional anesthetic is selected, epinephrine should not be added to the local anesthetic solution.

  2. Complications associated with thyroid surgery are numerous (Table 30-4).

   a. It is useful to evaluate vocal cord function in the early postoperative period by asking patients to say the letter "e".

   b. Postoperative airway obstruction caused by hematoma or tracheomalacia may require urgent reintubation of the trachea.

D. Hypothyroidism

  1. Clinical manifestations are slow in onset, making the diagnosis difficult (Table 30-5).

  2. Treatment and anesthetic considerations

   a. There is no evidence to support postponement of elective surgery (including coronary artery bypass graft surgery) in mild to moderate hypothyroid patients.

   b. There is no evidence to support a specific anesthetic technique or selection of drugs, although opioids and volatile anesthetics are often considered to have more depressant effects in these patients. There appears to be little if any decrease in anesthetic requirements as reflected by mini-

TABLE 30-4. Complications Following Thyroid Surgery

Thyroid storm (mimics onset of malignant hyperthermia)

Airway obstruction (computed tomography of neck)

Recurrent laryngeal nerve damage (hoarseness)

Hypoparathyroidism (symptoms of hypocalcemia develop in 24–48 hours and include laryngospasm)

TABLE 30-5. Manifestations of Hypothyroidism
Lethargy
Cold intolerance
Decreased cardiac output and heart rate
Peripheral vasoconstriction
Reduced platelet adhesiveness
Anemia (gastrointestinal bleeding)
Impaired renal concentrating ability
Adrenal cortex suppression

mal alveolar concentration (MAC). Meticulous attention must be paid to maintaining body temperature.

II. PARATHYROID GLANDS

A. **Calcium physiology.** Parathyroid hormone secretion is regulated by the serum ionized Ca^{2+} concentration (negative feedback mechanism) to maintain Ca^{2+} levels in a normal range (8.8–10.4 $mg \cdot dl^{-1}$).

B. **Hyperparathyroidism**
  1. Hypercalcemia is responsible for a broad spectrum of signs and symptoms (nephrolithiasis, confusion).
  2. **Treatment and anesthetic considerations.** Preoperative intravenous administration of normal saline and furosemide can lower serum Ca^{2+}. There is no evidence that a specific anesthetic drug or technique is preferable. A cautious approach to the use of muscle relaxants is suggested by the unpredictable effect of hypercalcemia at the neuromuscular junction. Careful positioning of osteopenic patients is necessary to avoid pathologic bone fractures.
  3. Serum Ca^{2+} should decrease within 24 hours following successful surgery.

TABLE 30-6. Manifestations of Hypocalcemia
Neuronal irritability
Skeletal muscle spasms
Congestive heart failure
Prolonged QT interval

TABLE 30-7. Comparative Pharmacology of Corticosteroids

| | Relative Potency (Cortisol = 1) | | Approximate Equivalent Dose (mg) |
	Anti-inflammatory	Mineralocorticoid	
Short-Acting			
Cortisol	1.0	1.0	20.0
Cortisone	0.8	0.8	25.0
Prednisone	4.0	0.25	5.0
Prednisolone	4.0	0.25	5.0
Methylprednisolone	5.0	±	4.0
Intermediate-Acting			
Triamcinolone	5.0	±	4.0
Long-Acting			
Dexamethasone	30	±	0.75

TABLE 30-8. Manifestations of Excess Glucocorticoid Therapy

Truncal obesity and thin extremities (reflects redistribution of fat and skeletal muscle wasting)
Osteopenia
Hyperglycemia
Hypertension (fluid retention)
Emotional changes
Susceptibility to infection

C. **Hypoparathyroidism.** Clinical features are manifestations of hypocalcemia, and treatment is with intravenous administration of Ca^{2+} gluconate, 10–20 ml of a 10% solution (Table 30-6).

III. ADRENAL CORTEX

A. Biologic effects of adrenal cortex dysfunction reflect **cortisol** or **aldosterone** excess or deficiency (Table 30-7).
B. **Glucocorticoid excess (Cushing's syndrome)**
 1. Signs or symptoms of glucocorticoid excess reflect known actions of glucocorticoids (Table 30-8).
 2. **Treatment and anesthetic management.** Adrenalectomy is the traditional treatment (Table 30-9).
C. **Mineralocorticoid excess** should be considered in nonedematous hypertensive patients who have persistent hypokalemia and are not receiving K^+-wasting diuretics.
D. **Adrenal cortex insufficiency (secondary to exogenous steroid therapy)**
 1. Pituitary-adrenal suppression may persist for 9–12 months after cessation of steroid therapy, necessitating supplemental glucocorticoid coverage during

TABLE 30-9. Management of Patients Undergoing Adrenalectomy

Normalize intravascular fluid volume (diuresis with spironolactone)
Glucocorticoid replacement (cortisol, 100 mg every 8 hours)
Reduce initial dose of muscle relaxant

**TABLE 30-10. Supplemental Steroid
Coverage Regimens**

Cortisol, 25 mg iv before induction of anesthesia, followed by
a continuous infusion (100 mg over 24 hours)
Cortisol 200–300 mg in divided doses on day of surgery

---

periods of increased stress (trauma, surgery, infection).
2. Recommended approaches for supplemental steroid
coverage (beyond the daily therapeutic dose) vary
greatly in the dose administered (Table 30-10).

IV. ADRENAL MEDULLA

A. The adrenal medulla is analogous to a postganglionic
neuron, although the catecholamines secreted by the
medulla function as hormones, not as neurotransmitters.
B. **Pheochromocytoma.** These tumors produce, store, and
secrete catecholamines that may result in life-threatening cardiovascular effects (Table 30-11).
1. **Diagnosis.** Determinations of plasma or urine catecholamine concentrations and urinary concentration of the catecholamine metabolite vanillylman-
delic acid are the most frequent screening tests.
2. **Anesthetic considerations**
a. **Preoperative preparation** consists of alpha
blockade (phentolamine, prazosin), restoration of
intravascular fluid volume, and institution of
beta blockade. Beta blockade is indicated only if
cardiac dysrhythmias or tachycardia persists after alpha blockade.
b. **Perioperative anesthetic management** (Table
30-12)

TABLE 30-11. Manifestations of Pheochromocytoma

Paroxysmal hypertension (headaches)
Cardiac dysrhythmias
Orthostatic hypotension (decreased blood volume)
Congestive heart failure
Cardiomyopathy

TABLE 30-12. Anesthetic Management of Patients With Pheochromocytoma

Continue preoperative therapy

Invasive monitoring (arterial and pulmonary artery catheters)

Adequate depth of anesthesia before laryngoscopy

Maintenance with opioids and isoflurane or enflurane

Select muscle relaxants with minimal cardiovascular effects (vecuronium, atracurium)

Control blood pressure with nitroprusside

Control tachydysrhythmias with propranolol, esmolol, or labetalol

Anticipate hypotension with ligation of tumor's venous supply (initially treat with intravenous fluids, vasopressors if necessary)

---

    c. Postoperatively, catecholamine levels return to normal over several days, and about 75% of patients become normotensive within 10 days.

V. DIABETES MELLITUS

Diabetes mellitus is the most commonly occurring endocrine disease in surgical patients.

A. Classification (Table 30-13)

B. Hyperglycemia reflects the normal response to stress (elevations in circulating concentrations of catecholamines, glucagon, and cortisol that inhibit insulin release); glucose control is even more difficult in diabetic patients.

TABLE 30-13. Classification of Diabetes Mellitus

Insulin-Dependent (Type I)

    Childhood onset

    Thin

    Ketoacidosis prone

    Always requires exogenous insulin

Non–insulin-Dependent (Type II)

    Maturity onset

    Obese

    Not prone to ketoacidosis

    May be controlled by diet or oral hypoglycemic drugs

TABLE 30-14. Manifestations of Hyperosmolar Nonketotic Coma

Elderly with impaired thirst mechanism
Minimal or mild diabetes
Profound hyperglycemia (>1000 mg·dl^{-1})
Absence of ketoacidosis
Hyperosmolarity (seizures, coma, venous thrombosis)

C. **Hypoglycemia.** In anesthetized patients, signs of sympathetic nervous system hyperactivity due to hypoglycemia can be misinterpreted as inadequate anesthesia.
   1. Diabetic surgical patients are more likely to develop hypoglycemia if renal disease prolongs the action of insulin or oral hypoglycemic drugs.
   2. An avoidable cause of accidental hypoglycemia is the administration of insulin to diabetic patients who are not receiving sufficient oral or intravenous glucose intake.
D. **Hyperosmolar nonketotic coma** (Table 30-14)
E. **Diabetic ketoacidosis** occurs when there is insufficient insulin to block the metabolism of fatty acids, resulting in the accumulation of acetoacetate and beta-hydroxybutyrate (Table 30-15).
F. **Perioperative monitoring.** Preoperatively determine blood glucose and serum K$^+$ concentrations and confirm the absence of ketones. Dehydration may be present as a result of osmotic diuresis. Glucose administered intravenously for an adult is usually 5–10 g·h^{-1} (100–200 ml of 5% dextrose in water). Positioning is important, as diabetic patients may have pre-existing peripheral vascular disease or neuropathy.
G. **Management regimens.** Regardless of the approach selected, the common goal is to prevent hypoglycemia

TABLE 30-15. Manifestations of Diabetic Ketoacidosis

Metabolic acidosis
Hyperglycemia (300–500 mg·dl^{-1})
Dehydration (osmotic diuresis and vomiting)
Hypokalemia (manifests when acidosis is corrected)
Skeletal muscle weakness (hypophosphatemia with correction of acidosis)

and to accept mild hyperglycemia that can be corrected gradually in the postoperative period.

1. A common approach is to administer a fraction (1/3–1/2) of a patient's usual morning NPH insulin dose plus 100–200 ml·h^{-1} of 5% dextrose.

2. An alternative approach is placement of 7–10 units of regular insulin in 1000 ml of 5% dextrose in water infused at 75–100 ml·h^{-1} (0.5–1.0 unit·h^{-1} of insulin). A small amount of insulin adheres to the wall of the containers and tubing, but this is not clinically significant.

VI. PITUITARY GLAND

The pituitary gland is divided into the anterior pituitary (thyroid-stimulating hormone, adrenocorticotropic hormone, gonadotropins, growth hormone) and posterior pituitary (vasopressin, oxytocin), which are under the control of the hypothalamus.

A. **Diabetes insipidus** reflects a relative or absolute deficiency of antidiuretic hormone that results in hypovolemia (inability to concentrate urine) and hypernatremia.

B. **Syndrome of inappropriate antidiuretic hormone** manifests as dilutional hyponatremia and decreased serum osmolarity; these typically occur in the presence of head injury or an intracranial tumor. Initial treatment is restriction of fluid intake to 800 ml·day^{-1}.

31

Obstetric Anesthesia

During pregnancy, alterations occur in nearly every maternal organ system, with associated important implications for anesthesiologists (Table 31-1) (Santos AC, Pedersen H, Finster M: Obstetric anesthesia. In Barash PG, Cullen BF, Stoelting RK [eds]: Clinical Anesthesia, pp 1267–1305. Philadelphia: JB Lippincott, 1992).

I. PHYSIOLOGIC CHANGES OF PREGNANCY

A. Increased alveolar ventilation along with decreased functional residual capacity (FRC) enhances maternal uptake and elimination of inhaled anesthetics.

B. Decreased FRC and increased basal metabolic rate predispose a parturient to arterial hypoxemia during periods of apnea, as associated with endotracheal intubation.

C. Vascular engorgement of the airway may predispose to bleeding on insertion of nasopharyngeal airways, nasogastric tubes, or endotracheal tubes.

II. FETAL EXPOSURE TO DRUGS USED IN OBSTETRIC ANESTHESIA

Most anesthetic drugs (opioids, local anesthetics, inhaled anesthetics) readily cross the placenta.

A. **Placental transfer** depends on several factors (Table 31-2).

B. **Fetus and newborn.** Several characteristics of the fetal circulation delay equilibration between fetal arterial and venous blood and thus delay the depressant effects of anesthetic drugs (Table 31-3).

III. ANESTHESIA FOR LABOR AND VAGINAL DELIVERY

Pain of the first stage of labor is caused by uterine contractions (T10–L1) and by distention of the perineum

TABLE 31-1. Physiologic Changes of Pregnancy

Hematologic Alterations

Increased plasma volume (40–50%)
Increased total blood volume (25–40%)
Dilutional anemia (hematocrit 35%)

Cardiovascular Changes

Increased cardiac output (30–50%)
Aortocaval compression (supine hypotensive syndrome occurs in about 10% of parturients)

Ventilatory Changes

Increased alveolar ventilation (70%)
Decreased FRC (20%)
Airway edema
Decreased $Paco_2$ (30%)

Gastrointestinal Changes

Delayed gastric emptying
Decreased lower esophageal sphincter tone (heartburn)

Altered Drug Responses

Decreased requirements for inhaled anesthetics (MAC)
Decreased local anesthetic requirements

TABLE 31-2. Determinants of Drug Passage Across the Placenta

Physical and Chemical Characteristics of the Drug

Molecular weight (<500)
Lipid solubility
Non-ionized vs. ionized

Concentration Gradient

Dose administered
Timing of intravenous administration relative to uterine contraction
Use of vasoconstrictors

Hemodynamic Factors

Aortocaval compression
Hypotension from regional blockade

> **TABLE 31-3. Characteristics of Fetal Circulation That Delay Drug Equilibration**
>
> The fetal liver is the first organ perfused by the umbilical vein.
>
> Dilution of umbilical vein blood by fetal venous blood from the gastrointestinal tract, head, and extremities (this phenomenon explains why thiopental, 4 mg·kg^{-1}, administered to the mother does not produce significant depressant effects in the fetus).

during the second stage of labor (S2–4). Analgesia relieves pain and anxiety and reduces maternal secretion of catecholamines.

A. **Psychoprophylaxis.** Parturients who are educated in the physiology of childbirth generally require less systemic medication.

B. **Systemic medication.** Time and method of administration must be chosen carefully to avoid maternal and neonatal depression.

   1. **Opioids**

      a. **Meperidine** appears to produce less neonatal ventilatory depression than morphine. Meperidine administered intravenously (analgesia in 5–10 minutes) or intramuscularly (peak effect in 40–50 minutes) rapidly crosses the placenta.

      b. **Fentanyl,** 1 μg·kg^{-1} iv, provides prompt pain relief (forceps application) without severe neonatal depression.

      c. **Naloxone,** 10 μg·kg^{-1}, may be administered directly to newborns to reverse excessive opioid depression.

   2. **Tranquilizers.** Promethazine provides sedation and does not accentuate neonatal depression when combined with meperidine.

   3. **Ketamine** provides adequate analgesia (0.2–0.4 mg·kg^{-1} iv) without neonatal depression.

C. **Regional anesthesia** when properly applied provides analgesia without interfering with the progress of labor (a mother's ability to bear down) or producing maternal or fetal depression.

   1. **Spinal anesthesia.** Because of the profound motor paralysis that it induces, spinal anesthesia is limited to delivery (lidocaine 5% using 30–50 mg injected with a patient in the sitting position). To reduce the incidence of postdural puncture headache, 25- or 26-gauge spinal needles are recommended.

2. **Epidural anesthesia.** Segmental epidural anesthesia by means of a catheter in the lumbar epidural space provides pain relief during labor (T10–L1) and can then be extended to provide analgesia during delivery (S2–4).

   a. This form of anesthesia does not usually interfere with the first stage of labor when initiated in the presence of active labor (cervix dilated 5–6 cm in primiparas and 3–4 cm in multiparas) and when aortocaval compression is avoided.

   b. Test dose with lidocaine 45 mg, plus epinephrine (EPI) 15 µg (isoproterenol 5µg an alternative), identifies accidental subarachnoid or intravascular injection. After a negative test dose, adequate first-stage analgesia is usually achieved with an additional injection of 5 ml of local anesthetic (1% lidocaine, 0.25% bupivacaine, 2% 2-chloroprocaine). This dose may be repeated as needed or followed immediately by a continuous epidural infusion of a more dilute infusion (0.33% lidocaine, 10–15 ml·h^{-1}; 0.125% bupivacaine, 8–12 ml·h^{-1}). **Patient-controlled epidural analgesia** is an alternative to intermittent injection or continuous infusion techniques. The addition of fentanyl (1 µg·ml^{-1}) to bupivacaine may reduce the local anesthetic requirement.

   c. For the second stage of labor, analgesia can be extended to include the sacral segments by administration of an additional 5–10 ml of the originally used local anesthetic solution with the parturient in a semirecumbent position. The second stage of labor may be lengthened by anesthesia.

3. The **most frequent complication** of spinal and epidural anesthesia is **maternal hypotension** (systolic blood pressure <100 mm Hg or a 20% decrease). In most instances, hypotension can be prevented by **prehydration** (intravenous infusion of 500–1000 ml of a balanced salt solution; avoid glucose-containing solutions unless the mother is hypoglycemic) and **positioning** (left uterine displacement to prevent aortocaval compression). If blood pressure is not restored in 1–2 minutes, **ephedrine** should be administered intravenously in 5- to 10-mg increments.

D. **Inhalation analgesia** makes pain of uterine contractions more tolerable and is useful for delivery in combination with a pudendal nerve block (S2–4).

IV. ANESTHESIA FOR CESAREAN SECTION

The choice of anesthesia depends on the urgency of the procedure and the condition of the fetus.

A. **Regional anesthesia.** Advantages include lessened risk of aspiration, fulfillment of the mother's wishes to remain awake, and avoidance of depressant drugs. The time required for induction of regional anesthesia makes the technique less suitable for urgent cesarean section. For example, time of induction to delivery averages 15–20 minutes with a spinal anesthetic and 30–40 minutes with an epidural anesthetic.

1. **Spinal anesthesia.** Despite a T4 level of anesthesia, a patient may still need supplemental analgesia (fentanyl, 25 μg iv), especially when the uterus is exteriorized (Table 31-4).

   a. Improved perioperative analgesia can be provided by the addition of fentanyl, 6.25 μg, or preservative-free morphine, 0.1 mg, to the local anesthetic solution.

   b. Oxygen should be routinely administered by face mask to improve fetal oxygenation.

2. **Lumbar epidural anesthesia.** Compared with spinal anesthesia, lumbar epidural anesthesia requires more time and drug to establish an adequate sensory level, but there is a lessened risk of postdural puncture headache, and the level of anesthesia can be adjusted by titration of local anesthetic solution injected through the indwelling catheter.

TABLE 31-4. Spinal Anesthesia for Cesarean Section

	Lidocaine* (5%)	Tetracaine* (1%)	Bupivacaine* (0.75%)
Height (cm)			
150–160	50	7	8
160–182	70	8	10
>182	75	9	12
Onset (min)	1–3	3–5	2–4
Duration (min)	45–75	120–180	120–180

*Dose (in milligrams).

TABLE 31-5. Epidural Anesthesia for Cesarean Section

2-Chloroprocaine 3%
Bupivacaine 0.5%
Lidocaine 2%

    a. Adequate anesthesia is usually achieved with
15–25 ml of local anesthetic solution with
1:200,000 EPI given in divided doses (Table
31-5).

    b. Addition of morphine (3–5 mg) to the local anesthetic solution provides postoperative analgesia.

B. General anesthesia. Advantages are rapidity and reliability, making it the **technique of choice for emergency cesarean section** and when substantial hemorrhage is anticipated (placenta previa). Situations in which uterine relaxation facilitates delivery (multiple gestations, breech) are most often managed with general anesthesia (Table 31-6).

    1. A newborn's condition after cesarean section with general anesthesia is comparable to that when regional techniques are used. The **uterine incision to delivery time (<180 seconds)** is more important to fetal outcome than is anesthetic technique.

TABLE 31-6. General Anesthesia for Cesarean Section

Premedication with a nonparticulate antacid, 15–30 ml within 30 minutes of induction

Maintain patients in left uterine displacement position while on operating table

Preoxygenation

Pretreatment (nondepolarizing relaxant)

Thiopental, 4 mg·kg^{-1} (or ketamine, 0.5^{-1}·mg·kg^{-1}), plus succinylcholine, 1.0–1.5 mg·kg^{-1}, during cricoid pressure (inject at the onset of contraction if in labor)

Skin incision after confirmation of tracheal tube placement

Maintenance in the predelivery interval with 50% nitrous oxide and 0.5 MAC of a volatile anesthetic

Avoid extreme hyperventilation of the lungs

Add oxytocin to the infusion after delivery and deepen anesthesia (opioids?)

Extubate the trachea when patients awaken

2. Usual amount of blood loss at cesarean section is 750–1000 ml, and transfusion is rarely necessary.

3. When tracheal intubation is unexpectedly difficult, it may be safer to let the mother awaken and pursue alternative approaches (awake fiberoptic tracheal intubation, regional anesthesia) rather than persist at unsuccessful and traumatic attempts at tracheal intubation.

V. MANAGEMENT OF HIGH-RISK PARTURIENTS

A. **Pre-eclampsia-eclampsia** is characterized by hypertension, proteinuria, and edema that may progress to oliguria, congestive heart failure, and seizures (eclampsia). In severe cases (blood pressure >160/110, proteinuria >5 g·day^{-1}, oliguria, intrauterine growth retardation), all major organ systems are affected because of widespread vasospasm.

1. **General management** (Table 31-7)

2. **Anesthetic management**

   a. In volume-repleted patients positioned with left uterine displacement, the institution of epidural anesthesia (assume no clotting abnormality) does not typically cause an unacceptable reduction in blood pressure and leads to significant improvements in placental perfusion.

   b. Spinal anesthesia may produce severe alterations in cardiovascular dynamics, resulting from sudden sympathetic nervous system blockade.

   c. General anesthesia is indicated in acute emergencies, remembering the probable exaggerated blood pressure responses to induction of anesthesia and intubation of the trachea and interaction of Mg^{2+} with muscle relaxants.

TABLE 31-7. Considerations in the Management of Parturients With Pre-eclampsia or Eclampsia

Prevent or control seizures (magnesium sulfate potentiates muscle relaxants)

Restore intravascular fluid volume (central venous or pulmonary capillary wedge pressure 5–10 mm Hg; urine output 0.5–1.0 ml·kg^{-1}·h^{-1})

Normalize blood pressure (hydralazine, nitroprusside)

Correct coagulation abnormalities

    d. Reduced doses of ephedrine are used to treat hypotension, as patients with pre-eclampsia or eclampsia exhibit increased sensitivity to vasopressors.

B. Antepartum hemorrhage

    1. Placenta previa (painless bright red bleeding after the seventh month of pregnancy) is the most common cause of antepartum hemorrhage.

    2. Abruptio placentae typically manifests as uterine hypertonia and tenderness with dark red vaginal bleeding. Maternal and fetal mortality rates are high.

    3. General anesthesia (often with ketamine induction, 0.75 kg·mg^{-1} iv) is used in view of the high risk of hemorrhage and clotting disorders.

C. Heart disease. Cardiac decompensation and death occur most commonly at the time of maximum hemodynamic stress. For example, cardiac output increases during labor, with the greatest increase immediately after delivery of the placenta. These changes in cardiac output are blunted by regional anesthesia.

D. Preterm delivery is defined as birth before the 37th week or term weight more than 2 standard deviations below the mean (small for gestational age). Such infants account for 8–10% of all births and nearly 80% of early neonatal deaths.

    1. Several problems are likely to develop in preterm infants (Table 31-8).

    2. Beta$_2$ agonists (ritodrine, terbutaline) used to inhibit labor may interact with anesthetic drugs or produce undesirable changes before induction of anesthesia (Table 31-9).

        a. Delay of anesthesia for at least 3 hours after the cessation of tocolysis allows beta-mimetic effects to dissipate, and K$^+$ supplementation is not necessary.

TABLE 31-8. Problems Associated With Prematurity

Respiratory distress syndrome (glucocorticoids administered to the mother for 24–48 hours may enhance fetal lung maturity)

Intracranial hemorrhage

Hypoglycemia

Hypocalcemia

Hyperbilirubinemia

TABLE 31-9. Side Effects of Beta₂ Agonists
Administered to Stop Premature Labor

Hypokalemia (cardiac dysrhythmias)
Hypotension (accentuated by regional anesthesia)
Tachycardia (avoid atropine, pancuronium)
Pulmonary edema (cautious prehydration)

b. Preterm infants are more sensitive to the depressant effects of anesthetic drugs. Regardless of the technique or drugs selected, the **most important goal is prevention of asphyxia and trauma to a fetus.**

VI. FETAL AND MATERNAL MONITORING

Pulse oximetry is a useful addition to routine monitoring of maternal blood pressure and electrocardiogram.

A. Biophysical monitoring. Ultrasound cardiography and measurement of uterine activity with a tocodynamometer provide noninvasive monitoring of fetal well-being (Table 31-10; Fig. 31-1).

B. Biochemical monitoring. Fetal scalp pH is a good predictor of **Apgar score** at 1–2 minutes after birth. When scalp pH is <7.16, 80% of babies have Apgar scores of 6 or less. Hemorrhage may occur at the fetal sampling site despite application of pressure.

VII. ANESTHETIC COMPLICATIONS

A. General anesthesia (Table 31-11)
B. Regional anesthesia (Table 31-12)

TABLE 31-10. Biophysical Monitoring of the Fetus

Baseline heart rate (normal 120–160 beats·min⁻¹)
Beat-to-beat variability (reflects variations in autonomic nervous system tone; disappears with fetal distress, opioids, local anesthetics)
Fetal heart rate deceleration

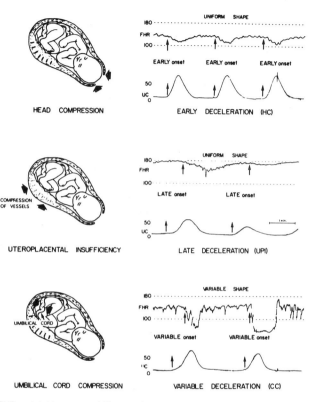

HEAD COMPRESSION

EARLY DECELERATION (HC)

UTEROPLACENTAL INSUFFICIENCY

LATE DECELERATION (UPI)

UMBILICAL CORD COMPRESSION

VARIABLE DECELERATION (CC)

FHR = fetal heart rate; UC = uterine contraction

Figure 31-1. Relationship and significance of fetal heart rate changes in association with uterine contractions.

TABLE 31-11. Risks of General Anesthesia in Parturients
Rapid desaturation (low FRC)
Laryngospasm/edema (mucosal congestion)
Pulmonary aspiration

TABLE 31-12. **Risks of Regional Anesthesia in Parturients**

Hypotension (decrease incidence by prehydration, left uterine displacement, ephedrine)

Total spinal anesthesia

Seizures (accidental intravascular injection of local anesthetics; treatment is thiopental, 50–100 mg, or diazepam, 5–10 mg)

Headache

Nerve injury (consider role of fetal compression of lumbosacral trunk)

VIII. NEONATAL RESUSCITATION IN THE DELIVERY ROOM

A. About 6% of all neonates require resuscitation. Several factors contribute to the likelihood of depression at birth, requiring neonatal resuscitation (Table 31-13).

B. **Resuscitation.** Every delivery room must be equipped with appropriate resuscitation equipment and drugs for newborn and maternal resuscitation (see Chapter 44 and Appendix E).

  1. **Initial treatment and evaluation of all infants.** The pharynx is suctioned, heart rate is quantitated, and ventilation is assessed. The scoring system introduced by Apgar is a useful method of clinically evaluating infants (Table 31-14).

  2. **Meconium staining** is treated by oropharyngeal suctioning at the time of delivery; tracheal intubation and airway suctioning are probably only

---

TABLE 31-13. **Events Associated With Neonatal Depression at Birth**

Prematurity (80% <1500 g need resuscitation)

Drugs used during labor or delivery

Trauma or precipitated labor

Birth asphyxia (reflects interference with placental perfusion)
  Tight umbilical cord
  Prolapsed cord
  Premature separation of placenta
  Uterine hyperactivity
  Maternal hypotension

TABLE 31-14. Calculation of Apgar Scores

	0	1	2
Heart rate	Absent	<100 beats·min⁻¹	>100 beats·min⁻¹
Respiratory effort	Absent	Slow and irregular	Crying
Muscle tone	Limp	Some flexion of extremities	Moving
Reflex irritability	No response	Grimace	Crying, cough
Color	Pale, blue	Body pink, extremities blue	Pink

**TABLE 31-15. Other Drugs and Fluids Used in
Neonatal Resuscitation**

Naloxone (avoid in infants born to opioid-addicted mothers)
Epinephrine (treat asystole or persistent bradycardia;
   administer intravenously or by tracheal tube)
5% Albumin (10 ml·kg^{-1})
Lactated Ringer's solution (10 ml·kg^{-1})
Type O-negative blood (10 ml·kg^{-1})

---

necessary in the presence of a low Apgar score and
evidence of mechanical airway obstruction.

3. **Use of cardiac massage.** Intermittent compression
of the middle third of the sternum is applied 100
times·min^{-1} with the middle and index fingers
until the heart rate is >100 beats·min^{-1}. During
chest compressions, positive-pressure ventilation
with 100% oxygen should be performed at a rate of
40–60 breaths·min^{-1}.

4. **Rapid correction of acidosis.** A newborn pH < 7.0
should be promptly corrected with sodium bicarbonate.

5. **Other drugs and fluids** (Table 31-15).

IX. NONOBSTETRIC SURGERY IN
PREGNANT WOMEN

A. When the necessity for surgery arises, anesthetic
considerations are related to multiple factors (Table
31-16).

**TABLE 31-16. Considerations in the Management
of Anesthesia for Nonobstetric Surgery
in Parturients**

Physiologic changes of pregnancy
   Decreased requirements for local and inhaled anesthetics
   Low FRC
   High basal metabolic rate
   Slowed gastric emptying
   Aortocaval compression
Teratogenicity of anesthetic drugs (period of organogenesis is
   15–56 days; single exposure seems unlikely to cause
   abnormalities)
Adequacy of uteroplacental circulation
Initiation of premature labor

B. Only perform emergency surgery during pregnancy, especially in the first trimester. It is logical to select drugs with a long history of safety (opioids, muscle relaxants, thiopental, nitrous oxide). The fetal heart rate should be monitored after the 16th week of pregnancy.

32

Neonatal Anesthesia

The neonatal period is often defined as the first 30 days of extrauterine life (Berry FA: Neonatal anesthesia. In Barash PG, Cullen BF, Stoelting RK [eds]: Clinical Anesthesia, pp 1307–1333. Philadelphia, JB Lippincott, 1992). The major transition of the pulmonary system occurs during the first hours of life, whereas the major transition of the circulatory system occurs during the first 48–72 hours of life.

I. TRANSITION OF THE CARDIOPULMONARY SYSTEM

A. **Fetal circulation** is characterized by three shunts (placenta, foramen ovale, and ductus arteriosus), with oxygenated blood leaving the placenta through the umbilical vein. After the lungs expand and the umbilical cord is clamped, dramatic circulatory changes follow, including reductions in pulmonary vascular resistance (Table 32-1).
   1. Pulmonary vascular resistance declines to neonatal levels after 3–4 days.
   2. The foramen ovale usually becomes permanently closed over the first several months of life. Nevertheless, about 30% of individuals <30 years of age and 20% of those >30 years of age have a foramen ovale that may become patent if the right atrial pressure exceeds the left atrial pressure.

B. **Transition of the pulmonary system**
   1. The primary initial event in the transition of the pulmonary system is initiation of ventilation, which changes the alveoli from a fluid-filled to an air-filled state. The initial negative intrathoracic pressures may be 40–60 cm H_2O.
   2. By 10–20 minutes, a newborn has achieved its almost normal functional residual capacity and arterial blood gases are stabilized (Table 32-2).

C. **Persistent pulmonary hypertension (persistent fetal circulation).** Hypoxemia and acidosis may cause pul-

TABLE 32-1. Circulatory Changes Associated With Initial Expansion of a Neonate's Lungs

Pulmonary blood flow increases
Foramen ovale closes (left atrial pressure > right atrial pressure)
Ductus arteriosus closes

TABLE 32-2. Arterial Blood Gas Values of Neonates

Age	Pa_{O_2} (mm Hg)	Pa_{CO_2} (mm Hg)	pH
10 minutes	50	48	7.20
1 hour	70	35	7.35
1 week	75	35	7.40

monary hypertension to persist or recur. As a result, there is a **right-to-left shunt** through the foramen ovale and ductus arteriosus. Persistence of pulmonary hypertension occurs in three situations (Table 32-3).

II. TRANSITION AND MATURATION OF THE RENAL SYSTEM

A. The limited ability of a neonate's kidneys to concentrate or dilute urine results from the low glomerular filtration rate at birth. By 3–4 days, this limited ability is largely overcome. The kidneys are approximately 70% mature by 1 month, and renal function is sufficient to handle almost any contingency. Immature renal tubular cells do not respond optimally to aldo-

TABLE 32-3. Events Associated With Persistent Pulmonary Hypertension

Meconium aspiration *in utero* (reflects chronic fetal hypoxia vs. acute hypoxia during delivery)
Respiratory failure of a neonate (treatment may include extracorporeal membrane oxygenation)
Congenital diaphragmatic hernia (often a "honeymoon period" during and soon after surgery)

sterone; neonates cannot conserve sodium (Na⁺) even
with a severe Na⁺ deficit **(obligate Na⁺ loser).**

B. **Fluid and electrolyte therapy in neonates.** Fluids must
contain Na⁺, as in lactated Ringer's solution. Fluid
therapy should be conservative (2–3 ml·kg⁻¹·h⁻¹
maintenance plus replacement for trauma or blood
loss) for premature infants and those with bronchopulmonary dysplasia (increased lung water).

III. **ANATOMIC AND MATURATIONAL FACTORS OF
NEONATES AND THEIR CLINICAL
SIGNIFICANCE** (Fig. 32-1)

IV. **ANATOMIC AND PHYSIOLOGIC FACTORS OF
THE PULMONARY SYSTEM** (Table 32-4)

A. Airway obstruction, breath-holding, coughing, or apnea (as during laryngoscopy) leads to rapid desaturation because of high oxygen consumption.

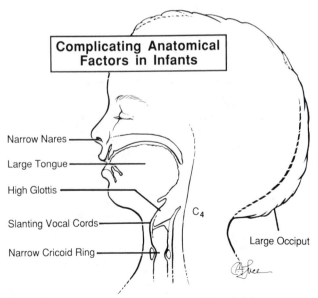

Figure 32-1. Complicating anatomic factors in infants.

TABLE 32-4. Comparison of Ventilation in Neonates and Adults

	Neonate	Adult
Oxygen consumption (ml·kg^{-1}·min^{-1})	7–9	3
Tidal volume (ml·kg^{-1})	7	7
Breathing rate (times·min^{-1})	30–50	12–16
Functional residual capacity (ml·kg^{-1})	27–30	30
Alveolar ventilation (ml·kg^{-1}·min^{-1})	100–150	60

    B. A rapid breathing rate (necessary because of high oxygen consumption) results in elevated alveolar ventilation with associated rapid induction of and recovery from anesthesia.

V. MATURATION OF THE CARDIOVASCULAR SYSTEM

Ventricular compliance is limited, and increases in cardiac output are achieved principally by increases in heart rate **(rate-dependent cardiac output).** Any slowing of heart rate results in decreased cardiac output. Hypoxemia and vagal stimulation are the principal causes of bradycardia. The sympathetic nervous system is immature, and cardiac output can increase by only 30–40%. The baroresponse is immature, as reflected by a reduced heart rate response to hypotension.

VI. ANESTHESIA FOR NEONATES

    A. Premedication. An anticholinergic drug (atropine, 0.02 mg·kg^{-1} im) is useful to reduce secretions and may be administered intravenously before succinylcholine. There is little need to administer sedatives or opioids to neonates.

    B. Endotracheal intubation. Routine tracheal intubation and controlled ventilation of the lungs are not mandatory for short, noninvasive operations. Decisions to intubate the trachea while a patient is awake must be tempered by the possibility that associated hypertension could rupture fragile cerebral vessels. The trachea should be extubated only when a neonate is awake and reacting to the tube.

TABLE 32-5. Anesthetic Requirements (MAC) in Very Young Infants

	Halothane MAC
Premature infant	0.6%
Full-term neonate	0.89%
Neonate 2–4 months	1.12%

C. **Does the neonate need anesthesia?** Even premature neonates perceive and react to pain (hypertension), emphasizing the need to titrate anesthesia to the needs of all patients regardless of age.

D. **Anesthetic dose requirements of neonates**
   1. Neonates and premature infants have a decreased anesthetic requirement (MAC) compared with older children (Table 32-5).
   2. **Possible explanations for lower MAC are multiple** (Table 32-6).

E. **Anesthetic management of the neonate** is determined by the requirements for surgery and the patient's condition (Table 32-7).
   1. **If extubation of the trachea** is anticipated at the end of surgery, the anesthetic is tailored to minimize residual effects from inhaled anesthetics and muscle relaxants.
   2. Regional anesthetic techniques (caudal, spinal) combined with general anesthesia facilitate early tracheal extubation and provide postoperative pain relief.
      a. Accidental total spinal anesthesia is manifested as a declining arterial oxygen saturation rather than as hypotension (reflects lack of sympathetic nervous system tone in neonates).

TABLE 32-6. Explanations for Decreased Anesthetic Requirements (MAC) in Neonates

Immature central nervous system
Progesterone
Elevated endorphins (enter central nervous system across an immature blood-brain barrier)

TABLE 32-7. Choice of Anesthetic Based on a Neonate's Underlying Condition

Systolic blood pressure <40 mm Hg (fluid bolus of 10 ml·kg^{-1}; controlled ventilation of the lungs with oxygen; nondepolarizing muscle relaxant)

Hemodynamically unstable (fentanyl, 10–12.5 μg kg^{-1} iv; select a muscle relaxant to offset opioid-induced bradycardia)

Stable cardiovascular system (factors that influence choice of anesthetic technique include anticipation of tracheal extubation at the conclusion of surgery, the need to control blood pressure, and the need for postoperative pain relief).

    b. A ring block of the penis (0.25–0.5% bupivacaine subcutaneously at the base of the penis) provides anesthesia for circumcision.

  F. Uptake and distribution of anesthetic in neonates. A more rapid induction (and greater hypotension, especially with "overpressurization") occurs when volatile anesthetics are administered to neonates, reflecting several differences from older children and adults (Table 32-8).

VII. SURGICAL PROCEDURES IN NEONATES

Two confounding factors in neonatal surgery are prematurity (respiratory distress syndrome) and associated congenital anomalies (especially cardiac). A history of maternal cocaine abuse is associated with premature birth and decreased cardiac output on the first day of life.

  A. Congenital diaphragmatic hernia is present in about 1 in every 4000 live births, and mortality (despite surgery) remains near 50% principally because of severe underdevelopment of the lungs. Abdominal contents

TABLE 32-8. Reasons for More Rapid Induction of Anesthesia in Neonates

Greater alveolar ventilation relative to the functional residual capacity

A greater proportion of the cardiac output goes to vessel-rich group tissues (heart, brain)

Lower blood:gas solubility

Lower MAC requirement

> #### TABLE 32-9. Manifestations of Congenital Diaphragmatic Hernia
>
> Scaphoid abdomen
> Decreased to absent breath sounds on affected side
> Arterial hypoxemia
> Radiographic confirmation

compress the developing lung buds and often result in hypoplastic lungs.

1. **Antenatal diagnosis.** Polyhydramnios is present in 30%, and ultrasonography can be used to make the diagnosis *in utero*.
2. **Clinical presentation** depends on the degree of the hernia and interference with ventilation (Table 32-9).
   a. Immediate supportive care is **tracheal intubation** and **decompression of the stomach.**
   b. Delivery of excessive airway pressure carries a high risk for pneumothorax.
   c. Associated congenital anomalies (often cardiac) should be sought.
3. **Anesthetic considerations for diaphragmatic hernia** (Table 32-10)
B. **Omphalocele-gastroschisis**
   1. An **omphalocele** is covered with a membrane (amnion), which protects against infection and loss of extracellular fluid. Affected neonates have a high incidence (about 20%) of other congenital anomalies, especially cardiac defects.

> #### TABLE 32-10. Anesthetic Considerations in the Presence of Congenital Diaphragmatic Hernia
>
> Consider delaying surgery 24–48 hours while the neonate is being stabilized (severe pulmonary dysfunction may be treated with extracorporeal membrane oxygenation)
> Avoid nitrous oxide
> Gentle attempts (<30 cm H_2O) to expand the lungs after hernia reduction
> Suspect contralateral pneumothorax if sudden hypoxemia occurs
> Anticipate the need for postoperative support of ventilation

TABLE 32-11. Perioperative Concerns Associated With Omphalocele-Gastroschisis

Fluid loss (requires balanced salt solutions; monitor central venous pressure and urine output)

Control infection

Avoid nitrous oxide

Skeletal muscle relaxation (primary closure and ventilation; Dacron silo a consideration if intragastric pressure >20 mm Hg)

Hypertension (renin release in response to mechanical decrease in renal blood flow)

Leg edema

Anticipate the need for postoperative ventilation of the lungs

2. **Gastroschisis** is not covered with a membrane (infection, hypothermia, and fluid loss are likely), but associated congenital anomalies are less probable.
3. **Antenatal diagnosis.** High levels of alpha-fetoprotein in the maternal serum (closure of the abdominal wall and neural tube reduces release into the amniotic fluid) suggest the diagnosis, which may be confirmed by ultrasonography. Cesarean section may be considered when the diagnosis is known.
4. **Perioperative concerns** (Table 32-11)
C. **Tracheoesophageal fistula** occurs in about 1 in every 3000 live births, and 85% have a fistula from the distal trachea to the esophagus and a blind proximal esophageal pouch. About 50% have associated congenital anomalies (especially cardiac), and prematurity may be associated with respiratory distress syndrome.
1. **Clinical presentation** (Table 32-12)
2. **Anesthetic considerations.** A gastrostomy may be performed initially to protect the lungs from aspi-

TABLE 32-12. Manifestations of Tracheoesophageal Fistula

Polyhydramnios

Inability to pass a nasogastric tube

Cyanosis and choking with oral fluids

Aspiration pneumonitis

TABLE 32-13. Anesthetic Considerations in the Presence of Tracheoesophageal Fistula

Leave the gastrostomy tube open to air

Awake vs. asleep tracheal intubation

Position the tracheal tube distal to the fistula (breath sounds; gas bubbles out of gastrostomy tube cease)

Consider migration of the tracheal tube into the fistula with sudden changes in compliance or oxygen saturation

Anticipate the need for postoperative ventilation of the lungs

ration and allow an infant's general condition to improve before surgery (Table 32-13).

D. **Intestinal obstruction**
   1. **Upper gastrointestinal tract obstruction** usually manifests in the first 24 hours of life (Table 32-14).
   2. **Lower gastrointestinal tract obstruction** usually manifests 2–7 days after birth (Table 32-15).

E. **Meningomyelocele** introduces unique management problems (Table 32-16).

TABLE 32-14. Perioperative Concerns Associated With Upper Gastrointestinal Obstruction

Vomiting and electrolyte losses (Na^+)

Awake tracheal intubation (consider topical anesthesia if a concern is that associated hypertension could cause intracranial hemorrhage in a premature infant)

Adequate skeletal muscle relaxation

Nitrous oxide is acceptable if minimal gas is in the bowel

Anticipate the need for postoperative ventilation of the lungs

TABLE 32-15. Perioperative Concerns Associated With Lower Gastrointestinal Obstruction

Fluid loss into the gastrointestinal tract (delay anesthesia until $Na^+ > 130$ mEq·l^{-1} and urine output is adequate)

Consider awake tracheal intubation if a patient is vomiting

Avoid nitrous oxide

Provide adequate skeletal muscle relaxation

Anticipate the need for postoperative ventilation of the lungs

TABLE 32-16. Management Problems Associated With Meningomyelocele
Infection
Fluid and electrolyte losses
Positioning for tracheal intubation
Hydrocephalus

VIII. SURGICAL PROCEDURES IN THE FIRST MONTH

A. Necrotizing enterocolitis in premature infants carries numerous considerations for anesthetic management if surgery is needed to resect gangrenous bowel (Table 32-17).

B. Inguinal hernia repair in neonates. Hernia in an infant may progress to incarceration or obstruction, emphasizing the need for prompt surgical repair. A major concern in premature infants is **postoperative apnea.** It is recommended that outpatient hernia repair not be considered in infants <50 conceptual weeks (gestational age plus postnatal age). Postoperative apnea monitoring for about 18 hours is a consideration. Postoperative analgesia can be provided with caudal anesthesia or an ilioinguinal-iliohypogastric nerve block (3 mg·kg^{-1} of 0.5% bupivacaine with epinephrine).

C. Pyloric stenosis
   1. Pyloric stenosis is a medical emergency, and surgical therapy is considered only after correction of fluid and electrolyte deficits (Table 32-18).

TABLE 32-17. Anesthetic Considerations in the Presence of Necrotizing Enterocolitis
Peritonitis
Sepsis
Acidosis
Hypovolemia (replace with balanced salt solution, whole blood)
Tolerate minimal anesthesia (ketamine, 0.5–1.0 mg·kg^{-1} iv; avoid nitrous oxide)
Invasive monitoring (blood pressure, central venous pressure, arterial blood gases)
Anticipate the need for postoperative ventilation of the lungs

TABLE 32-18. **Indications That Patients With Pyloric Stenosis Are Adequately Prepared for Surgery**

Normal skin turgor
$Na^+ > 130$ mEq·l^{-1}
$K^+ > 3$ mEq·l^{-1}
Chloride > 85 mEq·l^{-1}
Urine output 1–2 ml·kg^{-1}·h^{-1}

   2. **Anesthetic management.** The major concern is aspiration (Table 32-19).
D. **Ligation of a patent ductus arteriosus** may be necessary in a small premature infant with congestive heart failure and respiratory distress syndrome. Administration of fentanyl, 20–25 µg·kg^{-1} iv, and pancuronium provides adequate analgesia and surgical working conditions. The need for continued ventilation of the lungs postoperatively is predictable.
E. **Placement of a central venous catheter** requires tracheal intubation, a motionless patient, and a high index of suspicion for bleeding and pneumothorax.

IX. RESPIRATORY DISTRESS SYNDROME

The use of exogenous surfactant is associated with decreased mortality in this syndrome, and the incidence of bronchopulmonary dysplasia (characterized by decreased lung compliance and hyper-reactive airways) has decreased.

TABLE 32-19. **Perioperative Concerns Associated With Pyloric Stenosis**

Orogastric tube (empty the stomach and instill 5–7 ml sodium bicarbonate)
Awake vs. asleep (inhalation or intravenous) intubation of the trachea
Skeletal muscle relaxation (anesthesia or short-acting muscle relaxant)
Extubate the trachea when patient is awake
Consider caudal anesthesia (1.25 ml·kg^{-1} of 0.25% bupivacaine) after the induction of general anesthesia

X. THE RETINOPATHY OF PREMATURITY

The retinopathy of prematurity is of greatest risk in neonates weighing <1000 g, whereas the incidence is low in neonates weighing >1500 g without other complicating medical conditions. An arbitrary recommendation is to maintain SaO_2 near 95% in infants <40 weeks of conceptual age.

XI. SUDDEN INFANT DEATH SYNDROME

Sudden infant death syndrome is the most frequent cause of death in infants 1–12 months of age. The causes are unknown, but premature infants and those with bronchopulmonary dysplasia may be at increased risk.

33

Pediatric Anesthesia

Appropriate anesthetic management of pediatric surgical patients must be considered within the context of a patient's maturity and the severity of the surgical problem (Cook DR: Pediatric anesthesia. In Barash PG, Cullen BF, Stoelting RK [eds]: Clinical Anesthesia, pp 1335–1351. Philadelphia, JB Lippincott, 1992). By 3 months of age, the most significant part of maturation has occurred (Table 33-1).

I. PREANESTHETIC EVALUATION AND PREPARATION

The primary purpose of taking a preanesthetic history is to assess a child's medical condition and level of anxiety. A simple explanation of what the child can expect before induction of anesthesia reduces the element of surprise and facilitates the induction of anesthesia.

A. Minimum hemoglobin values. Use of an arbitrary hemoglobin value (10 g·dl^{-1} if >3 months of age) is useful as a screening procedure but should not be used as the final criterion for deciding if a child may be anesthetized for elective surgery.

1. Iron deficiency anemia should not delay elective surgery if the surgical procedure is not expected to result in significant blood loss.

2. Blood transfusion is never justified to treat uncomplicated iron deficiency anemia or increase the hemoglobin value to some arbitrary standard.

B. Hydration and restriction of fluids. Infants may have clear liquids up to 3–4 hours before surgery.

C. Preanesthetic medication (see Chapter 3). Between 6 months and 1 year of age, infants begin to show sufficient awareness of surroundings so that psychological aspects of hospitalization and the potential value of preanesthetic medication should be considered.

1. **Atropine and scopolamine**

a. Bradycardia induced by halothane and succinylcholine (SCh) is most prominent in infants,

TABLE 33-1. Comparison of Infant and Adult Body Composition

Body Component	% of Body Weight	
	Infant	*Adult*
Total body water	73	60
Extracellular fluid	44	15–20
Blood volume	8–10	7
	80–100 ml·kg^{-1}	65–70 ml·kg
Intracellular water	33	40
Muscle mass	20	50
Fat	12	18

especially those <3 months of age. A vagolytic dose of atropine (0.02 mg·kg^{-1} im or iv) provides protection against a cholinergic challenge in infants. It is a common practice to administer atropine after an infant is in the operating room.

   b. When sedation is the principal goal along with drying of secretions, scopolamine (0.1 mg im for 6–12 months of age, 0.15 mg for 1–5 years of age) is preferable.

2. **Route and time of administration.** When possible, the oral route of administration (with the exception of the anticholinergics) is preferred.

II. ANESTHETIC DRUGS AND RELATED DRUGS

Selection of drugs and techniques is based on an individual anesthesiologist's experience and preference and not a patient's age. Some anesthesiologists encourage parents' active participation in the induction of anesthesia.

A. Inhalation agents

1. Inhalation induction of anesthesia in infants is often complicated by breath-holding, laryngospasm, and distention of the stomach with anesthetic gases. Halothane (perhaps sevoflurane) allows the most rapid and uneventful induction. Isoflurane, enflurane, and desflurane are pungent ethers and may produce airway irritation.

2. The incidence of bradycardia, hypotension, and cardiac arrest during induction of anesthesia is greater in infants and small children than in adults. This greater incidence of untoward effects is attributed to a more rapid development of drug

concentrations owing to differences in pharmacokinetics and pharmacodynamics between children
and adults (see Table 32-8).

B. Intravenous drugs
1. Use of a small needle (27 gauge) preceded by a der-
mal lidocaine patch permits placement of a catheter for intravenous administration of drugs to induce anesthesia.
2. Methohexital ($15-25$ mg·kg^{-1}) can be administered rectally for rapid induction of anesthesia,
with recovery occurring in 30–40 minutes. Hiccups are a common side effect.

C. Opioids are used to reinforce nitrous oxide or in high
doses as the sole anesthetic in critically ill infants (Table 33-2).

D. Muscle relaxants. When allowances are made for differences in volume of distribution and anesthetic requirements (MAC), infants appear to be relatively
resistant to SCh and relatively sensitive to nondepolarizing muscle relaxants.

III. ENDOTRACHEAL INTUBATION (see Chapter 5)

A. Routine intubation of the trachea of infants and
children can be achieved with exceedingly low morbidity, keeping in mind the unique anatomic characteristics of this age group.

B. The tube should pass through the glottis and the area
of the cricoid cartilage without resistance, and air
should leak around the tube when positive airway
pressure of approximately 20 cm H_2O is applied.

C. Use of cuffed tracheal tubes in children <10 years of
age is not mandatory.

TABLE 33-2. Intravenous Opioid Doses in Infants		
	Adjuvant with Nitrous Oxide	**Sole Anesthetic**
Morphine	0.05–0.1 mg·kg^{-1}	1 mg·kg^{-1}
Fentanyl	3–5 µg·kg^{-1}	25–50 µg·kg^{-1}
Sufentanil	1–2 µg·kg^{-1}	10–15 µg·kg^{-1}
Alfentanil	100 µg·kg^{-1}	

IV. PEDIATRIC BREATHING CIRCUITS

An optimal breathing circuit for pediatric patients provides minimal dead space and resistance to breathing and is lightweight.

A. **The Jackson-Rees system (Mapleson D)** is a popular breathing circuit that requires fresh gas flow equivalent to 2.5–3.0 times a child's minute volume to prevent rebreathing during spontaneous ventilation (see Fig. 4-2F).

B. **The coaxial circuit (Bain circuit)** is a modification of the Jackson-Rees system in which lightweight disposable inspired and exhaled gas conduits are arranged coaxially with the inspiratory tubing running within the expiratory tubing (see Fig. 4-3). This arrangement permits heat exchange between the warm exhaled and unwarmed inspired gases, thus reducing the degree of heat loss from the airway. The coaxial circuit can be used for a patient of any age, provided suitable fresh gas flows are selected (Table 33-3).

C. **Magill system.** An advantage over the Jackson-Rees system is preferential venting of exhaled gases (containing carbon dioxide), thus eliminating the need for high fresh gas flows to prevent rebreathing during spontaneous ventilation (see Fig. 4-2A).

D. **Circle absorption.** Infant circle systems employ low-resistance valves with tubing and canisters that are reduced in size.

V. REGIONAL ANESTHESIA

Regional anesthesia is useful to supplement general anesthesia, as the sole anesthetic (may require heavy sedation), or to provide postoperative analgesia (Table 33-4).

VI. MONITORING (Table 33-5)

TABLE 33-3. Fresh Gas Flows Recommended for the Coaxial Circuit	
Infants <10 kg	$2 \: l \cdot min^{-1}$
Children 10–50 kg	$3.5 \: l \cdot min^{-1}$
>50 kg	$70 \: ml \cdot kg^{-1} \cdot min^{-1}$

TABLE 33-4. Regional Anesthesia Techniques
Applicable to Pediatric Patients

Brachial plexus block
  Supraclavicular approach (forearm and upper outer arm,
    including shoulder)
  Axillary (forearm and hand)
Intravenous regional block
Ilioinguinal and iliohypogastric nerve blocks (hernia surgery)
Penile block (bupivacaine 0.5%, 1 ml·kg^{-1} without
  epinephrine)
Spinal anesthesia (perform at L4 or L5–S1; tetracaine,
  0.4 mg·kg^{-1})
Epidural anesthesia (caudal technically easy; bupivacaine
  0.25%, not to exceed 3 mg·kg^{-1} with 1:200,000 epinephrine)

VII. PEDIATRIC FLUID THERAPY

A. **Maintenance fluids** are determined by body weight,
caloric expenditure, and loss (insensible, renal, and
gastrointestinal). A guideline is **4 ml·kg^{-1}·h^{-1} of 5%
dextrose in 0.25 normal saline** (alternatively, 2.5%
dextrose in 0.5 normal saline or 5% dextrose in lactated Ringer's solution).

B. **Intraoperative fluids and blood loss replacement**
may be as simple as replacing the deficits from the

TABLE 33-5. Monitoring Techniques Used for
Pediatric Patients

Precordial or esophageal stethoscope (evaluate changes in
  rate, quality, and intensity of heart sounds)
Electrocardiogram (useful for rate and rhythm; no indication
  of cardiac output)
Blood pressure (electronic oscillometers; arterial cannulation
  with 22- to 24-gauge catheter over needle)
Central venous pressure (adequacy of blood replacement or
  venous return; aspirate air)
Ventilation (clinical observation; arterial blood gases)
Pulse oximetry (oxygen saturation, heart rate, amplitude of
  blood pressure pulsation)
Capnography and mass spectrometry (confirm proper tracheal
  tube placement, analyze composition of inhaled and exhaled
  gases; detect venous air embolism)
Temperature

**TABLE 33-6. Guidelines for Third-Space
Loss Replacement**

Intra-abdominal surgery	$6–10 \ ml·kg^{-1}·h^{-1}$
Intrathoracic surgery	$4–7 \ ml·kg^{-1}·h^{-1}$
Superficial and neurosurgery	$1–2 \ ml·kg^{-1}·h^{-1}$

preoperative fast and providing maintenance fluids or
as complex as correcting pre-existing deficits and replacing intraoperative losses.

1. **Fasting deficit** is calculated as an infant's hourly
   maintenance fluid requirement times the number
   of hours since the last feeding. Half the calculated
   deficit is administered during the first hour of anesthesia and the remainder during the next 2 hours
   plus maintenance fluid.
2. **Third-space intraoperative losses** reflect seques-
   tration of fluid in a nonfunctional compartment,
   which varies in magnitude with the surgical procedure (Table 33-6).
3. Replacement solutions (maintenance and third
   space) depend on the magnitude of loss and duration of surgery (Table 33-7).

**TABLE 33-7. Fluid Replacement as Determined by Site
and Duration of Surgery**

*Short Surgical Procedure With Minimal to Moderate
Third-Space Loss*

5% Dextrose in lactated Ringer's solution for maintenance
and third-space loss (limit to $15–20 \ ml·kg^{-1}$ to avoid
hyperglycemia)

*Long Surgical Procedure With Moderate to Extensive
Third-Space Loss*

5% Dextrose in 0.25 normal saline for maintenance and
lactated Ringer's solution for third-space loss

Massive Third-Space Loss

5% albumin to restore 1/3 to 1/4 of the loss

Daily Fluid Maintenance Requirements

First 10 kg	$4 \ ml·kg^{-1}·h^{-1}$
Second 10 kg	$2 \ ml·kg^{-1}·h^{-1}$
>20 kg	$1 \ ml·kg^{-1}·h^{-1}$

4. **Blood replacement**
  a. Blood volume is about 100 ml·kg^{-1} in infants and about 80 ml·kg^{-1} in older children.
  b. Normovolemic hemodilution is commonly accepted, but blood replacement is usually considered when loss exceeds 20% of the calculated blood volume.
  c. Gradual blood loss can be replaced with lactated Ringer's solution equal to two to three times the estimated loss. Some, however, recommend three to four times the volume of crystalloid solution for each milliliter of blood loss.
  d. Packed red blood cells, 1 ml·kg^{-1}, increase the hematocrit by about 1.5%.

VIII. POSTANESTHESIA CARE

A. Infants and children generally recover more quickly from anesthesia and surgery and are less disturbed by minor complications than adults.

B. Management of subglottic edema
  1. Subglottic edema usually manifests as a brassy cough and stertorous breathing 2–4 hours after tracheal extubation.
  2. Mild cases require little or no therapy other than high inhaled concentrations of humidified oxygen.
  3. **Racemic epinephrine** (0.5 ml of a 2% solution diluted to a volume of 3.5 ml) administered in a nebulizer with intermittent positive-pressure ventilation is the most effective treatment.
  4. There is no evidence that steroids are effective, but they seem to be useful in some cases (**dexamethasone,** 4 mg iv for infants <1 year of age; 8 mg iv for older children as a single injection).
  5. Tracheostomy may be required in severe cases that do not respond to conventional treatment.

34

Anesthesia for
the Geriatric Patient

More important than chronologic age is a patient's physiologic age, which varies from person to person and from one organ system to another (McLeskey CH: Anesthesia for the geriatric patient. In Barash PG, Cullen BF, Stoelting RK [eds]: Clinical Anesthesia, pp 1353–1387. Philadelphia, JB Lippincott, 1992). There is little correlation between chronologic age and biologic age.

I. ANESTHESIA RISKS

Compared with younger patients, elderly patients may be at greater risk for perioperative complications because of age-related **concomitant diseases** and **declines in basic organ function** that are independent of disease.

A. **Effects of concomitant disease.** The presence of age-related concomitant diseases probably plays a greater role than does age itself in contributing to perioperative complications and mortality (Table 34-1).

B. **Effects of emergency procedures.** The risk of perioperative complications and death is increased in the elderly if surgery must be performed on an emergency basis, which allows little time for control of concomitant diseases and stresses organ systems that have deteriorated with age.

II. PATHOPHYSIOLOGY OF AGING

A. **Cardiovascular system.** Many of the changes previously thought to reflect aging (especially declines in cardiac output) now appear to be manifestations of age-related disease or a sedentary lifestyle resulting in prolonged deconditioning (Table 34-2).

  1. Patients >70 years of age have at least a 50% chance of developing significant ischemic heart disease with or without symptoms.

TABLE 34-1. Age-Related Concomitant Disease

Hypertension
Ischemic heart disease
Congestive heart failure
Peripheral vascular disease
Obstructive pulmonary disease
Renal disease
Diabetes mellitus
Arthritis
Dementia

2. **Cardiac output.** Age-related declines in cardiac output, when they occur, slow the onset of intravenously administered drugs (delayed unconsciousness) and speed establishment of inhaled anesthetic concentrations (unexpected hypotension).

3. **Cardiac reserve.** The concept that elderly patients have a reduced cardiac reserve, making them less capable of responding to stress, is not a consistent observation. For example, despite an age-related attenuation in maximum heart rate, an otherwise elderly nonsedentary patient is able to enhance cardiac output in response to increased demands.

4. **Heart rate and adrenoreceptor responsiveness of the elderly cardiovascular system.** An age-related decrease in target organ responsiveness to catecholamines may reflect a **decreased number of receptors or reduced receptor responsiveness.** Chronotropic and inotropic effects of drugs are reduced in elderly patients, as reflected by reduced heart rate responses

TABLE 34-2. Changes in the Cardiovascular System With Aging

	Change
Cardiac output	No change or decrease
Resting heart rate	Decrease
Maximum heart rate	Decrease
Arterial distensibility	Increase
Systemic vascular resistance	Increase
Systolic blood pressure	Increase

to atropine, isoflurane, propranolol, and isoproterenol. The dose of phenylephrine required to increase mean arterial pressure by 20 mm Hg is almost twice as great in the elderly.

5. **Dysrhythmias.** The prevalence of cardiac dysrhythmias (isolated supraventricular and ventricular beats), decreased T-wave amplitude, and first-degree heart block is increased in elderly patients.

B. **Ventilatory system.** Aging is associated with reduced ventilatory volumes and decreased efficiency of gas exchange as reflected by a decreased PaO_2 (see Appendix A). Age-induced parenchymal changes in the lungs mimic those of emphysema. The ventilatory response to hypoxemia or hypercapnia in elderly patients is about one half that in younger patients. This response is further impaired by opioid premedication and inhaled anesthetics.

C. **Central nervous system**
   1. Declines in mental (cognitive) function with age may be related more to nutrition and level of stimulation than to an intrinsic effect of aging.
   2. Dementia (Alzheimer's disease) is not uncommon in elderly patients and may be associated with cerebral atherosclerosis and a gradual reduction in cerebral blood flow.
   3. **Decreased requirement for anesthetics** may reflect pharmacokinetic (volume of distribution, clearance) or pharmacodynamic (receptor responsiveness, neuronal density, neurotransmitter synthesis) mechanisms (see Section III B) (Table 34-3).

D. **Changes in body compartments** (Table 34-4)

E. **Protein binding** of drugs is reduced in elderly patients (albumin production declines with age), making more

---

TABLE 34-3. Age-Related Decreases in Dose Requirements

Volatile anesthetics (MAC declines in parallel with increasing age)

Local anesthetics

Opioids (equivalent electroencephalogram suppression at lower plasma concentrations)

Barbiturates (thiopental induction dose 30% less)

Benzodiazepines

Etomidate

TABLE 34-4. Age-Related Changes in Body Composition
Loss of skeletal muscle mass
Increase in body fat (volume of distribution increased for lipid-soluble drugs; cumulative drug effects)
Decrease in total body water (reflects 20–30% reduction in blood volume by 75 years of age; a slowed rate of intercompartmental clearance results in unexpectedly high initial plasma drug concentrations)

free drug available to enter the central nervous system as well as available for hepatic metabolism.

F. **Renal function.** Glomerular filtration rate and renal tubular function decrease with age, most likely reflecting decreased renal blood flow owing to a decline in cardiac output or more important a reduction in the magnitude of the renal vascular bed. Serum creatinine level may remain normal despite advanced renal disease, reflecting the impact of concomitant loss of skeletal muscle mass. Renal reserve to withstand water or electrolyte imbalance is reduced in elderly patients and may be further compromised by perioperative changes in renal blood flow, as caused by dehydration or blood loss. A useful way to protect the kidneys during surgery is to maintain urine output above $0.5 \text{ ml·kg}^{-1} \cdot \text{h}^{-1}$.

G. **Hepatic function.** Reduced hepatic clearance of various substances parallels a reduction in the number of hepatocytes and hepatic blood flow with aging. Enzyme function appears to be maintained with aging.

H. **Basal metabolic rate and thermoregulation.** Basal metabolic rate declines about 1% per year after 30 years of age, resulting in slowed metabolism of drugs and an increased incidence of **intraoperative hypothermia.** Shivering in response to hypothermia increases oxygen consumption 400–500%, placing increasing demands on the cardiac and pulmonary systems, which in elderly patients may manifest as arterial hypoxemia or myocardial ischemia.

I. **Airway reflexes.** Laryngeal, pharyngeal, and airway reflexes are less active in elderly patients, making pulmonary aspiration more likely.

J. **Endocrine system.** Glucose intolerance in the absence of diabetes mellitus accompanies aging. This intolerance reflects peripheral resistance to the effects of insulin, emphasizing the importance of limiting glucose administration and perhaps measuring blood glucose concentrations in the perioperative period.

III. PHARMACOKINETICS AND PHARMACODYNAMICS RELATIVE TO AGING

The **elimination half-time ($T_{1/2\beta}$)** of injected drugs is **often prolonged** in elderly patients, reflecting **increased volume of distribution** (lipid-soluble drugs stored in increased total body fat content) and **decreased renal and hepatic clearance** that accompanies aging. For these reasons, **cumulative drug effects** with repeated injections are also more likely in elderly patients.

A. Intravenous agents

1. **Barbiturates.** The dose of thiopental required to induce anesthesia in elderly patients is reduced, most likely reflecting a slowed rate of clearance of drug from the central compartment to peripheral compartments. A decreased dose produces a plasma concentration similar to that resulting from a higher dose administered to younger patients. A prolonged duration of action of thiopental most likely reflects an increased volume of distribution and a resulting prolonged $T_{1/2\beta}$.

2. **Benzodiazepines.** The plasma concentration of diazepam required to achieve a desired pharmacologic effect is less in elderly patients (pharmacodynamic response). The $T_{1/2\beta}$ of diazepam in hours is about the same as a patient's age in years, reflecting an increased volume of distribution as a result of storage of this lipid-soluble drug in fat (pharmacokinetic response). Elderly patients also show enhanced sensitivity to midazolam.

3. **Opioids.** $T_{1/2\beta}$ of opioids is increased as a reflection of increased volume of distribution. Decreased dose requirements reflect increased brain sensitivity (pharmacodynamic mechanism) to the effects of opioids.

4. **Etomidate.** Plasma clearance is reduced as a result of decreased hepatic blood flow and metabolism. There is no change in pharmacodynamics, but a slowed rate of intercompartmental clearance results in the development of a higher initial plasma concentration and the need for a reduced dosage requirement.

5. **Propofol.** Clearance rates of propofol are decreased in geriatric patients, leading to a recommendation that both the induction dose and maintenance infusion rate be decreased.

B. Inhalation drugs
1. Minimal alveolar concentration (MAC) of volatile anesthetics decreases with age **(about 4% for each decade of life over age 40)**, paralleling declining cerebral metabolic oxygen requirements (pharmacodynamic mechanism) (Fig. 34-1).
2. Age-related changes in cardiac output, the ratio of ventilation to perfusion, and tissue and blood solubility could alter the pharmacokinetics of inhaled anesthetics in elderly patients, but clinically significant differences have not been observed.

C. Muscle relaxants
1. Despite deterioration of the neuromuscular junction and nerves with age, there is no age-related change in the plasma concentration (pharmacodynamics)

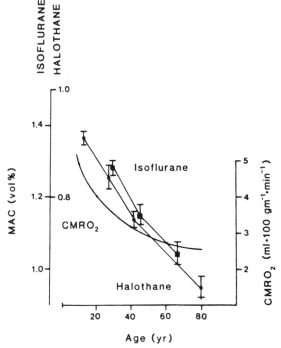

Figure 34-1. MAC for volatile anesthetics parallels age-related declines in cerebral metabolic requirements for oxygen ($CMRO_2$).

TABLE 34-5. Possible Reasons for Changes in Local Anesthetic Requirements With Aging

---

Decreased central nervous system neuronal population (only ⅓ of the total number of neurons remain by age 90)

Decreased number of axons in peripheral nerves

Deterioration of myelin sheaths

Narrowing of intervertebral spaces (reduces transforaminal escape and facilitates cephalad spread in the epidural space)

Reduced vertebral column height (influences dose for spinal anesthesia)

---

required to produce a specific muscle relaxant effect in elderly persons versus young adults.

2. Clearance of pancuronium or metocurine (renal) and vecuronium (hepatic) may be prolonged (pharmacokinetics) in elderly patients, emphasizing the need to adjust dosing intervals to avoid cumulative drug effects. Surprisingly, the clearance rates of doxacurium and pipecuronium, both of which are dependent on hepatic and renal elimination mechanisms, seem minimally changed by aging.

3. Clearance of atracurium is not influenced by aging, indicating that inactivation of this drug by Hofmann elimination or plasma ester hydrolysis is independent of age.

4. Dose requirements of succinylcholine seem to be little altered by age despite the possible presence of age-related declines in cardiac output and plasma cholinesterase activity.

D. **Local/regional anesthesia techniques.** Dose requirements for spinal, epidural, and peripheral nerve blocks may be reduced as a result of age-related changes (Table 34-5).

IV. UNIQUE ANESTHETIC CONSIDERATIONS

A. **Premedication.** Apprehension is less likely in elderly patients, and drugs selected for premedication should have short-lived effects, remembering the likelihood of increased sensitivity to sedative drug effects (especially with midazolam).

B. **Monitoring.** The need for invasive monitoring (arterial, central venous, pulmonary artery catheters) may be greater in elderly patients, considering their limited

---

**TABLE 34-6. Special Considerations in Airway
Management of Elderly Patients**

Edentulous (mask fit difficult)

Loose and/or diseased teeth

Temporomandibular joint dysfunction

Cervical arthritis

Avoid overextension of the neck (possibility of vertebrobasilar
arterial insufficiency)

Avoid lateral application of cricoid pressure (may dislodge
atherosclerotic plaque in carotid artery)

Increased risk of sympathetic nervous system stimulation
during laryngoscopy (pre-existing hypertension, ischemic
heart disease)

---

physiologic reserve and the frequent presence of concomitant diseases.

C. **Endotracheal intubation.** Age-related changes may introduce special considerations in airway management
of elderly patients (Table 34-6).

D. **Regional anesthesia versus general anesthesia.** No single anesthetic technique has been shown to be superior
for elderly patients, although regional anesthesia may
have some value for hip arthroplasty (decreased intraoperative blood loss and a reduced incidence of deep
vein thrombosis) and transurethral resection of the
prostate. Postoperative mental dysfunction is not different in elderly patients receiving general anesthesia
versus those receiving regional anesthesia plus intravenous sedation.

**TABLE 34-7. Drugs Likely to Be Taken by Elderly
Patients**

Antihypertensives

Antidepressants

Anticoagulants

Oral hypoglycemics

Corticosteroids

Beta blockers

Night-time sedatives

Alcohol

**TABLE 34-8. Postoperative Considerations in
Elderly Patients**

Supplemental oxygen (during transport and in postanesthesia
care unit)

Treat intraoperative hypothermia

Frequent reassurance to improve orientation

Return personal items to provide psychological security
(dentures, glasses, hearing aids)

E. **Positioning.** Osteoporosis, limited mobility owing to arthritis, and fragile skin dictate the need for careful positioning, placement of monitoring electrodes, and removal of tape.

F. **Drug interactions** most often reflect polypharmacy and
the additive or synergistic action of multiple drugs
(prescribed and over-the-counter). Preoperatively, a
list of likely drugs used should be investigated (Table
34-7).

G. **Outpatient anesthesia for elderly patients.** If elderly
patients pass routine preoperative screening tests, there
is no reason why age alone should prevent them from
being considered as candidates for outpatient procedures.

V. POSTOPERATIVE MANAGEMENT

Elderly patients require special attention to specific postoperative details (Table 34-8).

35

Outpatient Anesthesia

Outpatient anesthesia and surgery decrease medical costs, protect patients from hospital-acquired infections, and avoid disruption of the family unit, which is particularly important for pediatric patients (Wetchler BV: Outpatient anesthesia. In Barash PG, Cullen BF, Stoelting RK [eds]: Clinical Anesthesia, pp 1389–1416. Philadelphia, JB Lippincott, 1992). Unanticipated admission rates after outpatient surgery are usually <3%.

I. SELECTION CRITERIA FOR OUTPATIENT ANESTHESIA

Selection for outpatient surgery is based on a patient's characteristics and the planned surgical procedure.

A. Patient factors. The response to standard questions several days before the planned procedure (telephone interview is acceptable) facilitates determination of the need for laboratory tests in addition to those already ordered and whether a patient's medical condition warrants an anesthesiologist's evaluation a few days before surgery or if it can be done on the day of surgery (Tables 35-1 and 35-2).

  1. When medical problems are present, the most important decision is whether there is optimal control of such problems.

  2. In elderly patients, physiologic rather than chronologic age is the important consideration.

  3. There is no universal agreement about what constitutes an acceptable postconceptual age (gestation plus postnatal age) for an outpatient infant who was born prematurely. It is generally agreed that an increased incidence of apneic episodes after anesthesia in infants with a postconceptual age <50 weeks makes outpatient anesthesia a questionable selection.

  4. Explaining to the patient the reasons for not eating or drinking large amounts of fluid before surgery is important.

TABLE 35-1. Questionnaire Before Outpatient Anesthesia

Do you feel sick?

Do you have any serious illnesses (hypertension, diabetes)?

Do you get more short of breath on exertion than others your age?

Do you cough?

Do you wheeze?

Do you have chest pain on exertion?

Do you have ankle swelling?

Have you taken medication in the past 3 months?

Do you have allergies?

Have you or your relatives experienced difficulties with anesthesia?

Could you be pregnant?

     5. **Inappropriate candidates for ambulatory surgery.** Criteria must be individualized, but certain types of patients are unlikely candidates for outpatient anesthesia (Table 35-3).

  B. **Procedures** that are acceptable for outpatient anesthesia depend on a patient's characteristics and capabilities, the experiences of the surgeon and anesthesiologist, and the resources of the medical facility being used.

     1. Duration of surgery >90 minutes or the need for

TABLE 35-2. Questionnaire Before Pediatric Outpatient Anesthesia

Discussed With a Parent of a Pediatric Patient:

Breath-holding spells

Cardiac, respiratory, or other problems

History of prematurity and if yes:
    Was oxygen used?
    Was tracheal intubation required?
    Any lasting effects?

Muscular problems

Developmental delays

Asthma or frequent colds

Sickle cell disease/trait

Medications

Recent exposure to contagious diseases

**TABLE 35-3. Unlikely Candidates for
Outpatient Anesthesia**

Infant at risk
  Premature birth and <50 weeks postconceptual age
  Apneic episodes
  Failure to thrive
  Respiratory distress syndrome requiring ventilatory support
  Bronchopulmonary dysplasia
  Family history of sudden infant death syndrome and <6–12
    months of age
Malignant hyperthermia susceptibility
Uncontrolled seizure activity
Medically unstable
Morbidly obese and other systemic diseases
Acute substance abuse
Presence of infection
Uncooperative and/or unreliable
No responsible person at home

---

blood transfusion is not a contraindication to outpatient surgery.

2. Operations that require a major intervention in the
cranial vault, thorax, or abdomen are not considered
acceptable outpatient procedures. Emergency procedures are unlikely to be performed on an outpatient basis.

C. **Facility.** Outpatient surgical facilities are either in a
hospital or a free-standing clinic (Surgicenter) that has
an admission agreement with a nearby hospital in the
event that unexpected postoperative hospitalization is
required.

II. ANESTHESIA MANAGEMENT

A. **Premedication** (see Chapter 3). It is important to select
drugs, doses, and routes of administration that are practical and do not prolong recovery.

B. Drugs used for premedication of outpatients include
short-acting opioids (fentanyl, 1.5 $\mu g \cdot kg^{-1}$ iv), seda-
tive-hypnotics (oral diazepam, intramuscular midazo-
lam), anticholinergics, H_2 receptor antagonists, antacids, and metoclopramide.

C. For pediatric patients, oral administration of diazepam
or a combination of diazepam, meperidine, and atropine does not delay recovery.

III. TECHNIQUES AND DRUGS

Successful anesthesia for outpatient surgery is evidenced by prompt postoperative presence of alertness, ambulation, analgesia, and alimentation.

A. **Regional techniques.** A satisfactory outpatient regional anesthesia experience depends on appropriate selection of patients, sedatives, local anesthetics, and specific regional technique.

1. Time to perform the block and to permit its onset is a potential drawback when procedures are short and turnover time between cases is rapid. Residual skeletal muscle weakness delays patient discharge.

2. Short-acting drugs (midazolam, fentanyl, alfentanil) are indicated in selected patients (anxious; need for paresthesias during performance of block) but must be titrated to avoid oversedation.

3. Short-acting local anesthetics (2-chloroprocaine, lidocaine) reduce the likelihood of unwanted postoperative skeletal muscle weakness. Infiltration of the incision with bupivacaine provides prolonged postoperative analgesia.

4. Potential side effects must be considered when selecting regional anesthetic techniques for outpatient surgery (Table 35-4).

   a. There is no evidence that the incidence of postdural puncture headache is increased by early ambulation of an outpatient. Bed rest does not reduce the incidence of this type of headache.

   b. For outpatient surgery on the lower extremity or perineal area, spinal anesthesia may be preferable to epidural anesthesia because of the absence of sacral root sparing with the former technique.

B. **During conscious sedation,** a patient responds appropriately to commands **(take a deep breath)** and is able to maintain a patent upper airway unassisted. Selection of appropriate drugs and doses (slow titration through a small catheter in a large vein) is mandatory. Warning of coming events (injection of local anesthetic, inser-

---

TABLE 35-4. Complications of Regional Techniques for Outpatient Anesthesia

Sciatic-femoral (prolonged motor blockade)
Supraclavicular or interscalene (pneumothorax)
Spinal (headache)

tion of laparoscope, inflation of a tourniquet) makes the event less stimulating than if it were unanticipated. Pulse oximetry is an objective means of assessing oxygenation during conscious sedation.

C. **Injectable drugs** are more likely than inhaled anesthetics to influence the time of discharge after outpatient surgery. Desirable characteristics of injectable drugs emphasize patient safety, comfort, and rapid clearance (Table 35-5).

1. **Thiopental/methohexital.** Although both drugs have been successfully administered to outpatients, there is more rapid recovery of complete psychomotor function in patients receiving methohexital (1.0–1.5 mg·kg^{-1} iv) than thiopental (3–5 mg·kg^{-1} iv), presumably reflecting the more rapid metabolism of methohexital.

2. **Etomidate** has no apparent advantage over barbiturates and may be associated with an increased incidence of postoperative nausea and vomiting. Pain on injection and involuntary myoclonic movements are common side effects. Transient (about 8 hours) suppression of adrenocortical function after a single induction dose of etomidate does not necessitate exogenous steroid supplementation.

3. **Ketamine** administered to adults has not found wide acceptance for management of outpatient anesthesia because of its potential to produce prolonged effects and emergence delirium. Ketamine, in doses of 2–3 mg·kg^{-1} im, may be useful for improving acceptance of a mask induction of anesthesia in children 1–5 years of age.

TABLE 35-5. Desirable Characteristics of Injected Drugs for Outpatient Anesthesia

High therapeutic (safety) index
Water-soluble and stable in solution
Nonirritating after parenteral administration
No allergic reactions
Rapid and smooth onset of action
No cardiopulmonary depression
Rapid degradation to inactive and nontoxic metabolites
Short elimination half-time
Analgesia at subanesthetic levels
Rapid and smooth emergence without side effects

4. **Propofol.** Speed of recovery (time to open eyes) is more rapid following administration of propofol (2.5 mg·kg^{-1} iv) than following barbiturates, but onset of action is similar. There is a virtual absence of postoperative side effects (nausea, dizziness, drowsiness, pain at injection site) following administration of propofol, with little detectable evidence of impairment of psychomotor function 30 minutes later.

   a. Consistent with the rapid onset and prompt recovery following injection of propofol is its high lipid solubility and extensive hepatic metabolism (elimination half-time 1–3 hours).

   b. Hypotension and depression of ventilation may be greater following administration of propofol than barbiturates.

5. **Succinylcholine.** The possible occurrence of post-succinylcholine myalgia is a more important consideration than the rapid onset of drug effect in a patient undergoing an elective outpatient surgical procedure. Defasciculating doses of nondepolarizing muscle relaxants do not reliably prevent myalgia.

6. **Atracurium and vecuronium** are most useful in outpatient surgical procedures lasting >20 minutes. The onset and duration of equivalent doses of atracurium (0.25–0.30 mg·kg^{-1}) and vecuronium (0.04–0.05 mg·kg^{-1}) are similar and dose-dependent. Spontaneous or pharmacologic reversal of these drugs must be complete at the end of the procedure.

7. **Mivacurium** has an onset and duration (intubating doses of 0.2–0.25 mg·kg^{-1} produce maximum blockade in about 2.5 minutes and spontaneous recovery to 95% twitch height in about 30 minutes) that is shorter than those of atracurium or vecuronium but longer than succinylcholine. If a priming dose of mivacurium of 0.03 mg·kg^{-1} is followed by an intubating dose of 0.2 mg·kg^{-1} in a well-anesthetized patient, the time to tracheal intubation can be shortened to about 90 seconds. At the completion of surgery, residual blockade, if present, is easily antagonized.

8. **Opioids.** Long-acting opioids (morphine and meperidine) are less acceptable than shorter-acting drugs (fentanyl, sufentanil, alfentanil) for administration to outpatients. The incidence of nausea may be increased in patients receiving opioids.

   a. **Fentanyl.** Intraoperative anesthetic requirements and the postoperative need for analgesia as well as the time to discharge are decreased in adult outpatients receiving fentanyl, 1–3 $\mu g \cdot kg^{-1}$ (50–100 μg iv), just before the induction of anesthesia.

   b. **Sufentanil.** The preinduction adult dose of sufentanil is 10–15 μg iv.

   c. **Alfentanil.** Alertness may occur sooner and depression of ventilation may be less in adults receiving equal analgesic preinduction doses of alfentanil (0.5–1.0 mg iv) compared with fentanyl.

9. **Benzodiazepines.** Use of midazolam for induction of anesthesia is not popular because of delayed recovery and an amnesic effect, which may interfere with patients' remembering instructions. Flumazenil (0.2–1.0 mg iv at 0.2 $mg \cdot min^{-1}$) is a specific benzodiazepine antagonist, but its duration of action may be shorter than the undesired benzodiazepine sedative effect.

D. **Inhalation anesthetics** with low blood solubilities facilitate a rapid onset and prompt recovery from anesthesia that is useful for outpatients. No single drug or technique is ideal, and most anesthesiologists combine the advantages of injected and inhaled drugs. For short outpatient procedures (<90 minutes), there is probably no significant difference in awakening times following administration of halothane, enflurane, or isoflurane. For longer outpatient procedures, isoflurane may be associated with a more rapid awakening, perhaps reflecting its lower blood solubility. Pediatric patients may prefer an inhalation induction to the needle stick required for an intravenous induction of anesthesia.

1. **Nitrous oxide (N_2O)** remains the mainstay of inhalation anesthesia in the ambulatory setting despite concerns that it may increase the incidence of nausea and vomiting.

2. **Halothane** is the most commonly used volatile anesthetic for children, providing a mask induction with a low incidence of excitement. Cardiac dysrhythmias may be more likely to occur than during administration of other volatile anesthetics.

3. **Enflurane** in high concentrations can provide skeletal muscle relaxation sufficient for most outpatient surgical procedures.

4. **Isoflurane,** because of its pungent smell, is associated with a higher incidence of breath-holding, coughing, and laryngospasm than either enflurane or halothane. Like enflurane, isoflurane in high concentrations can provide skeletal muscle relaxation sufficient for most outpatient surgical procedures.

5. **Desflurane** is poorly soluble in blood and tissues, accounting for prompt psychomotor recovery following discontinuation of this drug.
6. **Sevoflurane** resembles desflurane in terms of rapid onset and prompt recovery following its discontinuation.

IV. POSTANESTHESIA CARE UNIT MANAGEMENT

A. Managing common postoperative problems is equal in importance to appropriate patient selection and choice of anesthetic for ensuring prompt discharge (usually <1.5 hours).

B. **Pain.** Appropriate control of postoperative pain includes supplementation of inhaled anesthetics with opioids, local or regional blockade, and intravenous administration of opioids (fentanyl, 0.35 $\mu g \cdot kg^{-1}$ every 5 minutes until pain is controlled). An elixir of acetaminophen and codeine is useful for treatment of mild pain in pediatric patients.

C. **Nausea and vomiting** are a common reason for delayed discharge or admission to the hospital after planned outpatient surgery. Contributing factors to postoperative nausea and vomiting are multiple (Table 35-6).
1. Nausea often accompanies postoperative pain and is relieved only when pain relief is achieved by intravenous injection of opioids.
2. **Antiemetics**
   a. **Droperidol** administered intravenously (10–25 $\mu g \cdot kg^{-1}$; 0.625–1.25 mg) to adults just before induction of anesthesia results in a decreased incidence of postoperative nausea and vomiting. Drowsiness becomes more noticeable when the

TABLE 35-6. Contributing Factors to Postoperative Nausea and Vomiting

History of motion sickness
History of emesis after previous anesthetics
Obesity
Site of surgery (laparoscopy, eye)
Use of opioids
Sudden movement or position changes
Postoperative pain

dose of droperidol exceeds 1.25 mg. In pediatric patients undergoing strabismus surgery, intravenous administration of droperidol, 75 $\mu g \cdot kg^{-1}$, before manipulation of the extraocular muscles reduces the incidence of postoperative vomiting but prolongs the recovery time.

    b. Droperidol/metoclopramide. A combination of droperidol (0.5–1.0 mg iv) administered 3–6 minutes before induction of anesthesia and metoclopramide (10–20 mg iv) administered 15–30 minutes before droperidol is effective in reducing the incidence of postoperative nausea and vomiting.

    c. Nausea and vomiting that develop postoperatively may be treated with intravenous administration of droperidol (0.25–1.0 mg) or metoclopramide (5–10 mg).

V. DISCHARGE CRITERIA (Table 35-7)

    A. Discharge criteria after epidural or spinal anesthesia include normal sensation, ability to walk (return of motor function and proprioception), and ability to urinate (return of sympathetic nervous system function).

    B. Before being discharged home, patients should be given diet instructions (clear liquids initially and avoid alcohol for at least 12 hours) and told to **expect minor annoyances** such as sore throat, headache, nausea, dizziness, incisional pain, and myalgia for about 24 hours. It is probably prudent not to drive an automobile or

---

TABLE 35-7. Discharge Criteria Following Outpatient Anesthesia

Responsible adult present to take patient home and provide subsequent observation

Stable vital signs

No nausea or vomiting

Pain is controllable with oral analgesics

No evidence of bleeding

No evidence of upper airway obstruction (laryngeal edema usually manifests within 1 hour after tracheal extubation)

Ability to recognize time and place

Ability to ambulate unassisted

nake important decisions for at least 24–48 hours. Patients are given the telephone number of the person to contact regarding significant postoperative complications.

C. A patient's condition is verified the next day, most often by a telephone interview.

36

Trauma and Burns

Trauma and burns are major health hazards, and anesthesiologists play a prominent role in the care of these acutely injured patients (Priano LJ: Trauma and burns. In Barash PG, Cullen BF, Stoelting RK [eds]: Clinical Anesthesia, pp 1417–1429. Philadelphia, JB Lippincott, 1992).

I. EPIDEMIOLOGY

A. Trauma is the **leading cause of death** of young persons. Approximately 50,000 people die each year from motor vehicle accidents, and 30,000 die from gunshot wounds. **Penetrating trauma** is usually associated with easily diagnosed isolated injuries. **Blunt trauma** may be associated with diffuse hidden injuries.

B. About 50% of victims die at the scene of trauma as a result of massive injury, and 30% will die after 1–2 **"golden" hours** if hemorrhage, pneumothorax, cardiac tamponade, or an expanding intracranial mass is not treated. Death occurs in 20% after several days as a result of sepsis or multiple organ failure.

C. Regionalization of care to **trauma centers** improves survival from trauma. These centers require 24-hour in-house surgeons, anesthesiologists, and nurses, plus radiology support, a laboratory, and a blood bank.

II. PREHOSPITAL CARE

A. Survival from trauma requires **rapid transport** from the scene to the hospital, well-trained **paramedical** personnel, and constant **medical supervision.**

B. Paramedics must be capable of establishing an **airway** (including endotracheal intubation), beginning **intravenous infusions** of fluids, stabilizing the neck and obvious **fractures,** relieving tension **pneumothorax,** and administering **drugs** such as succinylcholine, atropine, lidocaine, nitroglycerin, epinephrine, and opioids.

III. EMERGENCY ROOM

A. Proper care of trauma patients requires adequate numbers of trained **personnel,** orderly **protocols,** and advanced **planning.**

B. The first priority is establishment of an **airway** and administration of **oxygen.** Indications for **endotracheal intubation** are listed in Table 36-1.

   1. Until the possibility of cervical fracture has been ruled out, orotracheal intubation should be undertaken with an assistant applying gentle axial traction and stabilizing the patient's head in a neutral position. All patients should be assumed to have full stomachs. Nasotracheal intubation should not be attempted if there is the possibility of a basal skull fracture, because the tube may enter the brain. If airway obstruction exists and tracheal intubation cannot be accomplished, emergency cricothyrotomy is indicated (see inside of front cover).

   2. Airway management is particularly complex and requires careful thought when there is hoarseness, stridor, blunt or penetrating injury to the neck, subcutaneous emphysema, or tracheal deviation on a chest radiograph. Under these circumstances, routine oral or nasal tracheal intubation may worsen a laryngeal or bronchial injury and cause total airway obstruction or disruption.

TABLE 36-1. Indications for Tracheal Intubation in Trauma Patients

Protection from aspiration of blood or gastric contents
Airway obstruction
Positive-pressure ventilation
Tracheal toilet
Hypoxemia
Coma
Shock
Immobilization with sedation and/or paralysis if a patient is uncooperative

C. Multiple sites of **vascular access** must be established with large-bore catheters. **Warm** crystalloid **fluids** should be administered if there is hypotension.

D. A brief **history** and **physical examination** should be performed, including a complete **neurologic** assessment.

E. **Radiographs** must be taken of the chest and cervical spine.

F. A **blood sample** should be taken for immediate analysis of arterial blood gases, electrolytes, glucose, hematocrit, coagulation screen, toxicology screen, ethanol, and blood typing and cross-match.

G. A **nasogastric** tube should be inserted if there is no evidence of a basal skull fracture.

H. A **urinary catheter** should be inserted if there is no evidence of a pelvic fracture or damage to the urethra.

I. When indicated, **special diagnostic procedures** should be performed, such as peritoneal lavage, computed tomography, thoracocentesis, intravenous pyelogram, or angiography.

J. Surgical subspecialists should be called in for **consultation** as needed.

IV. ASSESSMENT OF INJURIES

A. **Shock** (generalized inadequate tissue perfusion usually accompanied by hypotension) after trauma is most often caused by hemorrhage and hypovolemia (Table 36-2).

B. **Central nervous system**
   1. The Glasgow Coma Score is useful for quantitating a patient's level of consciousness (see Table 19-15).

TABLE 36-2. Causes of Hypotension in the Trauma Patient

Hypovolemia
Spinal cord injury
Cardiac tamponade
Tension pneumothorax
Anaphylaxis
Drug overdose
Neurogenic pulmonary edema
Sepsis (unlikely to be a factor immediately after injury)

2. **Intracranial hematoma** is a frequent cause of neurologic deficit after trauma. Early diagnosis with computed tomography and treatment with surgical decompression are mandatory. Temporizing pharmacologic and mechanical measures may be introduced in an attempt to decrease intracranial pressure (see Table 19-9).

3. **Spinal cord injury** frequently accompanies trauma. Until such injury is ruled out (lateral radiograph of the cervical spine), the patient's vertebral column is stabilized in a neutral position (cervical collar, transfer from bed utilizing "log-rolling" technique).

C. **Facial injury** is assumed to be associated with cervical spine injury until proved otherwise.

1. Establishing an airway can be difficult (consider techniques in an awake patient; avoid muscle relaxants).

2. Nasal instrumentation is not performed if there is evidence of a basal skull fracture or the cribriform plate is not intact.

D. **Thoracic injury** from blunt trauma (rib fracture, pneumothorax, cardiac contusion) may not be obvious on external examination. An early chest radiograph (showing fractures, widened mediastinum, hemothorax) is useful.

E. **Abdominal injury** after blunt trauma (splenic or liver laceration, bowel rupture, vessel laceration) is most likely to be diagnosed by peritoneal lavage or computed tomography.

V. OPERATING ROOM

The operating rooms of a level 1 trauma center must be in a constant state of preparedness for trauma. Many centers hold an operating room open at all times as a "crash room." **Trauma operating rooms** should have anesthesia equipment that is checked out and ready for immediate use (Table 36-3).

VI. ANESTHESIA PERSONNEL

A. Members of the anesthesia department must set forth a treatment plan **before** an injured patient arrives. There must be a mechanism to ensure that adequate help will be immediately available. For hemodynamically unstable patients, responsibility for specific functions should be assigned in advance, such as ven-

---

**TABLE 36-3. Immediately Available Equipment
in an Operating Room for Care of
Trauma Patients**

Anesthesia machine
Ventilator
Laryngoscopes and a selection of tracheal tubes
Electronic monitor with pressure transducers
Blood pumps and primed infusion sets in blood warmers
Prefilled labeled syringes
Defibrillator
Ready access to extra supplies (catheters, fluids)

---

      tilation of the lungs, monitoring drug administration,
record keeping, and fluid and blood administration.
  B. After arrival of a hemodynamically unstable patient
in the operating room, priorities for attention are commonly in the order listed in Table 36-4.

VII. SELECTION OF ANESTHETIC AGENTS
AND TECHNIQUE

  A. Regional anesthesia is frequently useful when there
are isolated limb injuries. It is also conducive for

**TABLE 36-4. Priorities for Evaluation of
Hemodynamically Unstable
Trauma Patients**

Ensure adequacy of ventilation and oxygenation
Measure blood pressure
Attach an electrocardiograph
Designate a functioning intravenous catheter for drug
  administration
Insert blood warmers into intravenous delivery systems
Begin transfusion as needed
Place an intra-arterial catheter
Measure arterial blood gases and hematocrit
Measure temperature
Measure urine output
Consider placement of a central venous or pulmonary artery
  catheter (rarely indicated for the acute resuscitation of
  traumatized patients)
Induce anesthesia only after fluid resuscitation is initiated

---

providing postoperative neuraxial opioid analgesia. Techniques associated with major sympathetic nervous system blockade are relatively contraindicated in the presence of hypovolemia. Continuous regional techniques can be of benefit for operations involving reimplantation of severed limbs and digits, when it is desirable to have pain relief, sympathectomy, and increased limb blood flow extended into the postoperative period.

B. **General anesthesia** is required for most traumatized patients, particularly those with multiple injuries.

   1. In cases of severe trauma with shock or a decreased level of consciousness, administration of anesthetic drugs may be detrimental; skeletal muscle **paralysis** and ventilation of the lungs with **oxygen** may be all that is necessary. However, anesthetic drugs should be administered as soon as possible to relieve pain and minimize patient recall.

   2. There is no ideal anesthetic agent or technique for a trauma patient. In the presence of hypovolemia, the use of anesthetics that stimulate the sympathetic nervous system (ketamine or nitrous oxide [N_2O]) is common, but there are no data to suggest that such drugs improve patient outcome. In fact, continuous sympathetic nervous system stimulation may aggravate the lactic acidosis associated with hypovolemic shock.

TABLE 36-5. Rapid Sequence Induction and Maintenance of Anesthesia in the Trauma Patient

Ketamine or etomidate (short-acting opioids may be an alternative; thiopental is acceptable only if hypovolemia has been corrected)

Succinylcholine is safe in the first few hours after trauma (mivacurium may be an alternative)

Carefully titrate dose of volatile anesthetics (consider opioids if unacceptable hypotension accompanies even low doses of volatile anesthetics)

N_2O may be avoided (limits inspired oxygen concentration; risk if pneumothorax a possibility)

Monitors (blood pressure not always a reliable index of blood volume, cardiac output, or tissue perfusion)

Intraoperative awareness a risk (alcohol, hypothermia, and hypotension do not reliably produce amnesia for young injured patients)

3. All traumatized patients should be assumed to have full stomachs. If a patient's trachea has not already been intubated, a rapid-sequence induction of anesthesia with cricoid pressure is indicated (Table 36-5).

VIII. FLUID AND BLOOD REPLACEMENT (Table 36-6)

IX. TEMPERATURE

A. **Hypothermia** is a frequent complication of trauma; it may be exacerbated by surgery with open body cavities, anesthesia, and fluid therapy. Hypothermia may cause myocardial dysfunction, cardiac dysrhythmias, a coagulopathy, and acidosis. All victims of trauma should have their core temperature monitored.

B. Measures to prevent hypothermia should include warming all blood and intravenous fluids, use of thermal blankets, heating and humidifying anesthetic gases, and warming the operating room. In cases of severe hypothermia, it may be necessary to use core rewarming with gastric lavage, peritoneal dialysis, and extracorporeal circulation.

X. PERSISTENT HYPOTENSION

A. Many traumatized patients must be rushed to the operating room without having been completely evaluated preoperatively. It therefore becomes the respon-

---

TABLE 36-6. Treatment of Hypovolemia in the Trauma Patient

Aggressive intravenous fluid therapy (warm crystalloid solutions until blood available; colloid solutions are rarely needed for initial resuscitation)

Repeated measurements to monitor adequacy of intravascular fluid volume replacement (urine output, cardiac filling pressures, hematocrit, arterial blood gases, electrolytes)

Type O–negative blood in rare circumstances

Warm all fluids and blood

Autotransfusion (cell-saver) systems

Coagulopathy may accompany massive transfusions (dilutional thrombocytopenia most likely; empirical administration of fresh frozen plasma not recommended)

sibility of an anesthesiologist to be alert for various intraoperative complications. Specifically, if **hypotension** persists despite apparently adequate intravascular fluid volume replacement, one should look for occult hemorrhage, hemopneumothorax, cardiac tamponade, an expanding intracranial mass, acidosis, hypocalcemia, fat embolism, or hypothermia.

B. Arterial blood gases and hematocrit should be analyzed at frequent intervals. Less frequently, blood should be analyzed for electrolytes, glucose, and a coagulation screen.

XI. POSTOPERATIVE CARE

A. Severely injured patients should be treated postoperatively in an **intensive care unit** (see Chapter 43). Because of thoracic trauma, extensive surgery, head injury, and hypothermia, it is common for patients to require continued positive-pressure ventilation of the lungs. In addition, traumatized patients may develop adult respiratory distress syndrome.

B. Trauma patients are in particular need of adequate postoperative **pain control.** Techniques that have proved successful include intrathecal or epidural opioids, patient-controlled analgesia, continuous brachial plexus blockade (for reimplantation surgery), intrapleurally administered local anesthetics, and the full spectrum of regional and isolated nerve block techniques (see Chapter 18).

XII. BURNS

A. The severity of a burn depends on the depth and area of body surface involved. Mortality increases with burn severity and advancing age. **Superficial** and **partial-thickness** burns are exquisitely painful but usually heal without the need for skin grafting. **Full-thickness** burns must be excised and replaced with grafts.

B. **Initial resuscitation** should begin with attention to the airway, breathing, and circulation. All patients should receive oxygen. A patient's trachea should be intubated if the face is burned, there is stridor or hoarseness, or if there has been significant inhalation of steam, smoke, or toxic fumes. It is much easier to accomplish tracheal intubation early as opposed to later, when there may be glottic or facial edema. It is safe to use succinylcholine in the first few hours after a burn. Inhalation of carbon monoxide is common.

Carboxyhemoglobin or oxygen saturation must be measured. The most effective treatment is administration of 100% oxygen; hyperbaric oxygen is rarely indicated.

1. After the airway has been secured and other life-threatening injuries have been treated, burned patients must be resuscitated with large volumes of intravenous fluid. A burn causes a generalized increase in capillary permeability, with considerable loss of fluid and protein into interstitial tissue. Fluid loss is greatest in the first 12 hours.

2. Several formulas exist for estimating fluid needs. The Parkland formula describes administration of $4 \, ml \cdot kg^{-1}$ of fluid during the first 24 hours for each percent of the body surface area burned. However, volume replacement is best guided by measurement of urine output and hemodynamic variables.

C. Within hours after a burn and until it is nearly healed, patients are **hypermetabolic.** This is manifested by hyperthermia, increased catabolism, increased oxygen consumption, tachypnea, tachycardia, and increased serum catecholamine levels.

D. Mortality, morbidity, and cosmetic outcome have been improved by early **excision and grafting** of burns. Provision of anesthesia for this operation should involve the following considerations:

1. Access for monitoring can be difficult. Needle electrodes may be required for the electrocardiogram and nerve stimulator. A blood pressure cuff may be placed over burned areas, but an arterial catheter is advised for patients with large burns.

2. Accurate measurement and maintenance of temperature are essential. The operating room should be warm, all intravenous fluids must be warm, and a heated humidifier should be placed in the anesthetic circuit.

3. Blood loss can be massive and should be anticipated. Pressurized rapid-infusion systems can be very helpful.

E. The selection of **anesthetic drugs** is not the prime goal. Opioids should be used as part of any technique, because excruciating pain can be expected. Halothane may be disadvantageous, because epinephrine-soaked sponges may be used to control bleeding. Mechanical **ventilation** of the lungs is usually necessary because patients are hypermetabolic and may have pulmonary damage from smoke inhalation.

F. Burn patients do not respond normally to **muscle relaxants.** From about 24 hours after the burn until it has healed, administration of succinylcholine can result in a rapid rise in serum K^+ and cardiac arrest. In contrast, burned patients are resistant to nondepolarizing muscle relaxants. The mechanism for these responses to muscle relaxants is not known, although a proliferation of extrajunctional cholinergic receptors is suspected.

G. The care of patients with an **electrical burn** is similar to that for a thermal burn, with two exceptions. First, the extent of the burn can be misleading, with considerable areas of devitalized skeletal muscle lying beneath normal-appearing skin. Myoglobinuria is common, and urine output must be kept high to avoid renal damage. Second, electrical energy may result in spinal cord damage.

37

Cancer Therapy and its Anesthetic Implications

Advances in cancer therapy (chemotherapy, surgery, radiotherapy, bone marrow transplantation), coupled with the increasing number of patients who survive longer or are cured of their disease, ensure that cancer patients will present for surgery with increasing frequency (Rinder CS: Cancer therapy and its anesthetic implications. In: Barash PG, Cullen BF, Stoelting RK [eds]: Clinical Anesthesia, pp. 1447–1464. Philadelphia, JB Lippincott, 1992). Anesthesiologists will be asked to manage not only patients currently undergoing chemotherapy for cancer but also those manifesting early or late toxicities associated with their treatment (Table 37-1).

I. PULMONARY COMPLICATIONS

A. Many chemotherapeutic drugs have been implicated as causes of pulmonary injury, often resulting in a high mortality rate. Risk factors predisposing to the development of pulmonary toxicity vary for the different agents (Table 37-2).

B. **Clinical syndromes** of pulmonary toxicity developing after exposure to chemotherapeutic drugs can be placed in one of three major categories (Table 37-3).

C. **Toxicities of Specific Agents** (Table 37-4)

1. **Bleomycin** is used primarily for treatment of lymphomas, testicular tumors, and squamous cell carcinomas.

   a. This drug is preferentially concentrated in the lung, and pulmonary fibrosis has been observed to occur as long as 1 year after the last bleomycin dose.

   b. Preoperatively, the presence of decreased forced vital capacity and diffusion capacity suggests pulmonary fibrosis, although these changes are not universally present.

TABLE 37-1. Classification of Chemotherapeutic Drugs

Class of Compound	Type of Agent	Drug
Alkylating agents	Nitrogen mustards	Cyclophosphamide Melphalan Chlorambucil
	Alkylsulfonates	Busulfan
	Nitrosoureas	Carmustine Lomustine
Antimetabolites	Folic acid analogues	Methotrexate
	Pyramidine analogues	Fluorouracil Cytosine
	Purine analogues	Mercaptopurine
Natural products	Vinca alkaloids	Vinblastine Vincristine
	Antibiotics	Dactinomycin Daunorubicin Doxorubicin Bleomycin Mithramycin Mitomycin
Miscellaneous agents	Substituted urea	Hydroxyurea
	Cisplatinum	Cisplatin
	Hydrazine derivative	Procarbazine

TABLE 37-2. Risk Factors Predisposing to Development of Cytotoxic Drug-Induced Pulmonary Disease

Risk Factor	Drugs Implicated
Cumulative dose	Bleomycin Busulfan Carmustine
Age	Bleomycin
Concurrent or previous radiotherapy	Bleomycin Busulfan Mitomycin
Oxygen therapy	Bleomycin Cyclophosphamide Mitomycin
Other cytotoxic drug therapy	Carmustine Mitomycin Cyclophosphamide Bleomycin Methotrexate
Pre-existing pulmonary disease	Carmustine

TABLE 37-3. Pulmonary Syndromes Developing After Exposure to Chemotherapeutic Drugs
Chronic Pneumonitis and Progressive Pulmonary Fibrosis
Progressive dyspnea on exertion
Nonproductive cough
Fatigue
Single-breath carbon monoxide diffusion capacity decreased (most sensitive indicator of early pulmonary fibrosis)
Decreased forced vital capacity (evidence of restrictive lung disease)
Acute Hypersensitivity Reaction
Noncardiogenic Pulmonary Edema

2. **Nitrosoureas** as represented by carmustine (BCNU) are used largely in the treatment of intracranial tumors, melanomas, and gastrointestinal and hematologic malignancies.

3. **Alkylating agents** (busulfan, cyclophosphamide, chlorambucil, melphalan) are useful in the treatment of myeloproliferative disorders, particularly chronic myelogenous leukemia.

4. **Cyclophosphamide** is an alkylating drug that is commonly used in combination chemotherapy regimens for the treatment of a wide range of cancers and inflammatory diseases. Massive doses may be used in the therapy of some solid tumors and for bone marrow ablation in preparation for bone marrow transplantation.

5. **Methotrexate** is an antimetabolite that is widely used in the treatment of malignant and some nonmalignant disorders (rheumatoid arthritis).

6. **Thoracic radiation** may produce lung damage independently or act synergistically to enhance drug-induced pulmonary toxicity.

II. CARDIAC COMPLICATIONS

A. Chemotherapeutic drugs have the potential to produce a wide spectrum of **cardiac toxicity** (Table 37-5). The interaction of drug-induced cardiac toxicity with volatile anesthetics has not been well studied.

B. **Toxicities of Specific Agents** (Table 37-6)

1. **Doxorubicin** is an anthracycline chemotherapeutic drug with significant antitumor effects against leu-

TABLE 37-4. Pulmonary Toxicity of Specific Agents

Bleomycin

Pulmonary fibrosis the dose-limiting side effect (incidence increases exponentially above a cumulative dose of 450–500 mg)

Chest radiation may increase the incidence of pulmonary fibrosis

Hyperoxia or excessive crystalloid fluid administration may exacerbate pulmonary fibrosis (controversial but a common recommendation is to administer the lowest acceptable oxygen concentration as based on pulse oximetry)

Carmustine

Interstitial pneumonitis and fibrosis (incidence increases above a cumulative dose of 1200–1500 mg·m^{-2})

Chest radiation and oxygen therapy may have synergistic toxicity

Mitomycin (as for Bleomycin)

Busulfan

Progressive pulmonary fibrosis

Dose-dependent effect not proved

Enhanced toxicity with oxygen therapy not noted

Cyclophosphamide

Hypersensitivity reaction and fibrosing pneumonitis (both responses rare)

Risk of oxygen therapy not proved

Symptoms of dyspnea and cough may develop months to years after initiation of therapy

Methotrexate

Fulminant noncardiogenic pulmonary edema or inflammation with interstitial infiltrates and pleural effusions

No known risk factors

Mortality is low and symptoms generally respond to corticosteroids

Thoracic Radiation

Pneumonitis independent of concurrent chemotherapy (dyspnea and arterial hypoxemia typically occur 6–12 weeks after radiation treatment and in most cases resolve spontaneously over a few months)

Radiation fibrosis (develops progressively beginning 6–12 months after radiation)

TABLE 37-5. **Manifestations of Cardiac Toxicity Produced by Chemotherapeutic Drugs**

Electrocardiographic changes
Life-threatening cardiac dysrhythmias
Pericarditis
Myocardial ischemia
Cardiomyopathies
Congestive heart failure

kemias, lymphomas, and solid tumors such as breast cancers and soft-tissue sarcomas.
   a. Endomyocardial biopsy is the most accurate method for determining subclinical cardiomyopathy.

TABLE 37-6. **Cardiac Toxicity of Specific Agents**

Doxorubicin
   Cardiomyopathy the dose-limiting side effect (incidence increases above a total dose of 550 mg·m^{-2})
   Prior or concurrent mediastinal radiation may increase the incidence of cardiomyopathy
   Nonspecific ST-T wave changes and premature ventricular and atrial contractions are generally transient and benign

Daunorubicin (as for Doxorubicin)

Cyclophosphamide (massive doses)
   Pericarditis and pleural effusion
   Cardiac tamponade
   Hemorrhagic myocarditis with symptoms of congestive heart failure

5-Fluorouracil
   Myocardial ischemia (may reflect coronary artery spasm)
   Myocardial infarction

Thoracic Radiation
   Acute pericarditis with effusion
   Chronic constrictive pericarditis
   Myocardial fibrosis
   Valvular dysfunction
   Cardiac impulse conduction disturbances
   Accelerated coronary atherosclerosis with myocardial infarction

       b. In patients being evaluated preoperatively for surgery, exercise radionuclide angiography appears to be the most sensitive test for the detection of impaired cardiac reserve.

    2. Daunorubicin is an anthracycline used in antileukemic regimens.

    3. Cyclophosphamide (see Section I C 4)

    4. 5-Fluorouracil is most likely to produce evidence of myocardial ischemia in patients with underlying ischemic heart disease.

    5. Thoracic radiation and its adverse effects on the heart (especially accelerated atherosclerosis) may be decreased with the use of subcarinal shields and equally weighted anterior and posterior radiation fields.

III. CENTRAL NERVOUS SYSTEM COMPLICATIONS

  A. Neurologic toxicities arising from chemotherapy, radiotherapy, or the malignancy itself often occur in cancer patients. Assessment of neurologic status remains an important part of the preoperative evaluation of all cancer patients on any therapeutic regimen.

  B. Toxicities of Specific Agents (Table 37-7)

IV. HEMATOLOGIC COMPLICATIONS (Table 37-8)

V. METABOLIC COMPLICATIONS (Table 37-9)

  A. In patients with tumors that have a rapid rate of growth (acute lymphocytic leukemia), chemotherapy may cause significant cell death **(lysis),** resulting in the release of intracellular contents into the extracellular fluid.

  B. Multiple myeloma and solid tumors with skeletal metastases (cancers of the breast, kidney, lung) are often accompanied by **hypercalcemia.**

    1. Serum calcium levels may be measured in the preoperative preparation of the patient with certain cancers.

    2. Patients with moderate hypercalcemia have no special perioperative difficulties. Hypovolemia is common with severe hypercalcemia and requires preoperative hydration.

    3. If hypercalcemia is chronic, there is an increased incidence of renal calculi and loss of renal concentrating ability.

TABLE 37-7. Central Nervous System Toxicity of Specific Agents

Methotrexate

Meningeal irritation and rarely paraplegia following intrathecal administration

Encephalopathy following intravenous or intrathecal administration

Vinca Alkaloids (vincristine, vinblastine)

Loss of Achilles tendon reflex

Paresthesias that may progress to skeletal muscle weakness and sensory impairment

Cranial nerve toxicity

Laryngeal nerve palsy

Bilateral facial nerve and oculomotor palsies

Autonomic neuropathy (paralytic ileus, bladder atony, orthostatic hypotension)

Encephalopathy (may be accompanied by seizures attributed to drug-induced hyponatremia)

L-*Asparaginase*

Encephalopathy

Procarbazine

Mild drowsiness to stupor (potentiates sedative effects of other drugs)

Peripheral neuropathy (paresthesias and proximal skeletal muscle myalgias)

Orthostatic hypotension (attributed to monoamine oxidase inhibition; potential for hypertension with administration of indirect sympathomimetics)

Platinum

Ototoxicity

Peripheral neuropathies (stocking and glove sensory impairment)

TABLE 37-8. Hematologic Complications of Cancer and Chemotherapy

Anemia

Bone marrow suppression

Fibrinolysis (more likely following prostatic surgery for cancer)

Platelet dysfunction (hypercoagulable state or bleeding diathesis)

Disseminated intravascular coagulation (intracranial hemorrhage the major complication)

TABLE 37-9. Metabolic Complications of Cancer and Chemotherapy

Tumor Lysis Syndrome
 Hyperuricemia
 Hyperkalemia
 Hyperphosphatemia
 Acute renal failure

Hypercalcemia (bone metastases)
 Hypovolemia
 Renal calculi
 Loss of renal concentrating ability

Paraneoplastic Syndromes
 Humoral hypercalcemia
 Ectopic Cushing's syndrome (hypokalemia, hyperglycemia, hypertension, skeletal muscle weakness)
 Secretion of inappropriate antidiuretic hormone (hyponatremia)
 Impaired neurologic function
  Dementia
  Myelopathy
  Neuropathies
  Autonomic nervous system dysfunction
  Eaton-Lambert syndrome

C. **Paraneoplastic syndromes** refers to manifestations of cancer at sites not directly affected by malignant disease.
   1. Small-cell lung cancer is the malignancy most commonly associated with tumor synthesis of adrenocorticotropic hormone (ectopic Cushing's syndrome) and inappropriate secretion of antidiuretic hormone.
   2. **Eaton-Lambert syndrome** differs from true myasthenia gravis in that it predominantly involves peripheral skeletal muscle weakness rather than facial or bulbar muscles.
   3. Profoundly debilitated cancer patients may experience prolonged responses to succinylcholine owing to decreased synthesis of pseudocholinesterase or depression of pseudocholinesterase activity associated with cyclophosphamide.

VI. RENAL COMPLICATIONS

A. **Renal toxicity** is a major side effect of several chemotherapeutic agents, especially cisplatin.

  B. Cisplatin is a common component of combination chemotherapy of ovarian, testicular, bladder, and head and neck cancers.

   1. Beginning as early as 3 to 5 days after administration of cisplatin, there may be a progressive decrease in glomerular filtration rate (increasing blood urea nitrogen and creatinine levels; magnesium wasting) and development of acute tubular necrosis.

   2. Implications of recent cisplatin administration for anesthesiologists include attention to hydration and possible electrolyte abnormalities, especially hypomagnesemia (cardiac dysrhythmias, prolonged responses to neuromuscular blockers).

  C. Methotrexate in high doses may be associated with renal toxicity.

VII. LIVER COMPLICATIONS (Table 37-10)

  A. Hepatic toxicity from chemotherapeutic drugs may be difficult to distinguish from metastatic disease and infectious complications of the cancer.

  B. Methotrexate is clearly implicated in hepatic complications, emphasizing the importance of preoperative evaluation of liver function tests.

TABLE 37-10. Chemotherapeutic Agents Producing Hepatic Toxicity

Drug	Effect
Nitrosoureas	
BCNU (carmustine)	Increased liver enzyme levels
CCNU (lomustine)	Increased liver enzyme levels
Streptozocin	Increased liver enzyme levels
Antimetabolites	
Methotrexate	Cirrhosis
6-Mercaptopurine	Cholestasis, necrosis
Azathioprine	Cholestasis, necrosis
Cytosine arabinoside	Increased liver enzyme levels
Antibiotics	
Mithramycin	Acute necrosis
Enzymes	
L-Asparaginase	Fatty metamorphosis

VIII. VASCULAR COMPLICATIONS (Table 37-11)

A. **Pulmonary vascular occlusive disease** may reflect chemotherapeutic drug-induced vascular endothelial injury.

B. **Hepatic veno-occlusive disease** is most likely to follow high doses of chemotherapeutic drugs for bone marrow ablation and manifests as jaundice, hepatomegaly, and ascites.

1. **Treatment** is as utilized for the management of ascites and includes sodium restriction, use of spironolactone, and attempts to maintain plasma oncotic pressure.

TABLE 37-11. Vascular Complications Associated With Antineoplastic Agents

Complications	Drugs
Pulmonary veno-occlusive disease	Bleomycin Mitomycin
Hepatic veno-occlusive disease	Cyclophosphamide Carmustine Cisplatin Dacarbazine Mitomycin Azathioprine 6-Thioguanine
Cerebrovascular accidents	Cisplatin
Raynaud's phenomenon	Bleomycin Vinca alkaloids Cisplatin
Myocardial infarction	Vinca alkaloids Bleomycin Cisplatin 5-Fluorouracil
Hypotension	Vincristine Carmustine
Hypertension	Cisplatin Procarbazine
Acral erythema	Cytosine Hydroxyurea 5-Fluorouracil Doxorubicin
Retinal toxicity	Carmustine Cisplatin

TABLE 37-12. Complications of Bone Marrow Transplantation That May Impact on the Management of Anesthesia

---

Conditioning Regimen Used for Bone Marrow Ablation
High-dose chemotherapy (cyclophosphamide most commonly used; associated with pulmonary, gastrointestinal, hepatic, and renal toxicity)
Total body radiation (hypothyroidism)

Graft-Versus-Host Disease (multiple organ system dysfunction and sepsis)

Acute Pulmonary Complications
Interstitial pneumonitis (may require tracheal intubation and mechanical support of ventilation)
Evidence of restrictive lung disease
Evidence of obstructive lung disease

---

   2. These patients are often hypovolemic, and invasive monitoring with a central venous or pulmonary artery catheter may be necessary to ensure adequate filling pressures during surgery.

IX. BONE MARROW TRANSPLANTATION

   A. Allogeneic bone marrow transplantation is now well established as a therapy for malignant or genetic disease.
   B. **Marrow harvest** may result in significant depletion of intravascular fluid volume, requiring treatment as if it were hemorrhagic blood loss.
      1. Typically, bone marrow is aspirated from the anterior and posterior superior iliac spines, necessitating utilization of both the supine and prone positions.
      2. There is no evidence that the use of nitrous oxide during harvesting adversely affects marrow engraftment or subsequent hematopoiesis. Nevertheless, it may be prudent to avoid nitrous oxide in harvests lasting >2 hours.
      3. Postoperative difficulties include nausea, vomiting, hypotension (volume depletion), and pain at the aspiration site.
   C. **Anesthetic care of the marrow transplant recipient.** Complications following bone marrow transplantation may have significant influence on the anesthetic management of recipients presenting for subsequent surgery (Table 37-12).

38

Anesthesia Outside the Operating Room

Technologic advancements and new equipment requiring specialized environments have provided an expansion of anesthetic care to nonoperative locations (Gillies BS: Anesthesia outside the operating room. In: Barash PG, Cullen BF, Stoelting RK [eds]: Clinical Anesthesia, pp 1465–1477. Philadelphia, JB Lippincott, 1992).

I. GENERAL PRINCIPLES

A. In addition to routine anesthesia equipment, self-inflating bags, a defibrillator, and emergency drugs must be readily accessible.

B. The usual standards for monitoring should be followed, just as in the operating room (see Appendix F).

C. The possibility of increased exposure to radiation during radiologic procedures and the need for scavenging waste anesthetic gases should be considered.

II. ANESTHESIA FOR EXTRACORPOREAL SHOCK WAVE LITHOTRIPSY (ESWL)

A. ESWL is the most common noninvasive form of treatment for urinary calculi and may become an alternative therapy for cholelithiasis (Table 38-1).

B. Both immersion (introduces unique features) and non-immersion techniques have been used (Table 38-2).

C. **Anesthetic considerations** are similar to those for any patient scheduled to undergo an elective procedure requiring anesthesia (electrohydraulic lithotripsy is painful).

1. A good quality signal from the electrocardiogram (ECG) is essential as the shock wave is triggered from the R wave (waterproof ECG pads or occlusive dressings are recommended).

2. Temperature monitoring is useful, since shivering may accompany a decrease in body temperature.

447

TABLE 38-1. Extracorporeal Shock Wave Lithotripsy
for the Biliary System

Contraindications
  Bleeding disorders
  Pregnancy
  Aortic or renal artery calcifications
  Aortic or renal artery aneurysms
  Unstable medical status
  Acute cholecystitis
  Cholangitis
  Biliary obstruction
  Gastric or duodenal ulcers
  Pancreatitis

Relative Contraindications
  Pacemakers
  Obesity
  Abnormalities of body habitus
  Ectopic kidney or other anatomic anomaly

3. **Intravenous hydration** that results in modest diuresis throughout the procedure is helpful for passage of stone fragments.
4. Some method of attenuating the noise emitted from the lithotriptor during shock wave generation is recommended for the patient and anesthesiologist.
5. In order to obtain adequate imaging and focusing of the shock wave, the patient must remain motionless.
6. Several different methods of anesthesia have been used to facilitate performance of ESWL (Table 38-3).
D. **Complications of Extracorporeal Shock Wave Lithotripsy** (Table 38-4)

TABLE 38-2. Features Unique to Immersion
Extracorporeal Shock Wave Lithotripsy

Increased central blood volume (500–700 ml)
Enhanced stroke volume and cardiac output
Decreased systemic vascular resistance
Increased airway resistance and work of breathing
Possible hypothermia and shivering
Cardiac dysrhythmias (not likely if shock wave is initiated
  0.2–0.22 msec after the R wave)

TABLE 38-3. Methods of Anesthesia for Extracorporeal Shock Wave Lithotripsy

---

Continuous Epidural Anesthesia (T6 sensory level)
    Choice of local anesthetic a consideration, as many procedures are outpatient
    Waterproof occlusive dressings
    Loss of resistance technique without air
    Adequate hydration

General Anesthesia
    Avoids discomfort of immersion and noise
    High-frequency jet ventilation versus conventional controlled mechanical ventilation of the lungs

Intravenous Sedation and Analgesia
    Balance adequate analgesia with potential for depression of ventilation

---

TABLE 38-4. Complications of Extracorporeal Shock Wave Lithotripsy

---

Hematuria
Perirenal hematoma
Renal damage leading to hypertension
Sepsis

III. RADIOLOGY AND RADIATION THERAPY

  A. Most adult patients are able to tolerate noninvasive procedures without sedation. Anesthesia may be required for pediatric patients or confused or combative patients and for patients with neuromuscular movement disorders.

  B. Frequently, anesthesiologists are asked to monitor or to care for patients at risk for adverse reactions to contrast dye (history of atopy or allergy to seafood, prior reaction, high-risk procedures such as coronary artery or cerebral angiography) (Table 38-5).

    1. The incidence of adverse reactions to intravascular injection of contrast dye is approximately 5–8%.

    2. Nausea and vomiting occur as prodromal symptoms in as many as 20% of all anaphylactoid and fatal reactions to contrast dye.

TABLE 38-5. Manifestations of Allergic Reactions

Mild	Moderate	Severe
Urticaria	Tissue edema	Prolonged hypotension
Chills	Bronchospasm	Cyanosis
Fever	Hypotension	Arterial hypoxemia
Facial flushing	Seizures	Pulmonary edema
Nausea		Angina pectoris
Vomiting		Cardiac dysrhythmias

3. Patients undergoing contrast dye procedures usually have an induced diuresis from the osmotic load introduced by the dye (adequate hydration is important to prevent aggravation of pre-existing renal dysfunction).
4. **Treatment** of adverse reactions often depends on their severity (Table 38-6).

C. The greatest source of radiation exposure is during fluoroscopy (cardiac angiography). Exposure to ionizing radiation emitted from computed tomography (CT) scanners is low because the radiation is highly focused.
1. Radiation intensity decreases with the inverse square of the distance from the emitting source (a minimum of 1–2 meters is recommended).
2. Use of a lead apron and thyroid shield for the patient may be indicated.

D. Management of children during **cardiac catheterization** introduces several important considerations (Table 38-7).

TABLE 38-6. Treatment of Adverse Reactions to Contrast Dye

Supportive Care (intravenous fluids, oxygen)

Resuscitation Drugs
  Epinephrine
  Atropine
  Diphenhydramine
  Steroids

Prophylaxis
  Diphenhydramine, 25–50 mg iv
  Methylprednisolone, 100–1000 mg iv

TABLE 38-7. Considerations in Management of Children During Cardiac Catheterization

---

Premedication and sedation important for alleviating fear and anxiety that may exacerbate pre-existing heart disease (atropine important)

Level of sedation and analgesia provided must not alter underlying cardiac function or magnitude of intracardiac shunt (arterial blood gas determination useful)

Oxygen may cause closure of a patent ductus arteriosus (prostaglandin E_1 may prevent this response)

High hematocrit reading may predispose to coagulopathy and thrombosis

Onset of drug action may be influenced by direction of intracardiac shunt and pre-existing congestive heart failure

Cardiac dysrhythmias common (prompt access to a defibrillator and resuscitative drugs is required)

Protective clothing against ionizing radiation is required.

E. **Angiography** can usually be accomplished in the adult using local anesthesia with or without sedation (monitored anesthesia care). The exceptions are children, who usually require general anesthesia.
   1. Standard monitors are utilized in these patients.
   2. Many patients who present for **cerebral angiography** are at risk for intracranial hypertension. In these patients, control of arterial blood pressure and $Paco_2$, institution of tracheal intubation, and administration of volatile anesthetics may be influenced by effects on cerebral blood flow and intracranial pressure.
   3. Hypotension and bradycardia can occur during cerebral angiography with contrast dye injection and usually respond to volume replacement and atropine.
   4. Passage of large amounts of dye into the brain can result in seizures.
F. **Embolization procedures** (vascular malformations, aneurysms, tumors) may be painful and require sedation or regional or general anesthesia.
   1. Patients must be watched carefully for disruption of vessel integrity and flow in other vascular beds.
   2. Hydration is necessary because of the high dose of contrast dye injected.
   3. Nausea and vomiting are common (consider prophylaxis with metoclopramide and/or antiemetics).

G. **Computed tomography** is noninvasive and painless, requiring participation by the anesthesiologist only for patients who cannot cooperate (most frequently pediatric patients and head trauma patients).

1. Temperature monitoring is especially helpful in pediatric patients because CT suites are often colder than 25°C to allow for optimal functioning of the equipment.

2. During CT scanning of patients requiring sedation or general anesthesia, the primary concerns of the anesthesiologist are airway management (movement of the gantry may result in kinking or disconnection of the anesthesia circuit) and oxygenation.

3. Sterotactic-guided surgery using CT scanning is most often for biopsy or aspiration of intracranial masses. Placement of a radiolucent frame around the head may require deep sedation or general anesthesia in conjunction with local anesthesia to allow placement of the pins on the frame (necessary to ensure a motionless field for precise localization).

H. **Magnetic resonance imaging (MRI)** entails placing the patient in a magnetic field in an area that is also devoid of ferromagnetic equipment near the scanner (equipment must be made of aluminum or nonmagnetic steel).

1. The imaging capabilities of MRI are similar to those of CT with the advantage that no ionizing radiation is produced.

2. Contraindications for MRI scanning include patients with pacemakers, aneurysm clips, or intravascular wires. Patients with large metal implants should be monitored for implant heating.

3. Anesthesia is needed primarily to provide patient immobility and for children.

4. Heating of the pulse oximeter probe may result in burns.

5. Laryngoscopy may be difficult in the MRI suite because of the magnetic properties of batteries.

I. **Radiation therapy** requiring anesthesia care includes **external beam radiation** (patient immobility is the primary reason), usually in children, and **intraoperative radiation therapy.**

1. A series of external beam radiation treatments extended over several weeks requires repeated anesthetics, utilizing drugs associated with prompt awakening.

2. Intraoperative radiation may require transport of the patient from the operating room to the radiation therapy room while maintaining general anesthesia.

3. All personnel must leave the room during the treatment period because radiation doses are high (standard monitoring must be interfaced with a remote location).

IV. CARDIOVERSION

A. Anesthesiologists are often needed to manage the airway and to provide adequate sedation for patients undergoing elective cardioversion.

B. Intravenous sedation is most often provided with thiopental or methohexital. Avoid etomidate since associated mioclonus makes interpretation of ECG difficult.

V. ELECTROCONVULSIVE THERAPY is most often utilized for the treatment of major depressive illness in patients who have not improved on a trial of antidepressant medications, monoamine oxidase inhibitors, or lithium.

A. The electrically induced grand mal seizure produced by electroconvulsive therapy is responsible for the therapeutic effect.

B. The seizure causes a wide range of physiologic effects (Table 38-8).

TABLE 38-8. Physiologic Effects of Electroconvulsive Therapy

Cardiovascular Effects
Initial Phase
  Bradycardia
  Hypotension
Later Phase
  Tachycardia
  Dysrhythmia
  Hypertension
  Increased systemic and myocardial oxygen consumption

Cerebral Effects
Increased cerebral blood flow
Elevated intracranial pressure
Increased oxygen consumption

Systemic Effects
Elevated intraocular pressure
Increased intragastric pressure

TABLE 38-9. Anesthetic Considerations for
Electroconvulsive Therapy

Apply usual monitors
Oxygen before, during, and after the seizure
Methohexital, 0.5–1 mg·kg^{-1} iv, or thiopental, 1.5–3 mg·kg^{-1} iv
Succinylcholine, 0.5–1 mg·kg^{-1} iv
Consider isolation of an extremity with a blood pressure cuff
  so as to allow assessment of the duration of the seizure
Adequate monitoring, airway equipment, and suction
  available

C. **Anesthetic considerations** include amnesia, airway management, prevention of bodily injury from the seizure, control of hemodynamic changes, and a smooth, rapid emergence (Table 38-9).

VI. ANESTHESIA FOR DENTAL SURGERY

A. Mentally retarded patients may have associated medical diseases of importance to the anesthesiologist (congenital heart disease, aspiration, upper airway abnormalities).

B. The ideal technique for anesthesia should allow for a smooth, rapid induction, easy airway management, and prompt uncomplicated emergence.

  1. Ketamine has been recommended for sedation, induction, and maintenance of anesthesia. Acceptable alternative drugs include methohexital, propofol, and alfentanil, often supplemented with an inhalation drug.

  2. An anticholinergic drug may be useful to decrease salivary secretions.

  3. Tracheal intubation, usually through the nose, is recommended in lengthy or unusually bloody procedures.

  4. Because of bleeding and the routine use of oropharyngeal packing, close observation of the patient during emergence is essential.

VII. TRANSPORT OF PATIENTS who receive anesthesia or sedation outside the operating room should include monitoring during transfer to the postanesthesia care unit. Supplemental oxygen may be indicated.

39

Anesthesia for Organ Transplantation

Transplantation of a variety of tissues in order to permanently replace those with disease is now routine in clinical practice (Firestone L, Firestone S: Anesthesia for organ transplantation. In: Barash PG, Cullen BF, Stoelting RK, [eds]: Clinical Anesthesia, pp 1479–1511. Philadelphia, JB Lippincott, 1992).

I. ANESTHESIA CARE FOR ORGAN DONORS

A. The majority of viscera for transplantation are derived from brain-dead organ donors (usually as a result of catastrophic neurologic injury) who have not suffered prolonged periods of circulatory compromise or septicemia (Table 39-1).

B. Viscera for transplantation from living donors (principally kidneys) are designed to improve graft survival by improving HLA identity between donor and recipient.

II. BRAIN DEATH

A. **Diagnosis of Brain Death** (Table 39-2)

1. An electrically silent (flat) electroencephalogram is consistent with the diagnosis of brain death, although residual activity may still be present after cessation of cerebral blood flow.

2. An assessment of respiratory brain stem function is by the apnea test (mechanical ventilation of the lungs with 100% oxygen is stopped, and respiratory effort is judged by serial determinations of $Paco_2$, usually over 10 minutes).

3. Irreversibility is implicit in the diagnosis of brain death and is established by the lack of improvement in the neurologic examination for 12–24 hours (reversible events that may confound the diagnosis are seizures, centrally active drug effects,

---

TABLE 39-1. Screening Tests for Brain-Dead Organ Donors

Serologic Screening
  Hepatitis B
  Human immunodeficiency virus
  Toxoplasmosis
  Herpes
  Tuberculosis
  Cytomegalovirus (acceptable if recipient is also infected)

Potential Heart Donors
  Age <50 years
  Absence of pre-existing cardiac disease
  Myocardial contractility adequate as judged by
    echocardiography

Potential Liver Donors
  Liver function tests

Potential Kidney Donors
  Urinalysis and cultures
  Blood urea nitrogen
  Serum creatinine

---

hypothermia, cardiovascular or metabolic instability).
  B. **Physiologic Consequences of Brain Death** (Table 39-3)
    1. Treatment of hypotension is by restoration of intravascular fluid volume with colloid and crystalloid solutions, and if necessary, infusion of dopamine (phenylephrine may diminish splanchnic perfu-

---

TABLE 39-2. Criteria for the Determination of Brain Death

Loss of Cerebral Cortical Function
  No spontaneous movement
  Unresponsive to external stimuli

Loss of Brain Stem Function
  Absent respiratory reflex (apnea test)
  Absent cranial nerve reflexes (pupillary light reflex, corneal
    reflex, oculocephalic reflex, oculovestibular reflex)

Supporting Studies
  Electroencephalogram
  Cerebral blood flow studies (angiography, transcranial
    Doppler scan, xenon computed tomographic scan)

> **TABLE 39-3. Common Physiologic Consequences of Brain Death**
>
> | Condition | Cause |
> |---|---|
> | Hypotension | Hypovolemia (diabetes insipidus; hemorrhage) |
> | | Neurogenic shock |
> | Arterial hypoxemia | Neurogenic pulmonary edema |
> | | Aspiration pneumonitis |
> | | Fluid overload |
> | Hypothermia | Hypothalamic infarction |
> | | Exposure |
> | Cardiac dysrhythmias (especially bradycardia) | Intracranial injury or herniation |
> | | Hypothermia |
> | | Arterial hypoxemia |
> | | Electrolyte abnormality |
> | | Myocardial contusion |
> | | Myocardial ischemia |

sion and thereby jeopardize abdominal donor organs).
2. Bradycardia is resistant to atropine but often responds to dopamine or isoproterenol.

III. DONOR OPERATION

A. **Anesthesia care** for multiple organ retrieval is designed to maintain donor organ perfusion and oxygenation.

B. Visceral and somatic reflexes may be present, especially with surgical stimulation, requiring treatment with a vasodilator (general anesthetics are not necessary).

C. Neuromuscular activity mediated by spinal somatic reflexes is suppressed with muscle relaxants.

IV. ORGAN PRESERVATION

A. Preservation strategies are based on the control of adverse cellular events that follow ischemia and reperfusion (Table 39-4).

B. **Preservation of the kidney** is most often carried out with Euro-Collins solution.

C. **Preservation of the liver** in University of Wisconsin solution maintains viability for at least 24 hours.

D. **Preservation of the heart** in cardioplegia solutions provides an ischemic time of 4–6 hours.

TABLE 39-4. Organ Preservation Solutions in Widespread Clinical Use

	Euro-Collins Solution	University of Wisconsin Solution	Crystalloid Cardioplegia
Potassium (mEq·l⁻¹)	100	100*	30
Sodium (mEq·l⁻¹)	10		25
Chloride (mEq·l⁻¹)	15		30
Bicarbonate (mEq·l⁻¹)	10		25
Insulin (units)		100	
Penicillin (units)		40	
Dexamethasone (mg)		8	
Mannitol (g)			12.5
Osmolarity (mOsm·l⁻¹)	375	320–330	440
pH (4C)	7.25	7.4	8.1–8.4

*Potassium lactobionate

V. TRANSPLANT IMMUNOLOGY

A. Transplantation of tissue from the same species **(allograft)** into an immunocompetent recipient evokes an immune response (foreign antigens present on cell surfaces of the allograft include the major histocompatibility complex and major blood group antigens).

B. **Mechanism of allograft rejection.** Unless suppressed, the recipient's immune system recognizes donor antigens that interact with receptors on surfaces of T cells.

C. **Clinical Immunology in Visceral Transplantation**

1. **Renal allografts.** The importance of HLA histocompatibility is controversial.

2. **Cardiac allografts.** Donor-specific ABO histocompatibility is necessary, whereas short ischemic time limits full prospective histocompatibility matching.

3. **Liver allografts.** In contrast to the heart and kidneys, hyperacute rejection does not occur in liver allografts (ABO and HLA matching less critical).

D. **Immunosuppressants: Mechanisms of Rejection Control**

1. Antirejection regimens are nonspecific and usually combine low doses of several drugs to provide superior immunosuppression and to minimize side effects (Table 39-5).

TABLE 39-5. Effects of Immunosuppressants on the Immune Response

Drug	Effect
Corticosteroids	Decrease interleukin 1 production from macrophages, which decreases effectiveness of T-helper cells Decrease interleukin 2 production from T cells
Azathioprine	Inhibits DNA and RNA synthesis, which decreases lymphocyte proliferation
Cyclosporine	Prevents T-helper cell activation by antigen
Antilymphocyte globulin	Diminishes populations of both T- and B-cell lymphocytes
OKT 3	Inactivates T cells and prevents reactivation

2. **Transfusion and Immunosuppression.** Multiple blood transfusions may induce immunologic non-reactivity and improve graft survival after renal transplantation.

VI. PREANESTHETIC EVALUATION OF TRANSPLANT CANDIDATES

A. **Kidney transplantation** is the treatment of choice for end-stage renal disease (Table 39-6).

1. **Pathophysiology of end-stage renal disease and dialysis.** In addition to uremia (unable to regulate volume and composition of body fluids), end-stage renal disease results in evidence of secondary dysfunction in other organ systems (Table 39-7).

2. **Specific Indications and Contraindications** (Table 39-8)

3. **Preanesthetic considerations.** Since the tolerable ischemic time for kidneys is at least 48 hours, cadaver allografts may be transplanted semielectively (Table 39-9).

4. **Harvesting and Related Donor Considerations**

   a. The donor is hydrated with crystalloid solutions to promote an active diuresis, and at the time of nephrectomy, a minimum urine output of 1 ml·min^{-1} is achieved by means of mannitol and furosemide.

   b. Heparin is administered systemically before removal of the organ from the donor, the organ is then flushed free of blood with a cold crystalloid solution.

TABLE 39-6. Etiologies of End-Stage Renal Disease in Renal Transplant Recipients

Etiology	Percent of Total Cases
Diabetic glomerulonephropathy	43.6
Other glomerulonephritides	23.2
Polycystic kidney disease	5.8
Chronic pyelonephritis	5.4
Obstructive uropathy	3.4
Alport's syndrome	2.1
Lupus nephritis	1.6
Miscellaneous, including unknown	14.9

TABLE 39-7. Common Pathophysiologic Manifestations of End-Stage Renal Disease

Organ System	Manifestations
Nervous system	Peripheral neuropathy Lethargy Coma
Hematologic	Anemia Diminished erythrocyte survival Platelet dysfunction Shift in the P_{50} of the oxyhemoglobin dissociation curve
Cardiovascular	Congestive heart failure Pericarditis Hypertension Dysrhythmias (abnormal electrolytes) Capillary fragility
Pulmonary	Pleural effusion Pulmonary edema
Musculo-skeletal	Generalized skeletal muscle weakness Renal osteodystrophy Metastatic calcification Gout Pseudogout
Gastrointestinal	Nausea Vomiting Ileus Peptic and colonic ulceration
Endocrine	Pancreatitis Glucose intolerance
Integument	Pruritus Hyperpigmentation
Immunologic	Impaired cellular immunity

TABLE 39-8. General Contraindications to Transplantation of Viscera

Incurable malignancy

Other major systemic illness

Old ("physiologic") age

Active systemic or incurable infection

Current alcohol, drug, or tobacco abuse

Evidence of emotional instability or lack of supportive social milieu

TABLE 39-9. **Preanesthetic Considerations for Renal Transplantation**

Hemodialysis prior to transplantation (correct electrolyte and volume derangements)

Status following hemodialysis (intravascular fluid volume, hematocrit, electrolytes, residual heparin)

Consider treatment of anemia

Supplement corticosteroids

Evaluate for presence of pleural or pericardial effusion

Possibility of ischemic heart disease (many of these patients are diabetic)

Protect arteriovenous fistula

      c. The timing of the donor and recipient procedures is coordinated so that the ischemic interval for the kidney is minimized.
    5. **Anesthetic Considerations for the Renal Transplant Recipient** (Table 39-10)
  B. **Liver transplantation** is the only treatment for end-stage liver disease, since medical management is only supportive and does not prolong life.

TABLE 39-10. **Anesthetic Considerations for the Renal Transplant Recipient**

Anesthetic Induction

  Delayed gastric emptying in the presence of diabetes mellitus

  Volume depletion likely after hemodialysis

  Consider interactions between vasodilating anesthetics and antihypertensive drugs

  Place central venous pressure catheter

Anesthetic and Surgical Procedures

  General anesthesia most often selected (may omit N_2O to avoid bowel distention, especially in children)

  Atracurium or vecuronium the preferred muscle relaxant

  Clamping of common iliac artery results in lower extremity ischemia

  Promote renal perfusion after unclamping (light anesthesia, crystalloids, dopamine)

Postoperative Management and Complications

  Oliguria (administer fluids judiciously)

  Pain and hypertension (neuraxial opioids)

  Bleeding and thrombosis of vascular anastomoses

1. **Pathophysiology of End-Stage Liver Disease** (Table 39-11)
2. **Orthotopic liver transplantation** is most often performed to treat benign parenchymal diseases (postnecrotic cirrhosis, biliary atresia). The presence of alcoholic cirrhosis, hepatitis B virus, or age >50 years is no longer considered an absolute contraindication to orthotopic liver transplantation.
3. **Preanesthetic considerations.** Many physiologic derangements (encephalopathy, coagulopathy) are not correctable until after transplantation.
   a. Arterial hypoxemia may reflect the presence of a pleural effusion, which is treated with thora-

---

TABLE 39-11. Common Pathophysiologic Manifestations of End-Stage Liver Disease

Organ System	Manifestations
Central nervous system	Encephalopathy (mild confusion to coma) Cerebral edema
Cardiovascular	Hyperdynamic circulation Decreased systemic vascular resistance Increased plasma volume Pericardial effusion
Pulmonary	Pleural effusion Atelectasis Ventilation-to-perfusion mismatching Intrapulmonary shunting
Gastrointestinal	Esophageal varices Ascites Portal hypertension Delayed gastric emptying
Hematologic	Decreased clotting factor levels Anemia Thrombocytopenia (hypersplenism) Decreased clearance of fibrinolytic substances and tissue plasminogen activators
Endocrine	Glucose intolerance Decreased glycogen stores
Renal	Oliguria Hyponatremia (diuretics, increased antidiuretic hormone activity) Hypokalemia (diuretics, gastrointestinal losses, poor nutrition)

centesis despite the likely presence of a clotting abnormality.

 b. Preparations to avoid intraoperative hypothermia are often instituted prior to induction of anesthesia (fluid warming units, warming blankets, nonconductive wraps).

 c. A thromboelastogram is useful to elucidate a need for specific blood product replacement.

 d. Positive recipient serologic studies emphasize the need for health care personnel to take appropriate precautions.

 4. Anesthetic considerations for the liver transplant recipient (Table 39-12). The orthotopic procedure is divided into three stages (Table 39-13).

C. Heart Transplantation

 1. Pathophysiology of end-stage heart disease. The leading causes of end-stage heart disease include ischemic and valvular heart disease and primary cardiomyopathy. Progression of the underlying pathophysiology eventually reduces ejection fraction and results in severe congestive heart failure that is refractory to conventional drug therapy.

TABLE 39-12. Anesthetic Considerations for the Liver Transplant Recipient

Anesthetic Induction

Ability to transfuse rapidly (at least two large-bore peripheral venous cannulas; rapid transfusion device)

Invasive monitoring (includes pulmonary artery catheter, as reperfusion of donor liver may be associated with cardiovascular depression; radial and femoral artery catheters)

Consider risk of pulmonary aspiration (ascites)

Anesthetic and Surgical Procedures

Volatile anesthetic or opioid combined with a muscle relaxant (avoid N_2O)

Rapid transfusion may result in hypocalcemia and hyperkalemia

Inotrope support (dopamine)

Oliguria

Air embolism

Postoperative Management and Complications

Metabolic alkalosis

Pneumonia

Primary nonfunction (retransplantation necessary)

TABLE 39-13. Overview of the Orthotopic Liver Transplantation Procedure

Phase	Surgical Procedures	Common Physiologic Changes
Preanhepatic	Dissection of porta hepatis Release of hepatic attachments	Third-space losses (ascites) Hemorrhage (venous collaterals)
Anhepatic	Clamp hepatic artery and portal vein Venovenous bypass (adults) Clamp inferior vena cava Retraction on diaphragm	Obstruction of venous return Oliguria Venous congestion Atelectasis
Neohepatic	Anastomosis of inferior vena cava Flush hepatic allograft Anastomosis of portal vein and hepatic artery Biliary drainage procedure	Hemorrhage (coagulopathy) Hyperkalemia Citrate intoxication Hypothermia Metabolic acidosis

2. **Indications and contraindications.** The typical candidate is a 40–60-year-old male with ischemic cardiomyopathy and a left ventricular ejection fraction <20%. Severe, irreversible pulmonary hypertension remains one of the few absolute contraindications to orthotopic heart transplantation (consider heart-lung transplantation).
3. **Preanesthetic Considerations** (Table 39-14)
   a. Chronic anticoagulation with warfarin may be considered in patients with large dilated hearts and low cardiac output.
4. **Anesthetic Considerations for the Heart Transplant Recipient** (Table 39-15)
D. **Heart-lung transplantation** is the procedure of choice for patients with end-stage lung disease complicated by right ventricular failure or end-stage congenital heart disease with pulmonary hypertension (Eisenmenger's syndrome).
   1. Air trapping and fixed pulmonary hypertension distinguish these patients from those undergoing heart transplantation procedures.
   2. Re-expansion of the transplanted lung may require bronchoscopy to relieve mechanical obstruction owing to secretions and occasionally bronchodilators to treat bronchospasm.
   3. Positive end-expiratory pressure is often required after bypass.
   4. Postoperative complications include pneumonia, dehiscence of the tracheal suture line, and development of broncholitis obliterans.

TABLE 39-14. Pathophysiologic Manifestations of Dilated Cardiomyopathy

Organ or System	Manifestations
Lungs	Pulmonary venous congestion
	Interstitial pulmonary edema
Kidneys	Prerenal azotemia
	Oliguria
Liver	Chronic passive congestion
	Hepatosplenomegaly
	Ascites
Nervous system	Confusion (low cardiac output)
Endocrine system	Increased plasma catecholamines levels
	Increased plasma renin concentrations

TABLE 39-15. Anesthetic Considerations for the Heart Transplant Recipient

Anesthetic Induction
  Conventional aseptic techniques
  Invasive monitoring (some recommend avoidance of right
    internal jugular vein catheterization; use long sterile
    sheath, as pulmonary artery catheter must be pulled back
    to a central venous pressure position)
  Full stomach precautions
  May be exquisitely sensitive to changes in preload or
    afterload
  Filling pressures difficult to interpret because ventricles are
    noncompliant

Maintenance of Anesthesia (select drugs compatible with
  poor ventricular function)

Surgical Procedures and Cardiopulmonary Bypass
  Diuretics may be required to maintain urine flow
  Methylprednisolone (?)
  Isoproterenol to support heart rate
  Prostaglandin E_1 to treat pulmonary hypertension

Postoperative Management
  Acute rejection
  Pneumonia
  Heart block
  Bleeding

E. **Lung transplantation** is appropriate for treatment of
end-stage lung disease (interstitial fibrosis often with
pulmonary hypertension, smoking-induced emphysema, cystic fibrosis, bronchiectasis) characterized by
progressive exercise intolerance and increasing oxygen requirements.
  1. **Donor lungs** may be jeopardized by prior fluid resuscitation, aspiration, and arterial hypoxemia because most organ donors are trauma victims.
  2. **Preanesthetic considerations** (Table 39-16)
  3. **Single-lung transplantation** procedures involve
  pneumonectomy (left lung preferred for technical
  reasons) and mobilization of the omentum with its
  vascular pedicle for bronchial wrapping.
    a. Single-lung transplantation is not an option if in-
    fection or severe bullous emphysema is present.
    b. An advantage of single-lung transplantation is
    its feasibility without cardiopulmonary bypass

TABLE 39-16. Preanesthetic and Anesthetic Considerations in the Lung Transplant Recipient

Brief tolerable ischemic time (about 4 hours)

Prediction of difficulties during and after induction
  Diminished expiratory flow rates (air trapping and arterial hypoxemia)
  Elevated pulmonary artery pressures (may require cardiopulmonary bypass)
  Arterial blood gas values

Invasive monitoring

Left endobronchial tube (also allows split ventilation postoperatively)

Avoid N_2O

Anticipate deterioration in oxygenation and hemodynamics with institution of one-lung ventilation (may require cardiopulmonary bypass)

Bronchoscopy may be necessary to reinflate the allograft

---

and use of bronchial (better healing) rather than tracheal anastomosis.

    4. Postoperative management after lung transplantation involves intensive respiratory support and early diagnosis of lung infection as differentiated from graft rejection (Table 39-17).

  F. Pancreas transplantation is usually reserved for severe and complicated diabetes and is often combined with a renal transplant in hopes of preventing diabetic nephropathy in the transplanted kidney.

    1. Surgically, there is extraperitoneal pancreatic placement and exocrine drainage *via* duodenocystosomy.

TABLE 39-17. Postoperative Management of the Lung Transplant Patient

Mechanical ventilation of the lungs (use positive end-expiratory pressure and lowest acceptable inspired oxygen concentrations)

Split-lung ventilation *via* an endobronchial tube (use to avoid overinflation of the native lung)

Pneumonia (bacterial, cytomegalovirus, opportunistic) versus graft rejection (determine *via* biopsy)

Damage to recurrent laryngeal and vagal nerves

Tracheal anastomotic leak (mediastinitis)

---

2. Postoperatively, patients seldom require intensive care, although control of plasma glucose levels using an insulin infusion is recommended.

VII. VISCERAL TRANSPLANTATION IN CHILDREN

A. **Renal transplantation in children** may be recommended even before dialysis is required in an attempt to prevent adverse effects associated with medical management (growth and cognitive retardation).
   1. Intra-abdominal placement of an adult-sized kidney may sequester a relatively large proportion of the child's blood volume, leading to hypotension.
   2. Adult kidneys initially produce adult-sized volumes of urine, requiring adjustment of maintenance fluids.

B. **Orthotopic liver transplantation in children** is most often for biliary atresia and inborn errors of metabolism.

C. **Orthotopic heart transplantation in children** is most often for congenital heart disease (aortic atresia, hypoplastic left-sided heart syndrome).

VIII. EVALUATION OF PATIENTS WITH A PRIOR TRANSPLANT

A. **Immunosuppressant Side Effects and Toxicities** (Table 39-18)

B. **Other Preanesthetic Considerations**
   1. Immunosuppressant medication must be continued.
   2. The patient population receiving transplants is prone to bacterial pneumonia and cytomegalovirus sepsis. For these reasons, extubation of the trachea after any surgical procedure is an important goal.

C. **Anesthesia After Kidney Transplantation**
   1. It is important to ascertain the degree of any residual renal impairment. If the allograft is functional, renal excretion of drugs is normal.
   2. Diabetes mellitus is a common coexisting disease.
   3. Cyclosporine may render allografts susceptible to other drugs with nephrotoxic potential (maintain diuresis and avoid enflurane).

D. **Anesthesia After Liver Transplantation** does not differ from that for a normal patient if the allograft is functioning properly.

E. **Anesthesia After Heart Transplantation**
   1. Despite denervation, the stroke volume is nearly normal.

TABLE 39-18. Side Effects and Toxicities of Immunosuppressants

Drug	Toxicity
Corticosteroids	Adrenal suppression
	Glucose intolerance
	Cushingoid appearance
	Integument fragility
	Aseptic necrosis
	Peptic ulcer exacerbation
Azathioprine	Anemia
	Thrombocytopenia
	Leukopenia
	Pancreatitis
	Hepatitis
	Decreased nondepolarizing muscle relaxant requirements
Cyclosporine	Glomerulosclerosis
	Hypertension
	Hepatotoxicity
	Neurotoxicity
	Increased renal "sensitivity" to insults
Antilymphocyte globulin	Leukopenia
	Thrombocytopenia
	Systemic symptoms
OKT3	Systemic symptoms
	Increased susceptibility to cytomegalovirus infections

TABLE 39-19. Altered Responses to Common Cardioactive Drugs After Cardiac Denervation

Drug	Response
Atropine	No vagolytic effect
Pancuronium	No vagolytic effect
Edrophonium	No vagotonic effect
Ephedrine	Less cardiostimulatory effect
Nifedipine	No depression of nodal conduction
Digoxin	Lack of an acute vagotonic effect
Norepinephrine	Enhanced beta-stimulatory effect
Phenylephrine	Decreased vasoconstrictive effects with long-standing heart failure

2. Changes in heart rate, although delayed, can still occur in response to specific events (pain, arterial hypoxemia, hypotension) and drugs that act directly on the heart (isoproterenol, propranolol). Conversely, drugs that act indirectly on the heart will fail to produce their typical effects after denervation (Table 39-19).

3. Myocardial ischemia and infarction develop in many patients. Since afferent innervation is lacking, most but not all episodes of myocardial ischemia are silent (dyspnea may be the only symptom). Indeed, accelerated atherosclerosis often blunts the life span of the donor heart.

4. Diagnostic electrocardiographic monitoring is important for the detection of ischemia. As a consequence of the midatrial orthotopic surgical technique, the electrocardiogram may contain two P waves (native atria and transplanted atria).

V

POSTANESTHESIA AND CONSULTANT PRACTICE

40

Postoperative Recovery

Individualized, problem-oriented monitoring and assessment are essential for patients recovering from anesthesia and surgery in a postanesthesia care unit (PACU) (Mecca RS: Postoperative recovery. In Barash PG, Cullen BF, Stoelting RK [eds]: Clinical Anesthesia, pp 1515–1546. Philadelphia, JB Lippincott, 1992). A patient should be admitted to a PACU whenever doubt exists concerning his or her ability to recover safely in an unmonitored setting (see Appendix F).

I. ADMISSION CRITERIA

A. Anesthesiologists should provide an **admission report** to the PACU nurse and supervise care of patients until vital signs are obtained (Table 40-1).

B. A minimal level of monitoring must be provided (Table 40-2).

C. All patients should receive **supplemental oxygen** unless waived by the anesthesiologist.

II. DISCHARGE CRITERIA

A. Clinical judgment must always supercede **established guidelines for discharge** from a PACU (Table 40-3).

III. CARDIOVASCULAR COMPLICATIONS

A. **Postoperative hypotension**

1. A 20–30% reduction in blood pressure from chronic preoperative levels that results in **symptoms of organ hypoperfusion** (acidosis, myocardial ischemia, oliguria, sympathetic nervous system activation, central nervous system disturbances) requires prompt differential diagnosis and treatment (Table 40-4).

TABLE 40-1. Admission Report to Postanesthesia Care Unit Nurses

Preoperative History
   Chronic medications
   Pre-existing diseases
   Drug allergies
   Premedication

Intraoperative Factors
   Surgical procedure
   Type of anesthetic and drug doses
   Muscle relaxant and reversal status
   Intravenous fluids
   Estimated blood loss
   Urine output
   Unexpected surgical or anesthetic events
   Intraoperative vital signs and laboratory findings
   Nonanesthetic drugs (antibiotics, diuretics, vasopressors)

Postoperative Instructions
   Pain management
   Acceptable vital sign ranges, blood loss, and urine output
   Anticipated cardiopulmonary problems
   Diagnostic tests (arterial blood gases, hematocrit, electrolytes)
   Location of responsible physician

2. **Treatment** is determined by the mechanism responsible for hypotension. After confirming the adequacy of oxygenation, it is often most appropriate to administer an intravenous bolus of crystalloid solution (300–500 ml). If blood pressure does not improve, consider possible ventricular

TABLE 40-2. Monitoring in a Postanesthetic Care Unit

Pulse oximetry
Vital signs at least every 15 minutes
   Blood pressure
   Heart rate
   Breathing rate and airway patency
   Level of consciousness
Electrocardiogram
Body temperature

**TABLE 40-3. Assessment Before Discharge
from a Postanesthesia Care Unit**

General Condition

  Oriented and follows simple instructions

  Adequate skeletal muscle strength

  Absence of acute anesthetic/surgical complications (airway
    edema, neurologic compromise, bleeding, nausea and
    vomiting)

Cardiovascular System

  Blood pressure, heart rate, and cardiac rhythm
    within ± 20% of the preoperative value and stable for at
    least 30 minutes

  Acceptable intravascular fluid volume status

Ventilation and Oxygenation

  Acceptable oxygen saturation

  Breathing rate 10–30·min^{-1}

  Able to cough and clear secretions

Airway Maintenance

  Intact protective reflexes (swallow, gag)

  No evidence of airway obstruction (stridor, retraction)

  No need for artificial airway support

Control of Pain

Renal Function (urine output >30 ml·h^{-1})

Metabolic and Laboratory

  Acceptable hematocrit, electrolytes, glucose, and arterial
    blood gases

  Evaluation of electrocardiogram and radiographs

Ambulatory Patients

  Ambulate without dizziness or hypotension

  Control of nausea and vomiting

  Control of pain

---

dysfunction. If blood pressure improves only transiently, consider the possibility of continued surgical bleeding. Vasopressors are a temporizing measure to restore perfusion pressure while the underlying cause for hypotension is corrected.

B. Postoperative hypertension

  1. A 20–30% increase in blood pressure from chronic preoperative levels that produces symptoms (myocardial ischemia, bleeding, headache) or unusual

TABLE 40-4.   Differential Diagnosis of Hypotension in
Patients in a Postanesthesia Care Unit

Arterial hypoxemia
Hypovolemia (most common cause)
Spurious (cuff too wide, transducer not calibrated)
Pulmonary edema (excess fluids)
Myocardial ischemia
Cardiac dysrhythmias
Decreased systemic vascular resistance (regional blocks,
   drugs)
Pneumothorax
Cardiac tamponade

risk of morbidity (increased intracranial pressure,
valvular heart disease) requires prompt differential diagnosis and treatment (Table 40-5).

2. **Treatment** is determined by the mechanism responsible for hypertension. After confirming the
   adequacy of oxygenation, it is most often appropriate to direct therapy toward correction of events
   leading to **increased sympathetic nervous system
   activity.** If hypertension persists despite correction
   of factors promoting sympathetic nervous system
   activity, it may be necessary to administer **antihypertensive medications** (hydralazine, labetalol, nitroprusside).

C. **Cardiac dysrhythmias in the postoperative period**
   1. Prompt differential diagnosis of cardiac dysrhyth-
      mias requires monitoring of the electrocardiogram
      (Table 40-6).
   2. **Treatment** is determined by the hemodynamic sig-
      nificance of the cardiac dysrhythmia (Table 40-7).

TABLE 40-5.   Differential Diagnosis of Hypertension in
Patients in a Postanesthesia Care Unit

Arterial hypoxemia
Spurious (cuff too narrow, transducer not calibrated,
   transducer overshoot)
Pre-existing essential hypertension
Enhanced sympathetic nervous system activity (pain, carinal
   stimulation, bladder distention, pre-eclampsia)
Excess fluid administration
Hypothermia

TABLE 40-6. **Differential Diagnosis of Cardiac Dysrhythmias in Patients in a Postanesthesia Care Unit**

Asymptomatic electrocardiogram abnormalities (nodal rhythms usually resolve spontaneously in 3–6 hours)

Bradycardia (increased parasympathetic nervous system activity reflecting opioids or anticholinesterases; heart block)

Tachycardia (increased sympathetic nervous system activity, paroxysmal atrial tachycardia)

Premature contractions (atrial usually benign; ventricular may be life-threatening)

IV. POSTOPERATIVE PULMONARY DYSFUNCTION

Analysis of arterial blood gases and oxygen saturation facilitates recognition and treatment.

A. Inadequate postoperative ventilation (Table 40-8)

B. Inadequate postoperative oxygenation (Table 40-9)

   1. An acceptable Pao_2 must be defined for each individual patient. A common recommendation is to **maintain Pao_2 between 70 and 100 mm Hg** by adjusting the fractional inspired oxygen concentration (Fio_2) (ideally <0.6) with or without positive end-expiratory airway pressure (PEEP) or continuous positive airway pressure (5–10 cm H_2O by face mask).

   2. Splinting due to postoperative pain contributes to **detrimental loss of lung volume (especially functional residual capacity),** emphasizing the importance of adequate postoperative pain relief.

   3. Exposing an intubated trachea to ambient pressures eliminates a patient's ability to create expi-

---

TABLE 40-7. **Treatment of Cardiac Dysrhythmias in Patients in a Postanesthesia Care Unit**

Eliminate excessive parasympathetic nervous system activity (atropine, ephedrine)

Eliminate excessive sympathetic nervous system activity (analgesics, beta antagonists)

Reduce ventricular irritability (lidocaine)

Artificial pacemaker insertion vs. administration of isoproterenol

---

TABLE 40-8. Differential Diagnosis of Hypoventilation in Patients in a Postanesthesia Care Unit

Inadequate ventilatory drive (residual effects of anesthetics; lack of stimulation)

Ventilatory mechanics
  Increased airway resistance (obstruction)
  Decreased compliance (obesity, fluid overload)
  Residual neuromuscular blockade

Increased dead space (pulmonary embolus)

Increased carbon dioxide production (hyperthermia, hyperalimentation)

ratory resistance **(physiologic PEEP),** leading to possible loss of functional residual capacity and decreased PaO_2.

V. ASPIRATION

A. Inhalation of acid fluid **(pH <2.5)** in the perioperative period manifests as various degrees of arterial hypoxemia and fluffy infiltrates (immediately or within 24 hours) on a chest radiograph. **Airway obstruction** may accompany aspiration of solid food particles.

B. **Treatment** of aspiration is correction of arterial hypoxemia with supplemental oxygen. Tracheal intubation and PEEP may be required if hypoxemia persists despite supplemental oxygen.

  1. **Pulmonary edema** is usually secondary to pulmonary capillary damage, which may create hypovo-

TABLE 40-9. Differential Diagnosis of Arterial Hypoxemia in Patients in a Postanesthesia Care Unit

Distribution of ventilation (mismatch to perfusion because of loss of functional residual capacity is most likely cause of postoperative hypoxemia)

Distribution of perfusion (mismatch to ventilation due to impaired hypoxic pulmonary vasoconstriction or altered pulmonary artery pressure)

Inadequate alveolar oxygen partial pressure

Reduced mixed venous oxygen partial pressure (decreased cardiac output; increased tissue oxygen extraction owing to shivering or sepsis)

lemia and necessitate intravascular fluid replacement.

2. **Antibiotics** are prescribed only if bacterial infection develops.
3. There is **no evidence that corticosteroids** improve long-term outcome.
4. **Bronchoscopy** may be necessary to relieve airway obstruction caused by inhaled food particles.

VI. POSTOPERATIVE RENAL COMPLICATIONS

A. **Oliguria** (urine output <0.5 ml$\cdot$kg$^{-1}\cdot$h^{-1}) in spite of **adequate perfusion pressure, hydration** (300–500 ml iv crystalloid bolus to assess hypovolemia), and **a low-dose furosemide challenge** (5 mg iv offsets fluid retention caused by antidiuretic hormone) increases the possibility of **acute tubular necrosis.**

B. **Polyuria** is usually self-limited and most often is due to **generous intraoperative fluid administration** or **hyperglycemia** (osmotic diuresis). Sustained polyuria (urine output >4–5 ml$\cdot$kg$^{-1}\cdot$h^{-1}) may result in hypovolemia and electrolyte disturbances.

VII. METABOLIC COMPLICATIONS (Table 40-10)

VIII. ELECTROLYTES AND GLUCOSE (Table 40-11)

IX. MISCELLANEOUS COMPLICATIONS (Table 40-12)

A. **Droperidol** (0.25–1.0 mg iv), with or without **metoclopramide** (5–10 mg iv), is effective in treating persistent postoperative **nausea** and **vomiting.**

B. **Temperature** $<35°C$ is an indication for assisted rewarming (radiant lighting, heating blankets, warmed

---

TABLE 40-10. Classification and Likely Explanation of Metabolic Derangements in Patients in a Postanesthesia Care Unit

Respiratory acidosis (hypoventilation)

Metabolic acidosis (hypovolemia, tissue hypoxia, hypothermia, renal failure, ketoacidosis, sepsis)

Respiratory alkalosis (hyperventilation)

Metabolic alkalosis (prolonged gastric suctioning, K^+-wasting diuretics)

TABLE 40-11. Electrolyte and Glucose Changes in Patients in a Postanesthesia Care Unit

Hypokalemia (cardiac dysrhythmias)

Hyperkalemia (hemolyzed sample, renal failure)

Hyponatremia (following transurethral resection of the prostate)

Hyperglycemia (<300 mg·dl^{-1} usually resolves spontaneously)

Hypoglycemia (masked by residual effects of anesthesia)

TABLE 40-12. Miscellaneous Complications That May Manifest in Patients in a Postanesthesia Care Unit

Nausea and vomiting (see Table 35-6)

Incidental trauma
  Dental damage
  Corneal abrasion
  Oral soft-tissue trauma
  Hoarseness/pharyngitis (occurs in 20–50% and is usually benign)
  Peripheral nerve compression
  Electrical or chemical burns
  Extravasation of intravenous fluids

Skeletal muscle pain (usually manifests the day after surgery)

Inadvertent hypothermia (usually less than 2°C and benign)

Persistent obtundation

TABLE 40-13. Differential Diagnosis of Coma in Patients in a Postanesthesia Care Unit

Hypothermia ($\leq 33°C$)

Hypoglycemia

Electrolyte imbalance (hyponatremia, hypomagnesemia, hypocalcemia, hypo-osmolarity)

Central nervous system damage (hypoxia, increased intracranial pressure, cerebral vascular accident, air embolus)

Drug overdose (treat with naloxone, flumazenil, physostigmine)

intravenous fluids). As body temperature rises, there may be a need to increase the rate of intravenous fluid administration to offset increased venous capacitance. Resolution of metabolic acidosis often corresponds to rewarming. Supplemental oxygen is administered to offset the increase in oxygen consumption accompanying shivering.

C. **Persistent obtundation** is most likely caused by residual effects of anesthetics or muscle relaxants. Skeletal muscle paralysis mimics obtundation but is ruled out by spontaneous ventilation, purposeful movement, and normal response to nerve stimulator. Persistence of sedative effects (anesthetic effects usually wane in 60–90 minutes) requires a differential diagnosis of coma (Table 40-13).

41

Management of Acute Postoperative Pain

Acute postoperative pain is a complex physiologic reaction to tissue injury, visceral distention, or disease (Lubenow TR, McCarthy RJ, Ivankovich AD: Management of acute postoperative pain. In: Barash PG, Cullen BF, Stoelting RK [eds]: Clinical Anesthesia, pp 1547–1577. Philadelphia, JB Lippincott, 1992). Historically, the treatment of postoperative pain has been given a low priority by surgeons and anesthesiologists. As a result, patients previously accepted pain as an unavoidable part of the postoperative experience. With the development of an expanding awareness of the epidemiology and pathophysiology of pain, more attention is being focused on the management of pain in an effort to improve quality of care and reduce morbidity.

I. FUNDAMENTAL CONCEPTS

A. **Nociception** refers to the detection, transduction, and transmission of noxious stimuli. Stimuli generated from thermal, mechanical, or chemical tissue damage may activate **nociceptors,** which are free nerve endings. As a result of chronic inflammation or repeated tissue injury, nociceptors may be sensitized and thereby become responsive to innocuous stimuli.

B. **Peripheral nerve afferent fibers** are categorized into three groups (A, B, and C), depending on diameter, degree of myelination, rapidity of conduction, and distribution of fibers.

1. **A delta fibers** are large myelinated fibers that mediate pain sensation.

2. **C fibers** are slowly conducting unmyelinated fibers. Approximately 50–80% of C fibers modulate nociceptive stimuli.

C. **Spinal Cord and Brain Pathways**

1. The peripheral afferent neuron (first-order neuron) sends axonal projections into the dorsal horn and

other areas of the spinal cord (relay centers for nociceptive activity), where a synapse occurs with a second-order afferent neuron.

2. Projections from the second-order afferent neuron cross to the contralateral hemisphere of the spinal cord and ascend from that level in the lateral spinothalamic tract to synapse in the thalamus.

D. Modulation of nociception can occur in the periphery or at any point where synaptic transmission occurs.

1. **Peripheral** modulation occurs by the liberation of substances (potassium, lactic acid, serotonin, bradykinin, histamine, prostaglandins) that sensitize and excite nociceptors. Aspirin and nonsteroidal anti-inflammatory drugs (NSAIDs) exert an analgesic effect by inhibiting prostaglandin synthesis in the periphery.

2. **Spinal.** Modulation in the spinal cord results from the action of neurotransmitter substances (glutamate, aspartate, substance P).

3. **Supraspinal.** Descending inhibitory tracts (opioid pathways and alpha-adrenergic pathways) that originate at the brain stem level (cell bodies located in the region of the periaqueductal gray and reticular formation) descend and synapse in the dorsal horn, where they release inhibitory neurotransmitters (endorphins, norepinephrine) that regulate synaptic transmission between primary and secondary afferent neurons. **Cognitive** modulation of pain (pain experienced in a pleasant environment elicits less discomfort) and **attention** (biofeedback based on premise that only a fixed number of afferent stimuli can reach cortical centers) influence the perception of pain.

II. PATHOPHYSIOLOGY OF PAIN

A. Components of surgical stress. There is growing understanding of the deleterious effects of postoperative pain on specific organ systems (Table 41-1).

B. Influence of Anesthesia on the Surgical Stress Response

1. **General anesthesia** does not reliably attenuate the neuroendocrine stress response (exception may be high doses of opioids or >1.5 MAC of volatile anesthetics).

2. **Regional anesthesia and analgesia** may block the cortisol response to stress if the site of surgery is well below the level of sensory block. Myocardial

TABLE 41-1. Adverse Physiologic Sequelae of Pain

Organ System	Clinical Effect
Pulmonary	Arterial hypoxemia
	Hypoventilation
	Pneumonia
Endocrine	Protein catabolism
	Hyperglycemia
	Sodium and water retention
Cardiovascular	Dysrhythmias
	Angina pectoris
	Myocardial infarction
	Congestive heart failure
Immunologic	Decreased immune function
Coagulation Effects	Thromboembolic phenomena
Gastrointestinal	Ileus
Genitourinary	Urinary retention

oxygen consumption and the work of breathing may be decreased by regional anesthesia.

   a. Epidural anesthesia and analgesia decrease the incidence of deep venous thrombosis and pulmonary embolism in patients undergoing total hip replacement and reduce the degree of postoperative hypercoagulability in vascular surgery patients.

   b. There is some evidence that epidural analgesia can improve pulmonary function postoperatively, reduce the incidence of adverse cardiovascular events, and decrease overall morbidity and mortality.

III. PHARMACOLOGY OF POSTOPERATIVE PAIN MANAGEMENT

Agents administered orally for postoperative pain management can be divided into opioid and nonopioid analgesics.

   A. **Nonopioid analgesics** are represented by aspirin, acetaminophen, and the NSAIDs and are used to treat minor or moderate acute postoperative pain (Table 41-2).

      1. **The mechanism of analgesic effects** is most likely inhibition of prostaglandin-mediated amplification of chemical and mechanical irritants on the sensory pathways.

      2. **Absorption/biotransformation/elimination.** This class of drugs undergoes rapid and complete absorption

TABLE 41-2. Pharmacokinetic Parameters/Maximum Dosage Recommendations of Nonopioid Analgesics

	Route	Time to Peak levels (hours)	Analgesic Onset (hours)	Actions Duration (hours)	Maximum Daily Recommended Dose (mg)
Salicylates					
Aspirin	po	0.5–2	0.5–1	2–4	3600
Diflunisal	po	2–3	1–2	8–12	2000
Propionic Acids					
Fenoprofen	po	1–2	1	4–6	3200
Ibuprofen	po	1–2	0.5	4–6	3200
Naproxen	po	2–4	1	4–7	1500
Indoles					
Indomethacin	po	1–2	0.5	4–6	200
Sulindac	po	2–4			400
Ketorolac	im	1	0.5–1	4–6	120
Oxicams					
Piroxicam	po	3–5	1	48–72	20
p-Ampinophenols					
Acetaminophen	po	0.5–1	0.5	2–4	1200
Phenacetin	po	1			2400

TABLE 41-3. Pharmacokinetic Parameters/Maximum Dosage Recommendations for Oral and Parenteral Opioid Analgesics

	Dosage		Analgesic Action (hours)			Comment
	Route	mg	Onset	Peak	Duration	
Morphine	iv	2.5		0.125		Rapid onset, peak respiratory depression 10 minutes
Codeine	im	15–60	0.25–0.5	1–5	4–6	Intramuscular route has little advantage compared with morphine
	po	15–60	0.25–1	0.5–2	3–4	Oral potency due to low first-pass effect
Hydromorphone	im	1–4	0.3–0.5	1	2–3	Potent analgesic but short duration limits usefulness
Oxycodone	po	5	0.5	1–2	3–6	Short-acting, preparations contain acetaminophen

Drug	Route					Comments
Methadone	po	2.5–10	0.5–1	1.5–2	4–8	Long duration of effect
Propoxyphene	po	32–65	0.25–1	1–2	3–6	Weak opioid
Meperidine	im	50–100	0.12–0.5	1	2–4	Short duration of effect. One tenth as potent as morphine
Buprenorphine	im	0.3–0.6	0.12	1	6–8	High mu affinity, may precipitate withdrawal
Butorphanol	im	2–4	0.1–0.2	0.5–1	3–4	May precipitate withdrawal
Dezocine	im	5–20	0.25	0.5–1.5	2–4	Potency similar to that of morphine
Nalbuphine	iv	5–10	0.25			
	im	10–20	0.25	1	3–6	May precipitate withdrawal
	iv	1–5				
Pentazocine	im	30–60	0.12–0.5	1–3	3–6	Used primarily for cancer pain
	po	50			4–7	

after oral administration. Hepatic metabolism and renal excretion of conjugated metabolites are the primary modes of elimination of these drugs.

3. **Adverse effects** of short-term therapy as used for acute pain management include gastrointestinal discomfort, central nervous system disturbances (dizziness, drowsiness), and prolonged bleeding (usually reversible in 24–48 hours after discontinuation of NSAIDs; lasts about 1 week after discontinuation of aspirin).

4. **Clinical uses** of nonopioid analgesics are limited to treatment of events associated with sensitizing effects of prostaglandins (musculoskeletal, post-traumatic, and inflammatory pain).

B. **Opioid analgesics** represented by morphine are used most often to treat severe postoperative pain (Table 41-3).

1. **The mechanism of analgesic effects** is most likely attributable to interaction with stereoselective **opioid receptors** (same sites of action as for endogenous neuromodulators represented by endorphins) (Table 41-4). **Agonist-antagonist opioids** may exhibit altered affinity for opioid receptors, accounting for the potential of these drugs to reverse the effects of an agonist (Table 41-4).

2. **Absorption/biotransformation/elimination.** Oral absorption may be extensive, but availability of the drug may be limited by extensive first-pass metabolism. Distribution of the drug depends on its lipid solubility. Biotransformation followed by renal elimination of conjugated metabolites (morphine-6-glucuronide is an active metabolite) is the primary mode of elimination.

3. **Adverse Effects** (Table 41-5)
   a. Physical dependence and analgesic tolerance are not generally a problem when opioids are used short term.
   b. Respiratory depression is more likely when the opioid is administered intravenously in high doses and in the absence of pain.

4. **Clinical uses.** Opioids remain the primary pharmacologic therapeutic agents for moderate to severe postoperative pain.
   a. Agonist-antagonists can be effective analgesics in the postoperative period and have a ceiling effect for respiratory depression (often a ceiling effect for analgesia as well).
   b. Unlike the nonopioid analgesics, these drugs do not interfere with platelet function.

TABLE 41-4. Pharmacology of Opioid Receptors

Receptor	Mu₁	Mu₂	Delta	Kappa	Sigma
Analgesia	Supraspinal		Spinal	Spinal	
Affect	Euphoria			Sedation	Dysphoria
Pupil	Miosis	Sedation		Miosis	Mydriasis
Ventilation		Depression	Depression		Tachypnea
Gastrointestinal	Nausea	Constipation	Nausea		
	Vomiting		Vomiting		
Genitourinary	Urinary		Urinary	Diuresis	
	retention		retention		
Temperature	Increase				
Other	Pruritus		Pruritus		
Tolerance	Yes		Yes	Little	
Cross-tolerance	Delta		Mu	No	

491

TABLE 41-5. Adverse Effects of Short-Term and Moderate Dose Opioid Therapy

Central Nervous System (tolerance develops rapidly)
  Sedation
  Dizziness
  Miosis

Gastrointestinal Effects
  Nausea and vomiting
  Constipation
  Spasm of the sphincter of Oddi (can persist for up to 24 hours after a single therapeutic dose)

Urinary Retention

---

      c. Traditional therapeutic regimens that utilized on-demand administration are being replaced with continuous administration as the benefits of a reduced stress response in the postoperative period are becoming more apparent. As the patient's analgesic requirements diminish, the transition from parenteral to oral therapy is often empirical and generally involves replacing the opioid with an opioid-NSAID combination.

IV. METHODS FOR ANALGESIA may involve pharmacologic use of analgesics by various routes of administration or nonpharmacologic application of mechanical, electrical, or psychological techniques. The optimal combination of these techniques is dependent on the type and degree of pain, the patient's perception of the pain, and the underlying medical, social, and environmental conditions in which the pain is managed.

  A. Routes of Analgesic Delivery (Table 41-6)

  B. Patient-controlled analgesia (PCA) provides superior analgesia with less total drug dose, less sedation, and more rapid return to physical activity (Table 41-7).

    1. Patient acceptance of PCA is very high.

    2. Use of PCA in pediatrics and in older debilitated patients may be difficult because the technique requires patient understanding and cooperation.

  C. Central neuraxial analgesia (Tables 41-8 and 41-9)

    1. Intrathecal administration of opioids produces long-lasting analgesia after a single injection (morphine, 0.25–1 mg).

TABLE 41-6. Routes of Analgesic Delivery

Oral (unpredictable onset and duration; requires a functioning gastrointestinal tract)

Transdermal

Transmucosal

Intramuscular (administration of analgesics by this route on a 3–4 hour basis results in plasma concentrations that exceed the analgesic requirements for only about 35% of the dosing interval)

Intravenous (intermittent versus continuous; patient-controlled analgesia)

Central neuraxial analgesia
　Intrathecal
　Epidural analgesia

Peripheral nerve blocks (short duration limits usefulness)
　Local infiltration
　Intra-articular (bupivacaine up to 100 mg)
　Intercostal (bupivacaine with or without epinephrine; perform in the midaxillary or posterior axillary line; risk is pneumothorax; cryoanalgesia lasts 1–3 months)
　Ilioinguinal (pain relief following inguinal or femoral herniorrhaphy, appendectomy, procedures on the scrotum)
　Penile
　Brachial plexus (continuous analgesia using bupivacaine 0.25% at 6–10 ml·h^{-1})
　Intrapleural (bupivacaine 0.25–05% 20 ml every 6 hours)

Other Modalities
　Transcutaneous electrical nerve stimulation (TENS)
　Psychological interventions for postoperative analgesia

---

    a. The onset of analgesic effect following the intrathecal administration of an opioid is directly proportional to the lipid solubility of the opioid (fentanyl has a rapid onset). The duration of the effect is longer with the more hydrophilic compounds (morphine).

    b. A disadvantage of this technique is the inability to titrate the drug effect.

  2. Epidural analgesia by epidural administration of opioids reflects passage of the drug across the dura (2–10% of the injected dose) as well as systemic absorption of the opioid (morphine, 10 mg iv or epidurally produces peak serum levels and decay curves that are nearly identical).

TABLE 41-7. Guidelines Regarding the Bolus Doses, Lockout Intervals, and Continuous Infusions for Parenteral Analgesics When Using a Patient-Controlled Analgesia System

Drug	Bolus Dose (mg)	Lockout Interval (minutes)	Continuous Infusion (mg·h⁻¹)
Agonists			
Fentanyl	0.015–0.05	3–10	0.02–0.1
Hydromorphone	0.10–0.5	5–15	0.2–0.5
Meperidine	5–15	5–15	5–40
Methadone	0.5–3.0	10–20	
Morphine	0.5–3.0	5–20	1–10
Sufentanil	0.003–0.015	3–10	0.004–0.03
Agonist-Antagonists			
Buprenorphine	0.03–0.2	10–20	
Pentazocine	5–30	5–15	6–40

TABLE 41-8. Complications of the Use of Neuraxial Opioids

| Complication | Reported Incidence (%) | | Treatment |
	Spinal	Epidural	
Respiratory depression	5–7	0.1–2	Support ventilation, naloxone
Pruritus	60	1–100	Antihistamine; naloxone
Nausea and vomiting	20–30	20–30	Antiemetics; transdermal scopolamine; naloxone
Urinary retention	50	15–25	Catheterize; naloxone

TABLE 41-9. Postoperative Epidural Analgesia

Route	Group A (Bupivacaine 25 mg/5 ml, 0.5%) Epidural Bolus	Group B (Morphine 5 mg) Epidural Bolus	Group C (Morphine 100 μg·h^{-1}) Epidural Infusion
Urinary retention	30 (100%)	30 (100%)	2 (7%)
Hypotension	7 (23%)	0	0
Weakness of hands	12 (40%)	0	0
Pruritus	0	12 (40%)	1 (3%)
Depressed consciousness	0	8 (27%)	0

TABLE 41-10. Comparison of Types of Epidural Administration

Advantages	Disadvantages
Continuous Epidural Infusions	
Less rostral spread	Need for sophisticated infusion device
Unchanging level of analgesia	
Permits concomitant use of a local anesthetic solution	
Permits use of short-acting opioids	
Less risk of catheter contamination	
Eliminates need for anesthesia personnel to perform injections	
Intermittent Epidural Bolus	
Simple	Limited number of suitable opioids
No need for infusion devices	High incidence of side effects
	Personnel needed to reinject catheter
	Excludes use of local anesthesia
	More difficult to titrate dose

TABLE 41-11. Continuous Epidural Infusion Regimens

Composition of Solution

Morphine (0.1 mg·ml^{-1}) or fentanyl (100 µg·ml^{-1}) with bupivacaine (1 mg·ml^{-1})

Rate of Infusion

Initiate intraoperatively at 4–6 ml·h^{-1} if operation expected to exceed 3 hours

Precede infusion with 5–10-ml bolus of the solution if operation is expected to be of short duration

Placement of Epidural Catheter

Hydrophilic opioids (morphine) spread rostrally (lumbar epidural placement acceptable)

Lipophilic opioids (fentanyl) provide a segmental analgesic effect (epidural catheter placement at dermatome levels included in the surgical field)

TABLE 41-12. Epidural Opioids: Latency and Duration of Postoperative Analgesia

Agent	Bolus Dose	Analgesic Effect			Continuous Infusion	
		Onset (minutes)	Peak (minutes)	Duration (hours)	Concentration	Rate (ml·h⁻¹)
Meperidine	30–100 mg	5–10	12–30	4–6		
Morphine	5 mg	23.5	30–60	12–24	0.01%	1–6
Methadone	5 mg	12.5	17	7.2		
Hydromorphone	1 mg	13	23	11.4	0.05%	0–8
Fentanyl	100 mg	4–10	20	2.6	0.001%	4–12
Sufentanil	30–50 μg	7.3	26.5	3.9	0.0001%	10
Alfentanil	15 μg·kg⁻¹	15		1–2		

  a. Epidural opioids may be administered as **continuous epidural infusions** or as an **intermittent epidural bolus** (Table 41-10).

  b. The epidural catheter is often placed before the induction of anesthesia so that a test dose of local anesthetic can confirm proper placement of the catheter in an awake patient. This practice also allows for the start of the continuous epidural infusion intraoperatively (Table 41-11).

  c. **Selection of analgesics** for epidural analgesia is influenced by the duration of action (Table 41-12).

  d. **Management of Inadequate Analgesia** (Figure 41-1)

  e. **Safety Considerations** (Table 41-13)

 3. **Caudal** nerve blocks play a minor role in acute pain management in adults, since they are technically more difficult to perform than a lumbar epidural block. In contrast, palpation of the sacral hiatus is easy in the pediatric patient (use a short 22- or 23-gauge needle with the child in the lateral position to inject 0.75–1 ml·kg^{-1} of bupivacaine, which provides analgesia to T10).

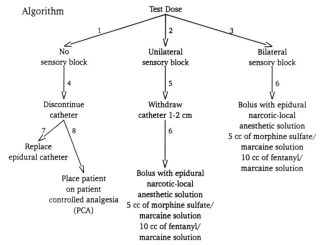

Figure 41-1. Test dose algorithm for inadequate analgesia. A 5-ml test dose of 2% lidocaine with 1:200,000 epinephrine is injected into the lumbar epidural catheter.

**TABLE 41-13. Safety Considerations in the
Management of a Continuous
Epidural Technique**

Subarachnoid Migration of the Catheter (add 0.1 bupivacaine
to solution and monitor for onset of sensory blockade)

Infection-Related Problems (monitor patient's temperature
and evaluate for signs of analgesia; remove catheter and
culture samples if signs of infection)

Epidural Hematoma (appears to be no risk if catheter placed
at least 1 hour before anticoagulation)

Respiratory Depression (monitor respiratory rate and sedation
every hour during the first 24 hours)

**TABLE 41-14. Factors Associated With Delayed
Depression of Ventilation Following
Neuraxial Opioids**

High opioid dose
Use of a water-soluble opioid (lipid solubility of fentanyl limits
drug available in cerebrospinal fluid for cephalad diffusion)
Lack of opioid tolerance
Concomitant systemic administration of opioids or other
central nervous system depressants
Increased abdominal or intrathoracic pressure
Advanced age

4. Delayed depression of ventilation following neuraxial opioids is more likely in the presence of specific circumstances (Table 41-14).

V. ORGANIZATION OF A POSTOPERATIVE
ANALGESIA SERVICE

A. The basic goals of the postoperative analgesia service
are (1) to administer and monitor postoperative analgesia, and (2) to identify and manage complications or
side effects of postoperative analgesic techniques.
B. The delivery of central neuraxial opioid analgesia requires cooperation among the anesthesiology, nursing,
surgery, and pharmacy staffs on a 24-hour basis.

TABLE 41-15. Postoperative Epidural Analgesia Order Sheet

(Please circle orders to be implemented and complete blanks where appropriate. Date and time for each procedure are to be noted.)

1. Admit to postoperative analgesia service.
2. Routine vital signs in postanesthesia recovery room (PAR) or intensive care unit.
3. Discharge from PAR by anesthesiologist.
4. On ward:
   a. Intravenous infusion maintained.
   b. Vital signs every 4 hours.
   c. Naloxone with syringe at bedside.
   d. Monitor for depression of ventilation.
      (1) Apnea monitor _____ during bed rest.
      (2) Breathing rate every hour for the first 24 hours and then every 4 hours.
      (3) If breathing rate <8 breaths·min^{-1}, administer naloxone, 0.4 mg iv, and immediately call the postoperative analgesia service.
5. Epidural solution (circle one):
   a. Morphine, 15 mg, with bupivacaine, 150 mg, in 150 ml normal saline, rate _____ ml·h^{-1}, as needed for pain for 72 hours.
   b. Fentanyl, 1.5 mg, with bupivacaine, 150 mg, in 150 ml normal saline, rate _____ ml·h^{-1}, as needed for pain for 72 hours.
   c. Sufentanil, 0.5 mg, with bupivacaine, 500 mg, in 500 ml normal saline, rate 8–10 ml·h^{-1}, as needed for pain.
6. Supplemental medications:
   a. Morphine, 2 mg iv or im, every 2–4 hours as needed for pain.
   b. Metoclopramide, 10 mg iv, every 4–6 hours as needed for nausea.
   c. Diphenhydramine, 25–50 mg orally, iv or im, every 4–6 hours as needed for pruritus.
   d. If pruritus is unresponsive to two doses of diphenhydramine, administer naloxone, 80 µg iv. May repeat once every 5 minutes.
7. Nursing staff on ward should call the postoperative analgesia service for any problems, questions, or the need to discontinue the infusion.
8. All other preoperative orders, medications, and diet per service with the exception of opioids.

Physician's
signature _____ Date _____

**TABLE 41-16. Postoperative Patient-Controlled
Analgesia Order Sheet**

Medication: Morphine, 30 mg per 30 ml prefilled syringe
            Loading dose = 2 mg
            Maintenance dose = 1 mg
            Lockout interval = 6 minutes
            4-hour time limit at 20 mg*
Disregard all other opioid orders during patient-controlled
analgesia use

Physician's signature

*If analgesia is inadequate, 4-hour limit dose may be increased to 30 mg.

    C. Written policy and procedure manuals for nursing staff
as well as preprinted epidural analgesia orders are useful (Table 41-15).
    D. Protocols outlining the initial parameters for starting
and maintaining PCA are useful (Table 41-16).
    E. A key aspect of the initiation of a postoperative anal-
gesia service is the identification of patient populations that are most likely to benefit from improved
postoperative pain management (Table 41-17).
        1. Patients may be aware of the neuraxial opioid con-
cept and request its use in their postoperative management.
        2. Despite the absence of confirmation that neurax-
ial opioid analgesia improves outcome, there is
sufficient evidence in the literature to support
the increased use of sophisticated techniques to
improve the quality of postoperative pain management.

**TABLE 41-17. Patient Population Most Likely to
Benefit from Improved Postoperative
Pain Management**

Thoracic surgery patients
Abdominal surgery patients
Orthopedic surgery patients
High-risk vascular surgical procedure patients

TABLE 41-18. **Pharmacologic Considerations for Pediatric Patients**

Drug	Dose (Age >3 months)	Interval (hours)	Route	Comments
Acetaminophen	5–15 mg·kg^{-1}	4–6	po	Overdose may cause hepatotoxicity
	20 mg·kg^{-1}	4–6	Rectal	
Ibuprofen	8 mg·kg^{-1}	6	po	
Naproxen	5 mg·kg^{-1}	8–12	po	
Codeine	0.5–1 mg·kg^{-1}	4–6	po	Most commonly combined with acetaminophen
Meperidine	1–1.5 mg·kg^{-1}	3–4	im	May cause less constipation and urinary retention than morphine
Morphine	0.8–1 mg·kg^{-1}	2–3	iv	
	0.1–0.15 mg·kg^{-1}	3–4	im	
	0.08–0.1 mg·kg^{-1}	2	iv	
	50–60 µg·kg^{-1}·h^{-1}		iv	Continuous infusion
	50 µg·kg^{-1}	12–24	Epidural	Abdominal surgery
	120–150 µg·kg^{-1}	12–24	Epidural	Thoracic surgery
	50–100 µg·kg^{-1}	12–24	Caudal	
Fentanyl	1–1.5 µg·kg^{-1}	1–2	iv	Minimum age 1 year
	2–4 µg·kg^{-1}·h^{-1}		iv	Continuous infusion

503

TABLE 41-19. Maximum Local Anesthetic Doses in Infants and Children

Agent	Infant Dose (mg·kg⁻¹):Age	Child Dose (mg·kg⁻¹)
Lidocaine	5:from birth on	5
Lidocaine with epinephrine	7:from birth on	7
Mepivacaine	4:<6 months	5
Bupivacaine	2:<3 months	3
Bupivacaine with epinephrine	2:<3 months	4
Chloroprocaine	4:<6 months	8
Chloroprocaine with epinephrine	5:<6 months	10

VI. SPECIAL CONSIDERATIONS IN PEDIATRIC ACUTE PAIN MANAGEMENT (see Section IV C 3)

A. A useful monitor of analgesic efficacy in children is **behavior observation.**

B. The selection and dosing of analgesic agents require special attention in the pediatric patient (Tables 41-18 and 41-19).

C. **Oral Analgesics**
   1. **Nonopioid.** NSAIDs are useful for acute postoperative pain management in children (ibuprofen, acetaminophen).
   2. **Opioids.** Codeine in combination with acetaminophen is commonly used for moderate postoperative pain in children.

D. Patient-controlled analgesia, often utilizing morphine (loading dose 0.1–0.2 mg·kg^{-1}, followed by 10–15 μg·kg^{-1}·h^{-1}), may be beneficial.

VII. RELATIONSHIP BETWEEN ACUTE AND CHRONIC PAIN (see Chapter 42)

A. It is generally agreed that pain persisting >6 months can be viewed as chronic pain.

B. Differentiation between acute and chronic pain is important because therapy is generally vastly different (opioids used to treat chronic pain may lead to tolerance and dependence).

42

Chronic Pain Management

Pain should be considered chronic not when it has reached a certain duration but when it has extracted a substantial toll on the individual in terms of functional loss, psychological distress, and social and vocational dysfunction (Abram SE, Haddox JD: Chronic pain management. In: Barash PG, Cullen BF, Stoelting RK [eds]: Clinical Anesthesia, pp 1579–1607. Philadelphia, JB Lippincott, 1992). Multiple environmental, psychological, and emotional factors (fatigue, anxiety, depression) also influence the intensity of pain.

   I. **PAIN PATHWAYS AND MECHANISMS** (see Chapter 41, Section I)

  II. **MANAGEMENT OF COMMON CHRONIC PAIN SYNDROMES**

   A. **Lumbosacral radiculopathy.** Epidural injection of corticosteroids (often with a local anesthetic) may produce beneficial effects (especially new onset pain), presumably by reducing the inflammation initiated by either mechanical or chemical insult to the nerve root.
      1. **Triamcinolone diacetate** (50 mg) or **methylprednisolone acetate** (80 mg) is injected into the epidural space as close to the affected nerve root as possible. The addition of 3–4 ml of local anesthetic (lidocaine) to the injected solution produces analgesia, confirming proper drug placement. Reassessment should be carried out 1–2 weeks after the initial injection. If symptoms are improved but still present, it is acceptable to repeat the epidural injection. Few patients obtain relief from repeated injections if the first epidural injection was of no help. Patients with chronic radicular low back pain or previous back surgery are unlikely to benefit from epidural injection of corticosteroids.

     2. Intrathecal injection of corticosteroids has been associated with symptoms consistent with aseptic meningitis.

B. Lumbosacral arthropathies (degeneration and inflammation of the lumbar facet joints and sacroiliac joints) may produce low back pain that is difficult to distinguish from radicular pain.

     1. Diagnosis is confirmed by injection of local anesthetic (1 ml) into the facet joint, often under fluoroscopic control. This injection may produce pain relief lasting 6 months.

     2. Nonsteroidal anti-inflammatory drugs, radiofrequency coagulation, and cryoanalgesia may be of some benefit.

C. Myofascial pain is characterized by marked tenderness of discrete points **(trigger points)** within affected skeletal muscles and the appearance of tight, ropy bands of skeletal muscle. Acute skeletal muscle strain with disruption of sarcoplasmic reticulum and release of Ca^{2+} and nociceptor-sensitizing substances (prostaglandins, bradykinin, serotonin) may play a role in the development of this pain.

     1. Scapulocostal syndrome. A trigger point is located just medial and superior to the upper portion of the scapula. Pain often radiates to the occipital region, shoulder, medial aspect of the arm, or anterior chest wall.

     2. Myofascial pain involving gluteal muscles produces pain referred to the posterior thigh and calf, mimicking S1 radiculopathy. Myofascial pain involving the piriform muscle, which overlies the sciatic nerve, can produce sciatic irritation that resembles radiculopathy.

     3. Treatment. The most important aspect of treatment for myofascial pain is physical therapy designed to restore skeletal muscle strength and elasticity. Infiltration of local anesthetic directly into the **trigger point** (daily if necessary) provides analgesia that confirms the diagnosis and permits initiation of physical therapy. Ultrasound therapy, transcutaneous electrical nerve stimulation (TENS), or vapocoolant spray applied over the affected area may also produce periods of analgesia during physical therapy.

D. Sympathetically Maintained Pain

     1. Reflex sympathetic dystrophy is a syndrome of pain, autonomic nervous system dysfunction, and dystrophic changes that usually occurs after trauma (crush injuries, lacerations) or surgery (carpal tunnel release, palmar fasciectomy) (Table 42-1). Reflex sympathetic dystrophy occasionally occurs after cerebrovascular accident or myocardial infarction.

    a. Diagnosis and treatment. Stellate ganglion block or lumbar sympathetic block confirms the diagnosis of reflex sympathetic dystrophy. Once the diagnosis is confirmed, treatment consists of a series of blocks until symptoms become minimal. Physical therapy and often TENS are carried out after each sympathetic block.

    b. Early treatment (within 1 month) with sympathetic blocks is successful in nearly 90% of patients. Delay of treatment to after 6 months is associated with success rates of about 50%.

    c. Surgical or neurolytic sympathectomy is reserved for patients who do not respond to sympathetic blocks. Success with sympathetic nerve ablation is usually transient.

    d. Temporary localized sympathetic nervous system (SNS) blockade using guanethidine injected intravenously into the extremity, isolated from the general circulation with a tourniquet, may be a useful alternative to SNS blockade produced by local anesthetics.

2. Causalgia refers to a syndrome of burning pain and autonomic nervous system dysfunction resulting from major nerve trunk injury such as gunshot wounds, which cause violent deformation of the brachial plexus, median nerve, or sciatic nerve.

    a. Pain often begins immediately after injury and is commonly accompanied by deep shooting or stabbing sensations. Movement or SNS activation (noise, anxiety) often exacerbates the pain. There is usually evidence of reduced SNS activity in

---

TABLE 42-1. Symptoms of Reflex Sympathetic Dystrophy

Burning pain

Hyperalgesia

Warm and erythematous skin followed by vasoconstriction and edema

Bone demineralization

Joint stiffness

the affected extremity (warm, dry, and venodilated). Dystrophic changes resemble reflex sympathetic dystrophy.
   b. **Treatment** with surgical sympathectomy (neurolytic lumbar sympathectomy is an alternative to surgical lumbar sympathectomy) seems to be more successful than local anesthetic–induced blockade.

III. PHARMACOLOGIC ADJUNCTS FOR CHRONIC PAIN

A. The use of opioids in the treatment of chronic pain that is not associated with malignancy is controversial.
B. **Antidepressants** are useful in the treatment of some chronic pain syndromes, presumably reflecting their blockade of presynaptic uptake of serotonin and/or norepinephrine.
   1. Differences among antidepressant drugs reside mainly in their potency and side-effect profiles (Table 42-2). There is no evidence that one drug is superior to any other in treating any given pain condition.
   2. Benefits of these drugs in patients with chronic pain syndromes include normalization of sleep patterns (drug-induced sedation), reduction in anxiety and depression, and decrease in the patient's perception of pain.
C. **Antipsychotic drugs** have been utilized to treat some chronic pain syndromes, presumably reflecting action

---

TABLE 42-2. Side Effects of Antidepressants

Antimuscarinic Effects
   Xerostomia
   Impaired visual accommodation
   Urinary retention
   Constipation

Antihistaminic Effects
   Sedation
   Increase in gastric fluid pH

Cardiovascular Effects
   Orthostatic hypotension
   Cardiac conduction defects (overdose)

TABLE 42-3. Side Effects of Antipsychotics

Extrapyramidal Symptoms
  Cogwheel rigidity and bradykinesia
  Oculogyric crisis
  Akathisia (restlessness and dysphoria)
  Tardive dyskinesia

Antihistaminic Effects

Alpha Blockade

Antimuscarinic Effects

---

of a nonspecific blockade of dopamine receptors (Table 42-3).
  D. **Anticonvulsants** (phenytoin, valproic acid, carbamazepine, clonazepam) may be efficacious in the treatment of certain chronic pain syndromes (Table 42-4).

IV. PSYCHOLOGICAL TREATMENTS FOR CHRONIC PAIN

  A. Chronic pain is often accompanied by psychological changes that may with time become more disabling than the somatic pain (Table 42-5).
  B. Psychological treatment requires a knowledge of psychoanalytic and therapeutic principles that are also time-consuming (Table 42-6).

V. CANCER PAIN

In assessing patients with malignant disease who seek treatment for pain, it is essential to determine the specific site and mechanism of their pain as well as the stage (prognosis) of their disease.

TABLE 42-4. Side Effects of Anticonvulsants

Nausea
Ataxia
Folate deficiency and gingival hyperplasia (phenytoin)
Increased liver transaminase enzyme levels (valproic acid)
Pancytopenia (carbamazepine)
Emotional lability (clonazepam)

TABLE 42-5. Psychological Factors Associated With Chronic Pain

Mental depression
Loss of appetite
Insomnia
Avoidance of social and vocational obligations
Constant complaining
Dependence on analgesics
Physician shopping

A. **Pharmacologic therapy.** Use of oral analgesics is the mainstay of treatment of cancer pain, keeping in mind several guidelines (Table 42-7).
B. When oral therapy is not possible or successful, a constant intravenous infusion technique is preferable to intermittent intramuscular injections.
C. **Intraspinal opioids.** Morphine is the drug most often selected for epidural or intrathecal administration. The drug may be administered as a bolus, by infusion *via* an external pump and catheter, or by infusion *via* a totally implanted pump and catheter.
   1. Marked resistance and tolerance to the effects of intraspinal opioids may develop (intermittent doses of local anesthetics or clonidine may allow opioid receptors to again become sensitive to their ligands).
   2. Withdrawal symptoms may result if neuraxial opioid doses are abruptly decreased or discontinued.
D. **Non-neurolytic nerve blocks** may be useful for controlling intractable pain from advanced malignancy without the risks associated with neurolytic (neurodestructive) nerve blocks (paresis, bowel and bladder dysfunction, painful neuritis) (Table 42-8).
E. **Neurolytic blocks** are usually reserved for patients with a terminal illness, in view of potential side effects such

---

TABLE 42-6. Psychological Treatments for Chronic Pain

Psychodynamic approaches
Cognitive therapies
Behavioral therapies
Biofeedback
Hypnosis

TABLE 42-7. Guidelines for the Treatment of Cancer Pain Using Oral Medications

Use drugs appropriate for the nature and severity of the patient's pain (codeine versus morphine; repeated administration of meperidine can result in accumulation of normeperidine, which is a central nervous system stimulant)

Use adequate doses (varies tremendously)

Maintain steady blood and tissue medication levels (administering analgesics by the clock as treatment on an as needed basis invariably results in periods of inadequate analgesia; transdermal fentanyl)

Consider the use of adjuvant drugs (tricyclic antidepressants, antiemetics, corticosteroids)

Promptly treat side effects

TABLE 42-8. Non-neurolytic Nerve Blocks for Treatment of Cancer-Related Pain

Sympathetic nervous system blockade (reflex sympathetic dystrophy, herpes zoster)

Local anesthetic injection of trigger points (myofascial pain)

Transcutaneous electrical nerve stimulation

Perineural injection of corticosteroids and/or local anesthetics (tumor compression of nerve roots)

Epidural corticosteroid injection (epidural tumor invasion)

---

as loss of motor function and loss of control of the bowels or bladder.

1. Drugs available for neurolysis are similar in efficacy but possess different characteristics (Table 42-9).
2. Intrathecal neurolysis requires precise positioning in order to place the affected sensory root uppermost (alcohol) or in the most dependent (phenol) position.

TABLE 42-9. Characteristics of Drugs Used for Neurolytic Block

Alcohol	Phenol
Pain on injection	No pain on injection
Prompt neurolysis	Neurolysis in about 15 minutes
Hypobaric	Hyperbaric

43

ICU—Critical Care

Critical care medicine is a multidisciplinary specialty based in the intensive care unit (ICU); its primary concern is care of patients with life-threatening illnesses (Brown M: ICU—Critical Care. In Barash PG, Cullen BF, Stoelting RK [eds]: Clinical Anesthesia, pp 1609–1632. Philadelphia, JB Lippincott, 1992). An average of 12% of adult hospital beds and 23% of children's hospital beds are ICU beds. ICU care consumes 20% of hospital costs.

I. CENTRAL NERVOUS SYSTEM

A. **Intracranial pressure (ICP) monitoring.** Untreated elevations in ICP (>20 mm Hg) can lead to global cerebral ischemia owing to reductions in cerebral perfusion. There is a correlation between clinical outcome and the level of ICP elevation after acute injury, emphasizing the importance of continuous monitoring of ICP and prompt intervention with treatment designed to lower ICP (see Table 19-8).

B. **Central nervous system trauma**
1. **The Glasgow Coma Scale** quantitates the severity of head injury and provides an estimate of prognosis (see Table 19-15).
2. **Somatosensory-evoked potentials,** if absent bilaterally, predict a vegetative state.
3. **Causes of seizures** (Table 43-1)
4. Management of patients with a severe head injury should include several steps (Table 43-2).

II. CARDIOVASCULAR SYSTEM

A. **Cardiogenic shock** is the most common cause of death among patients in coronary care units, occurring in 10–15% of those who experience an acute myocardial infarction. Prognosis is poor and mortality is high (Tables 43-3 and 43-4).

TABLE 43-1. Causes of Seizures

Febrile illness (children)
Head trauma
Brain tumor (30–50 years old)
Cerebral vascular disease (>50 years old)
Hypoglycemia
Hypocalcemia

TABLE 43-2. Management of Patients With a Head Injury

Secure airway
Stabilize blood pressure and ventilation
Consider cervical spine injury
Use computed tomography to detect surgically treatable lesions
Monitor and treat intracranial pressure
Evaluate fluids and electrolytes
Administer anticonvulsants
Administer prophylaxis for gastrointestinal bleeding
Assess coagulation status (5–10% develop disseminated intravascular coagulation)

TABLE 43-3. Manifestations of Cardiogenic Shock

Mental confusion
Peripheral vasoconstriction
Systolic blood pressure <80 mm Hg
Cardiac index <2 $l \cdot min^{-1} \cdot m^{-2}$
Left ventricular end-diastolic pressure >18 mm Hg

TABLE 43-4. Treatment of Cardiogenic Shock

Continuous monitoring of blood pressure, pulmonary capillary wedge pressure, and urine output
Inotropes (dopamine and/or dobutamine)
Mechanical assist devices (intra-aortic balloon counterpulsation)
Emergency coronary revascularization

TABLE 43-5. Manifestations of Cardiac Tamponade

Hypotension
Distant heart sounds
Electrical alternans
Distention of jugular veins on inspiration
Equalization of central venous pressure, pulmonary artery
 end-diastolic pressure, and pulmonary capillary wedge
 pressure

B. **Cardiac tamponade** is accumulation of fluid or blood
 in the pericardial space (in chronic renal failure or
 after cardiac surgery) that results in a decrease in cardiac output due to insufficient venous return (Table
 43-5). **Treatment** is surgical decompression or, if the
 condition is immediately life-threatening, pericardiocentesis at the patient's bedside.
C. **Pulmonary embolism** is a leading cause of morbidity
 and mortality, with emboli arising principally from
 the deep venous system of the lower extremities (Table 43-6). **Diagnosis** is confirmed by perfusion scans
 or pulmonary angiography. **Treatment** is initially with
 heparin. Fibrinolytic drugs may be considered.

III. RESPIRATORY SYSTEM

A. **Acute respiratory failure** is synonymous with **adult
 respiratory distress syndrome,** which is a descriptive
 term applied to many acute diffuse infiltrative lung
 lesions with diverse causes (Tables 43-7, 43-8, and
 43-9).
B. **Mechanical ventilation.** Standard positive-pressure
 ventilators permit several types of ventilatory modes.

TABLE 43-6. Manifestations of Pulmonary Embolism

Unexplained dyspnea of sudden onset
Substernal chest pain
Cardiac dysrhythmias
Congestive heart failure
Electrocardiographic evidence of right ventricular strain
Arterial blood gases (unchanged to decreased Pao_2 and $Paco_2$)

**TABLE 43-7. Injuries Associated With Adult
Respiratory Distress Syndrome**

Shock	Burns
Aspiration	Drug ingestion
Sepsis	Uremia
Trauma	Cardiopulmonary bypass
Head injury	Near-drowning

**TABLE 43-8. Manifestations of Adult Respiratory
Distress Syndrome**

Decreased lung compliance (lung water increases as a result
  of capillary permeability)
Refractory hypoxemia (shunt through fluid-filled alveoli)
Diffuse radiographic abnormalities

1. **Controlled mechanical ventilation** delivers gases
   at a preset rate and volume independent of patient
   effort or response. A patient with an intact ventilatory drive may require interventions (hyperventilation, sedation, muscle relaxants) to diminish
   the tendency to breathe asynchronously with the
   ventilator.
2. **Assist-control ventilation.** The patient creates a
   sub-baseline pressure in the inspiratory limb that
   triggers the ventilator to deliver a predetermined
   tidal volume. If a patient's ventilatory rate falls below a preset level, the machine enters the control
   mode.
3. In a form of **intermittent positive-pressure ventilation,** the ventilator delivers a preset tidal volume

**TABLE 43-9. Treatment of Adult Respiratory
Distress Syndrome**

Supplemental oxygen
Mechanical ventilation with positive end-expiratory pressure
Fluid replacement guided by pulmonary artery catheter and
  urine output
Antibiotics if infection is documented
Corticosteroids (unproven efficacy)

at a specified interval while providing a continuous flow of gas for a patient's spontaneous ventilation.

4. **High-frequency jet ventilation** is characterized by a small tidal volume (less than dead space), high ventilation rate (60–3000 breaths·min^{-1}), and low airway pressure.

5. **Pressure control ventilation** is characterized by a rapid rise to peak inspiratory pressure, thus removing the patient's desire to breathe (improved synchrony with the ventilator), decreasing the work of breathing, and potentially improving the distribution of ventilation.

6. **Pressure control inverse ratio ventilation** is characterized by an inspiratory-to-expiratory ratio >1:1, thus allowing alveoli with a slow time constant to fill (prolonged inspiratory phase) and improving oxygenation.

C. **Cystic fibrosis** is an inherited multisystem disease (pulmonary, pancreatic, hepatobiliary) characterized by abnormalities in exocrine gland function. Large amounts of airway mucus secretion predispose to bacterial infection. Treatment is directed toward mechanical drainage of secretions and control of bacterial infections.

IV. RENAL SYSTEM (See Chapter 25)

A. **Acute renal failure** is most often related to surgery or trauma associated with ischemia.

1. **Prerenal causes** of acute renal failure result from hypovolemia, leading to decreased renal blood flow.

2. **Intrinsic renal causes** of acute renal failure include nephrotoxins (antibiotics, especially aminoglycosides, contrast media, volatile anesthetics), renal ischemia, and glomerulonephritis.

3. **Postrenal causes** of acute renal failure include obstruction to urine flow from calculi, clots, and tumor compression. Cystoscopy and retrograde pyelography are the diagnostic procedures.

B. **Oliguric versus nonoliguric acute renal failure** (see Chapter 25)

1. Oliguric renal failure (urine output <400 ml·day^{-1}) has a less favorable prognosis than nonoliguric renal failure.

2. Drugs that increase solute excretion (mannitol or furosemide, 2–10 mg·kg^{-1} iv) may have the capacity to convert oliguric to nonoliguric renal failure.

TABLE 43-10. Complications of Acute Renal Failure

Hyperkalemia	Anemia
Metabolic acidosis	Platelet abnormalities
Hyponatremia	Sepsis
Pulmonary edema	Gastrointestinal hemorrhage
Pericardial effusion	

   3. In acute oliguric renal failure, daily increases in blood urea nitrogen (BUN) and creatinine levels average 10–20 $mg \cdot dl^{-1}$ and 0.5–1.0 $mg \cdot dl^{-1}$, respectively.
C. **Urinary indices.** A chemical profile of the urine aids in assessing the cause of acute renal failure (see Table 25-10).
D. **Complications of acute renal failure** (Table 43-10)
E. **Treatment** of acute renal failure, after ruling out correctable causes, is determined by the predictable complications that occur. **Hemodialysis** is indicated for treatment of symptomatic uremia (BUN > 100 $mg \cdot dl^{-1}$, creatinine > 8 $mg \cdot dl^{-1}$), hyperkalemia, acidosis, or fluid overload that is not responsive to conservative therapy.

V. INFECTIOUS DISEASES

A. **Nosocomial infections.** Hospital-acquired infections are the leading cause of death in most ICUs. These infections are often polymicrobial, involve multiple resistant strains of bacteria, and do not respond to antibiotic therapy.
   1. Several factors determine the incidence and outcome of nosocomial infections (Table 43-11).
   2. Sources of nosocomial infections are multiple (Table 43-12).

TABLE 43-11. Factors in Nosocomial Infections

Patient's age
Underlying diseases
Integrity of mucosal and integumentary surfaces
Status of immunologic defenses (acquired immunodeficiency syndrome, organ transplants)

TABLE 43-12. Sources of Nosocomial Infections

Urinary tract infections (gram-negative bacteria)
Wound infections (usually evident 3–10 days postoperatively)
Pneumonia (gram-negative bacteria and *Staphylococcus aureus*)
Intravascular devices
Intra-abdominal infections
Sinusitis (nasotracheal intubation)
Central nervous system infection (meningitis, brain abscess)
Fungal infection (diffuse microabscesses)

    B. Sepsis syndrome (Table 43-13). Progression from the sepsis syndrome to septic shock may be prevented by early intervention.

    C. Septic shock. Gram-negative bacteremia is present in 40% of patients who develop septic shock, with mortality occurring in 40–90%. *Escherichia coli* is the most common causative organism. **Endotoxins** contribute to clinical manifestations of septic shock. **Treatment** must be prompt and aggressive (Tables 43-14 and 43-15).

VI. NUTRITION

Adequate nutrition is essential to replace the nutrients being used to meet the energy needs of tissues and to repair tissues being catabolized.

VII. DISORDERS OF COAGULATION

Disorders of coagulation manifest as bleeding or thrombosis (see Chapter 10).

TABLE 43-13. Clinical Features of the Sepsis Syndrome

Clinical evidence of infection
Hypothermia or hyperthermia
Impaired organ function or evidence of inadequate perfusion
    Altered mentation
    Arterial hypoxemia
    Elevated plasma lactate level
    Oliguria

TABLE 43-14. Manifestations of Septic Shock

Early Shock	Late Shock
Increased cardiac output	Decreased cardiac output
Vasodilation	Vasoconstriction
	Disseminated intravascular coagulation
	Adult respiratory distress syndrome
	Acute renal failure

TABLE 43-15. Treatment of Septic Shock

Antibiotic therapy (do not await results of blood cultures)
Fluid resuscitation
Inotropes (dopamine, dobutamine)
Human monoclonal immunoglobulin antibody (binds to lipid portion of endotoxin)

    A. **Laboratory tests** provide a **hemostatic profile** and include platelet count, bleeding time, prothrombin time, and partial thromboplastin time.
    B. Disorders of hemostasis in critically ill patients are generally complex and represent **multiple acquired deficiencies** (Table 43-16).

VIII. POISONING

In the absence of a documented ingestion, it is important to maintain a high index of suspicion of poisoning in patients who present with central nervous system disturbances, acute renal failure, hepatic insufficiency, or bone marrow depression.

TABLE 43-16. Causes of Bleeding Disorders

Disseminated intravascular coagulation
Liver disease
Vitamin K deficiency
Anticoagulants
Massive blood transfusion

A. **Idenfication of the poison** requires analysis of gastric fluid, urine, and blood. Multiple drugs may be involved.

B. **Treatment** is supportive (cardiopulmonary resuscitation) and symptomatic (coma, acute renal failure, hepatic failure). In addition, attempts to reduce drug absorption (lavage, emetics, adsorbents) and to accelerate excretion (diuresis, dialysis, chelation) should be considered.

C. **Common poisons**

1. **Acetaminophen.** Hepatotoxicity is lessened by early administration of N-acetylcystine.

2. **Alcohols**

   a. **Ethanol.** Support of ventilation is usually sufficient.

   b. **Methanol and ethylene glycol.** Metabolites produce ocular and renal toxicity. Treatment is systemic alkalization followed by hemodialysis.

3. **Carbon monoxide** is the major cause of death in patients suffering smoke inhalation from fires. Hemoglobin has an affinity for carbon monoxide (carboxyhemoglobin) that is 200 times greater than for oxygen, resulting in profound tissue hypoxia (seizures, coma, death). Classic cherry-red color of the skin and mucous membranes is produced by the bright red cast of carboxyhemoglobin. Treatment is hyperventilation of the lungs with oxygen (shortens elimination half-time from 4 hours to 40 minutes), management of cerebral edema, and possibly hyperbaric oxygen.

IX. LEGAL AND ETHICAL ISSUES

A. **Brain death** is defined as irreversible cessation of all functions of the entire brain, including the brain stem. Brain death typically occurs when ICP exceeds systolic blood pressure within 12–24 hours of injury. There must be no evidence of hypothermia or depressant drugs (see Chapter 19).

B. **Do not resuscitate (DNR) orders** are controversial but are generally guided by the principle that resuscitation would not be "a treatment offering hope of restoration to normal integrated functioning cognitive existence."

44

Cardiopulmonary Resuscitation

Cardiopulmonary resuscitation (CPR) includes basic life support, advanced cardiac life support, and postresuscitation life support (Schwartz AJ, Campbell FW: Cardiopulmonary resuscitation. In: Barash PG, Cullen BF, Stoelting RK [eds]: Clinical Anesthesia, pp 1633–1672. Philadelphia, JB Lippincott, 1992). The professional responsibilities of an anesthesiologist include CPR. **See Appendix E for protocols.**

I. BASIC LIFE SUPPORT (EMERGENCY OXYGENATION)

The temporary delivery of oxygen to vital tissues is accomplished by providing effective airway management, ventilation, and artificial circulation (see Appendix E).

A. Airway Management During Cardiopulmonary Resuscitation

1. **Obstruction of the hypopharynx by the base of the tongue** (muscles supporting the tongue relax) is the most common cause of airway obstruction in unconscious patients (see Chapter 5). The cardinal principle for opening an obstructed upper airway is anterior displacement of the mandible (head-tilt-jaw-thrust), which pulls the tongue away from the posterior pharyngeal wall. The jaw thrust without head tilt is the preferred method for opening the airway in a patient with a suspected cervical spine injury.

B. Adjuncts for Artificial Ventilation

1. When airway obstruction persists despite maximal mandibular displacement, insertion of an oropharyngeal airway (not tolerated by responsive patients and may induce vomiting) or nasopharyngeal airway is a consideration.

2. **Tracheal intubation** is usually attempted only after oxygenation has been achieved by bag-and-mask ventilation.

C. Treatment of Airway Obstruction Due to Foreign Body
(see Appendix E)
   1. **Direct laryngoscopy** and instrumentation of the airway to extract the obstructing body may be useful.
   2. **Cricothyrotomy and Transtracheal Ventilation** (see description on inside front cover).
D. Artificial Ventilation
   1. Mouth-to-mask ventilation is being substituted for mouth-to-mouth techniques, reflecting increased concern about transmission of infection between patient and rescuer.
      a. Exhaled air ventilation provides an F_{IO_2} of 0.15–0.18. P_{AO_2} is <80 mm Hg and P_{aO_2} is even lower because of the effect of reduced cardiac output and increased venous admixture during CPR. Mild hypercarbia (P_{aCO_2} about 55 mm Hg) is also likely to be present.
      b. Because hypoxemia and hypercarbia occur during exhaled air ventilation, the use of ventilating devices that provide supplemental oxygen and allow increased alveolar ventilation should be instituted as soon as available (manually powered ventilators, oxygen-powered ventilators).
E. Artificial Circulation
   1. **External chest compression.** An absent **carotid** or **femoral artery pulse** (these persist when peripheral pulses are no longer palpable because of vasoconstriction) is an indication to initiate artificial circulation by external chest compressions. The sternum of an adult must be depressed 4–5 cm by the heel of a rescuer's hand placed over the lower half of the sternum. A rescuer's shoulders should be directly over his or her hands, with elbows locked so that the vector of compression force is applied straight downward onto the sternum. A compression duration equal to 50–60% of the cycle length at 80–100 compressions-min^{-1} (more rapid in infants) produces maximum pressure and flow.
      a. A rescuer must release the pressure completely during the relaxation phase to allow the heart to fill, but the hand must not lose contact with the sternum so that correct hand position is maintained.
      b. Blood flow provided by external compressions will temporarily sustain cerebral and cardiac viability only if oxygenation is effective. Nevertheless, cerebral blood flow is probably less than one-third normal, and coronary blood flow may

be even lower (low diastolic blood pressure) during external compressions.

2. **Mechanisms of blood flow** during external chest compressions are controversial. The development of modifications in technique to improve oxygen delivery during external compressions depends on the predominant mechanisms that produce blood flow.

   a. **Cardiac pump theory.** External chest compression squeezes the heart between the sternum and spine to force blood into the aorta. Blood flow depends on the rate of compression.

   b. **Thoracic pump theory.** Phasic changes in intrathoracic pressure result in venous inflow into the thorax and forward blood flow into the aorta. A prolonged compression time (50–60% of cycle time) favors flow produced by changes in intrathoracic pressure.

3. Survival from CPR is directly related to coronary perfusion pressure produced during chest compressions.

4. Measurement of the exhaled carbon dioxide concentration (PET_{CO_2}) provides an index of cardiac output and allows prediction of outcome. In patients, a PET_{CO_2} <10–15 mm Hg during closed chest compressions and ventilation *via* a tracheal tube points to a poor prognosis.

II. DRUG THERAPY DURING ARTIFICIAL CIRCULATION (Table 44-1)

A. Initial drug therapy is intended to correct arterial hypoxemia and elevate cerebral and coronary perfusion pressures **(epinephrine).** Sodium bicarbonate is no longer recommended as an initial drug to correct the metabolic acidosis that invariably accompanies cardiac arrest. Alveolar ventilation corrects acidosis by removing carbon dioxide without the side effects inherent in sodium bicarbonate administration (Table 44-2).

B. Once spontaneous circulation has been achieved, drugs with specific actions on heart rate, cardiac rhythm, cardiac contractility, and systemic vascular resistance may be used to provide a stable cardiac output and blood pressure.

III. ADVANCED CARDIAC LIFE SUPPORT (see Appendix E)

A. **Recognition of dysrhythmias**
   1. **Sudden death** frequently results from cardiac dys-

TABLE 44-1. Drug Therapy During Cardiopulmonary Resuscitation

Drug	Indications	Dose
Oxygen	Hypoxemia	100%
Epinephrine	Ventricular fibrillation	5–10 $\mu g \cdot kg^{-1}$ iv
	Asystole	1 mg in 10 ml in TT*
	Electromechanical dissociation	
Sodium bicarbonate	Not recommended except in selected patients	0.5 $mEq \cdot kg^{-1}$ iv every 10 minutes of continued resuscitation or by pH measurement
Lidocaine	Recurrent ventricular fibrillation or ventricular tachycardia	1 $mg \cdot kg^{-1}$ iv or TT* 1–4 $mg \cdot min^{-1}$ iv (adult)
Bretylium	When lidocaine not effective	5 $mg \cdot kg^{-1}$ iv every 5 minutes not to exceed 30 $mg \cdot kg^{-1}$
Atropine	Bradycardia	70 $\mu g \cdot kg^{-1}$ iv or TT*
	Heart block	
	Asystole	1 mg iv or TT*
Isoproterenol	When atropine not effective	2–20 $\mu g \cdot min^{-1}$ (adult)
Verapamil	Paroxysmal atrial tachycardia	70 $\mu g \cdot kg^{-1}$ iv
Calcium (Ca^{2+})	Not recommended	

*TT = tracheal tube.

TABLE 44-2. Adverse Effects of Sodium Bicarbonate

Leftward shift of the oxyhemoglobin dissociation curve
Hypernatremia
Hyperosmolarity
Paradoxical acidosis due to carbon dioxide production
Extracellular alkalosis
Possible inactivation of simultaneously administered
  catecholamines

rhythmias, especially in the presence of myocardial ischemia. ECG monitoring must be instituted early in CPR.

    2. Synchronized cardioversion is the indicated treatment for hemodynamically significant tachydysrhythmias. The cardioversion dose is 75–100 joules.

B. External defibrillation is applied as soon as possible in the treatment of ventricular fibrillation. Asystole is not responsive to external defibrillation.

    1. The defibrillator delivers an electrical current that uniformly **depolarizes the entire myocardium,** which subsequently repolarizes in a coordinated fashion with a supraventricular pacemaker.

    2. Initial adult dose is 200–300 joules followed by a repeat dose if ventricular fibrillation persists. A third dose of 360 joules is administered if the prior two doses are not successful. The initial pediatric dose is 2 joules·kg^{-1}. Excessive doses may produce myocardial damage and postshock cardiac dysrhythmias.

C. Intravenous Therapy During Cardiopulmonary Resuscitation

    1. Central (internal jugular, subclavian, femoral) venous catheters provide a more rapid onset of drug effect compared with administration through a peripheral catheter.

    2. Administration of drugs (epinephrine, atropine, lidocaine) into the **tracheal tube lumen** allows prompt absorption across the tracheal mucosa and serves as an alternative to intravenous injection. Intracardiac administration of epinephrine is rarely indicated.

D. Invasive therapeutic techniques during cardiopulmonary resuscitation. Cardiac pacing (myocardial infarction with heart block), pericardiocentesis, and treatment of tension pneumothorax may be lifesaving during CPR.

TABLE 44-3. Causes of Electromechanical Dissociation
Extensive myocardial damage
Impaired venous return
Cardiac tamponade
Tension pneumothorax
Pulmonary embolism
Hypovolemia
Volatile anesthetic overdose

1. **Cardiac pacing** is most effectively provided by the central venous placement of a pacing electrode (pacing pulmonary artery catheter) attached to an external pulse generator (settings for amperage, heart rate, and synchronous vs. asynchronous pacing). For treatment of heart block, the pacing electrode must be in the right ventricle.
2. **Pericardiocentesis** is performed by **subxiphoid insertion** of a spinal needle guided by attachment to and monitoring of the ECG.
3. **Tension pneumothorax** (compromises ventilation and venous return) is relieved by insertion of a needle into the **second or third intercostal space.** Insertion of the needle at the **midclavicular line** and no further medially avoids the internal mammary artery. Intercostal artery puncture is unlikely if the needle is passed **over the top of the rib.**

E. **Electromechanical dissociation** is recognized by an organized electrocardiographic pattern in the absence of a pulse. Causes of electromechanical dissociation are often life-threatening unless prompt intervention restores cardiac output (Table 44-3).

IV. SPECIAL SITUATIONS IN CARDIOPULMONARY RESUSCITATION (Table 44-4)

V. POSTRESUSCITATION LIFE SUPPORT

A. All patients resuscitated from cardiopulmonary arrest are placed in an intensive care environment where an evaluation is initiated to determine the degree of cerebral, cardiovascular, pulmonary, and renal damage that may have occurred as well as the underlying mechanism of the cardiopulmonary arrest (myocardial infarction may require thrombolytic therapy).

TABLE 44-4. Special Situations in Cardiopulmonary Resuscitation

Cause of Arrest	Pathophysiology	Treatment
Trauma	Irreversible—massive head trauma and visceral injury Reversible—hemorrhage, tension pneumothorax, cardiac tamponade Associated injuries—cervical spine, hypothermia	Cervical spine precautions for airway opening Rapid survey of reversible causes and specific treatment Restore blood volume
Exsanguination	Loss of cerebral and coronary perfusion External chest compression in absence of venous return	Control hemorrhage Restore blood volume
Electrocution	Apnea leading to hypoxemia Asystole or ventricular fibrillation Burns Skeletal muscle destruction and myoglobinuria	Artificial ventilation and circulation
Near-drowning	Asphyxiation leading to hypoxemia Gastric distention Pulmonary edema Hypothermia	Artificial ventilation and circulation
Hypothermia	Bradycardia Asystole or ventricular fibrillation Metabolic acidosis Diuresis	Electrocardiographic monitoring Core warming Cardiac pacing
Carbon monoxide poisoning	Decreased oxygen-carrying capacity of blood Seizures	Artificial ventilation with oxygen

B. **Postresuscitation Care for Ischemic-Anoxic Cerebral Injury**

   1. Cerebral injury is the result of the primary ischemic **insult** and **secondary postischemic changes** that begin with reperfusion and reoxygenation.

   2. Cessation of cerebral circulation owing to cardiac arrest results in depletion of oxygen stores and unconsciousness in 15 seconds. When oxygen is depleted, anaerobic glycolysis continues as long as glucose is available (about 4 minutes), resulting in lactate production and intracellular acidosis.

      a. Lactate production is greater and intracellular pH is lower if hyperglycemia is present at the time of cardiac arrest.

      b. The energy-dependent cell membrane ion pump fails, resulting in influx of Na^+ and Ca^{2+}, with the development of intracellular edema.

      c. It is unknown when irreversible cerebral injury occurs. This may be influenced by the body temperature and blood glucose level present at the time of the cardiac arrest. Histologic changes occur after 5–7 minutes. Ischemic anoxia sufficient to disrupt the blood-brain barrier requires 30–60 minutes.

   3. Restoration of cerebral blood flow after more than 5–10 minutes of circulatory arrest leads to secondary brain changes characterized by **regional hypoperfusion.** This nonhomogeneous restoration of cerebral blood flow may reflect vascular obstruction by edematous cells, aggregates of red blood cells, or vasospasm.

   4. With the occurrence of cerebral ischemia, there is **loss of autoregulation of cerebral blood flow.**

   5. Intracranial compliance may be reduced by cerebral edema, although intracranial pressure usually remains near normal unless the ischemic result is severe or of long duration. Increases in intracranial pressure sufficient to interfere with cerebral blood flow are more likely to occur after head injury or inflammatory insults.

   6. Postresuscitation management is aimed at optimizing cerebral blood flow and controlling cerebral metabolic requirements for oxygen (Table 44-5).

      a. There is no evidence that **barbiturates** improve neurologic outcome when administered after global cerebral ischemia.

      b. There is no evidence that **hypothermia** improves neurologic outcome when induced after global cerebral ischemia.

TABLE 44-5. **Goals for Optimizing Cerebral Blood Flow and Cerebral Metabolic Oxygen Requirements**

Normotension
Moderate hyperventilation ($Paco_2$ 25–35 mm Hg)
Normothermia
Maintain normal intracranial pressure (barbiturates, diuretics, corticosteroids)
Suppress seizures

      c. It is uncertain whether glucose-containing solutions should be avoided after successful CPR.

VI. MEDICOLEGAL CONSIDERATIONS

    A. Decisions to begin or end CPR must consider cardiac and brain function and responsiveness to therapy.
    B. A prospective diagnosis of irreversible brain damage is almost impossible to make.
    C. CPR is often begun to evaluate cardiovascular responsiveness. Often it is only by a trial of CPR that the heart can be diagnosed as irreversibly damaged and unresponsive to further therapy.

VI

APPENDIXES

A

Formulas

HEMODYNAMIC FORMULAS

Hemodynamic Variables: Calculations and Normal Values

Variable	Calculation	Normal Values
Cardiac index (CI)	CO/BSA	$2.5-4.0 \ l \cdot min^{-1} \cdot m^{-2}$
Stroke volume (SV)	CO × 1000/HR	$60-90 \ ml \cdot beat^{-1}$
Stroke index (SI)	SV/BSA	$40-60 \ ml \cdot beat^{-1} \cdot m^{-2}$
Mean arterial pressure (MAP)	Diastolic pressure + ⅓ pulse pressure	80–120 mm Hg
Systemic vascular resistance (SVR)	$\dfrac{MAP - CVP}{CO} \times 79.9$	$1200-1500 \ dynes \cdot cm \cdot sec^{-5}$
Pulmonary vascular resistance (PVR)	$\dfrac{\overline{PAP} - \overline{PCWP}}{CO} \times 79.9$	$100-300 \ dynes \cdot cm \cdot sec^{-5}$
Right ventricular stroke work index (RVSWI)	$0.0136 \, (\overline{PAP} - \overline{CVP}) \times SI$	$5-9 \ g \cdot m \cdot beat^{-1} \cdot m^{-2}$
Left ventricular stroke work index (LVSWI)	$0.0136 \, (MAP - PCWP) \times SI$	$45-60 \ g \cdot m \cdot beat^{-1} \cdot m^{-2}$

HR = heart rate; CVP = mean central venous pressure; BSA = body surface area; CO = cardiac output; $\overline{PAP}$ = mean pulmonary artery pressure; $\overline{PCWP}$ = pulmonary capillary wedge pressure; MAP = mean arterial blood pressure.

RESPIRATORY FORMULAS

	Normal Values (70 kg)
Alveolar oxygen tension $PAO_2 = (P_B - 47) FIO_2 - PACO_2$	110 mm Hg ($FIO_2 = 0.21$)
Alveolar-arterial oxygen gradient $A-aO_2 = PAO_2 - PaO_2$	<10 mm Hg ($FIO_2 = 0.21$)
Arterial-to-alveolar oxygen ratio, a/A ratio	>0.75
Arterial oxygen content $CaO_2 = (SaO_2) (Hb \times 1.34) + PaO_2 (0.0031)$	21 ml $\cdot$ 100 ml^{-1}
Mixed venous oxygen content $C\bar{v}O_2 = (S\bar{v}O_2) (Hb \times 1.34) + P\bar{v}O_2 (0.0031)$	15 ml $\cdot$ 100 ml^{-1}
Arterial-venous oxygen content difference $a-v \; O_2 = CaO_2 - C\bar{v}O_2$	4–6 ml $\cdot$ 100 ml^{-1}
Intrapulmonary shunt $\dot{Q}s/\dot{Q}_T = (CcO_2 - CaO_2)/(CcO_2 - C\bar{v}O_2)$ $CcO_2 = (Hb \times 1.34) + (PAO_2 \times 0.0031)$	<5%
Physiologic dead space $V_D/V_T = (PaCO_2 - P_{ECO_2})/PaCO_2$	0.33
Oxygen consumption $\dot{V}O_2 = CO \, (CaO_2 - C\bar{v}O_2)$	240 ml $\cdot$ min^{-1}
Oxygen transport $O_2T = CO \, (CaO_2)$	1000 ml $\cdot$ min^{-1}

Abbreviations:

CaO_2	Arterial oxygen content
$C\bar{v}O_2$	Mixed venous oxygen content
CcO_2	Pulmonary capillary oxygen content
CO	Cardiac output
FIO_2	Fraction inspired oxygen
O_2T	Oxygen transport
P_B	Barometric pressure
$\dot{Q}s/\dot{Q}_T$	Intrapulmonary shunt
$PACO_2$	Alveolar carbon dioxide tension
$PaCO_2$	Arterial carbon dioxide tension
PAO_2	Alveolar oxygen tension
PaO_2	Arterial oxygen tension
P_{ECO_2}	Expired carbon dioxide tension
V_D	Dead space gas volume
V_T	Tidal volume
$\dot{V}O_2$	Oxygen consumption (minute)

LUNG VOLUMES AND CAPACITIES

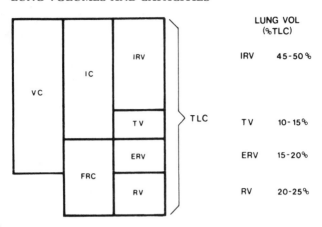

LUNG VOL
(%TLC)

IRV	45-50%
TV	10-15%
ERV	15-20%
RV	20-25%

		Normal Values (70 kg)
Vital capacity	VC	4800 ml
Inspiratory capacity	IC	3800 ml
Functional residual capacity	FRC	2400 ml
Inspiratory reserve volume	IRV	3500 ml
Tidal volume	TV	500 ml
Expiratory reserve volume	ERV	1200 ml
Residual volume	RV	1200 ml
Total lung capacity	TLC	6000 ml

Electrocardiography Atlas

LEAD PLACEMENT

	Electrode	
Bipolar leads	Positive	Negative
I	LA	RA
II	LL	RA
III	LL	LA
Augmented unipolar		
aVR	RA	LA, LL
aVL	LA	RA, LL
aVF	LL	RA, LA
Precordial	Position	
V_1	4 ICS–RSB	
V_2	4 ICS–LSB	
V_3	Midway between V_2 and V_4	
V_4	5 ICS–MCL	
V_5	5 ICS–AAL	
V_6	5 ICS–MAL	

We wish to thank Dr. Malcom S. Thaler for graciously permitting reproduction of electrocardiographic tracings from his book, The Only EKG Book You'll Ever Need, JB Lippincott, Philadelphia, 1988.

THREE-LEAD SYSTEMS

MCL = Modified central lead
CB = Central back
CS = Central subclavian

Bipolar Lead System	Electrode Placement	*ECG Lead	Advantage
II	RA R—clavicle LA L—10th rib (Midclavicular line) LL Ground	II (II)	Dysrhythmias
MCL 1	RA Ground LA L—clavicle LL V_1	III (V_1)	Dysrhythmias and conduction defects
CS 5	RA R—clavicle LA V_5 LL Ground	I (V_5)	Precordial ischemia
CB 5	RA R—scapula LA V_5 LL Ground	I (V_5)	Precordial ischemia and dysrhythmias

*Selected lead on monitor: ( ) = simulated ECG lead.

PACEMAKER DESIGNATIONS

1 Chamber paced	2 Chamber sensed	3 Response	4 Programmability	5 Antitachycardia function
<u>A</u>trium	<u>A</u>trium	<u>I</u>nhibit	<u>P</u>rogrammable (rate/output)	<u>B</u>ursts
<u>V</u>entricle	<u>V</u>entricle	<u>T</u>rigger	<u>M</u>ultiprogrammable	<u>N</u>ormal rate
				<u>C</u>ompetition
<u>D</u>ouble (A/V)	<u>D</u>ouble	<u>D</u>ouble	<u>C</u>ommunicating	<u>S</u>canning
	<u>O</u>/None	<u>O</u>/None <u>R</u>everse	<u>O</u>/None	<u>E</u>xternal

Note: The original pacemaker designation used a three-position code. Subsequently, expanded positions were added (4, 5). For example, the presence of atrial fibrillation may require a pacemaker with the code **VVI**. This designation indicates (1) <u>V</u>entricle is sensed, (2) <u>V</u>entricle is paced and the pacemaker is (3) <u>I</u>nhibited if a cardiac event is sensed.

THE NORMAL ELECTROCARDIOGRAM—
CARDIAC CYCLE

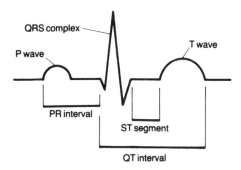

In this section the ECG complex is divided into the atrial (PR interval) and ventricular (QT interval) components.

ASHMAN BEATS

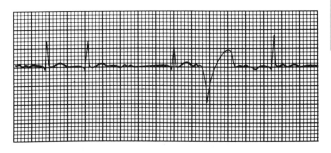

Rate: Variable.
Rhythm: Irregular.
PR interval: P wave may be present if supraventricular premature beat.
QT interval: QRS prolonged (>0.12 second) and altered, revealing bundle-branch pattern, most commonly right bundle. ST segment abnormal.

Note: Ashman beats are often confused with ventricular premature contractions. Ashman beats, usually seen with atrial fibrillation, have no compensatory pause and are a benign ECG finding requiring no treatment.

ATRIAL FIBRILLATION

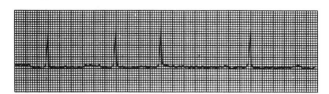

Rate: Variable (~150–200 bpm).
Rhythm: Irregular.
PR interval: No P wave, and PR interval not discernible.
QT interval: QRS normal.

Note: Must be differentiated from atrial flutter: (1) absence of flutter waves and presence of fibrillatory line; (2) flutter usually associated with higher ventricular rates (>150 bpm). Loss of atrial contraction reduces cardiac output (10–20%). Mural atrial thrombi may develop. Considered controlled if ventricular rate <100 bpm.

ATRIAL FLUTTER

carotid massage begins

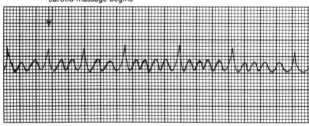

Rate: Rapid, atrial usually regular (250–350 bpm); ventricular usually regular (<100 bpm).
Rhythm: Atrial and ventricular regular.
PR interval: Flutter (F) waves are saw-toothed. PR interval cannot be measured.
QT interval: QRS usually normal; ST segment and T waves are not identifiable.

Note: Carotid massage will slow ventricular response, simplifying recognition of the F waves.

ATRIOVENTRICULAR BLOCK (First-Degree)

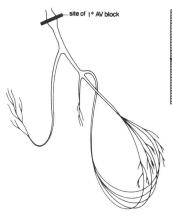

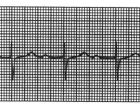

Rate: 60–100 bpm.
Rhythm: Regular.
PR interval: Prolonged (>0.20 second) and constant.
QT interval: Normal.

Note: Usually clinically insignificant; may be early harbinger of drug toxicity.

ATRIOVENTRICULAR BLOCK (Second-Degree), Mobitz Type I/Wenckebach Block

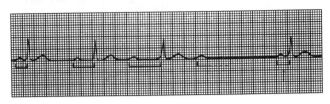

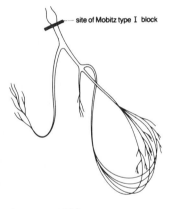

site of Mobitz type I block

Rate: 60–100 bpm.

Rhythm: Atrial regular; ventricular irregular.

PR interval: P wave normal; PR interval progressively lengthens with each cycle until QRS complex is dropped (dropped beat). PR interval following dropped beat is shorter than normal.

QT interval: QRS complex normal but dropped periodically

Note: Commonly seen (1) in trained athletes, and (2) with drug toxicity.

ATRIOVENTRICULAR BLOCK (Second-Degree), Mobitz Type II

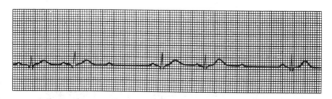

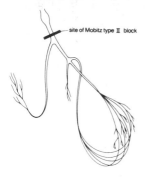

site of Mobitz type II block

Rate: <100 bpm

Rhythm: Atrial regular; ventricular regular or irregular.

PR interval: P waves normal, but some are not followed by QRS complex.

QT interval: Normal, but may have widened QRS complex if block is at level of bundle branch. ST segment and T wave may be abnormal, depending on location of block.

Note: In contrast to Mobitz type I block, the PR and RR intervals are constant and the dropped QRS occurs without warning. The wider the QRS complex (block lower in the conduction system), the greater the amount of myocardial damage.

ATRIOVENTRICULAR BLOCK (Third-Degree), Complete Heart Block

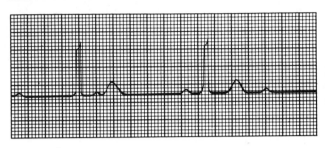

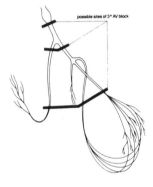

possible sites of 3° AV block

Rate: <45 bpm.

Rhythm: Atrial regular; ventricular regular; no relationship between P wave and QRS complex.

PR interval: Variable because atria and ventricles beat independently.

QT interval: QRS morphology variable, depending on the origin of the ventricular beat in the intrinsic pacemaker system (atrioventricular junctional versus ventricular pacemaker). ST segment and T wave normal.

Note: Immediate treatment with atropine or isoproterenol is required if cardiac output is reduced. Consideration should be given to insertion of a pacemaker. Seen as a complication of mitral valve replacement.

ATRIOVENTRICULAR DISSOCIATION

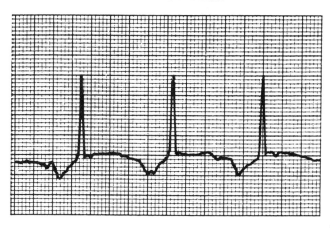

Rate: Variable.

Rhythm: Atrial regular; ventricular regular; ventricular rate faster than atrial rate; no relationship between P wave and QRS complex.

PR interval: Variable because atria and ventricles beat independently.

QT interval: QRS morphology depends on location of ventricular pacemaker. ST segment and T wave abnormal.

Note: Digitalis toxicity can present as atrioventricular dissociation.

BUNDLE-BRANCH BLOCK—LEFT (LBBB)

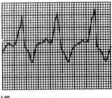

V6

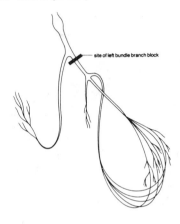

site of left bundle branch block

Rate: <100 bpm.
Rhythm: Regular.
PR interval: Normal.
QT interval: Complete LBBB (QRS > 0.12 second); incomplete LBBB (QRS = 0.10–0.12 second). Lead V_1 negative rS complex; I, aVL, V_6 wide R wave without Q or S component. ST segment and T wave defection opposite direction of the R wave.

Note: LBBB does not occur in healthy patients and usually indicates serious heart disease with a poorer prognosis. In patients with LBBB, insertion of a pulmonary artery catheter may lead to complete heart block.

BUNDLE-BRANCH BLOCK—RIGHT (RBBB)

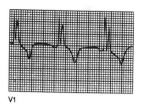

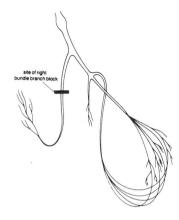

site of right
bundle branch block

V1

Rate: <100 bpm.
Rhythm: Regular.
PR interval: Normal.
QT interval: Complete RBBB (QRS > 0.12 second); incomplete RBBB (QRS 0.10–0.12 second). Varying patterns of QRS complex: rSR (V$_1$); RS, wide R with M pattern. ST segment and T wave opposite direction of the R wave.

Note: In the presence of RBBB, Q waves may be seen with a myocardial infarction.

ELECTROLYTE DISTURBANCES

	↓ Ca^{2+}	↑ Ca^{2+}	↓ K^+	↑ K^+
Rate:	<100 bpm	<100 bpm	<100 bpm	<100 bpm
Rhythm:	regular	regular	regular	regular
PR interval:	normal	normal/increased	normal	normal
QT interval:	increased	decreased	T flat	T peaked
			U wave	QT decreased

Note: ECG changes usually do not correlate with serum calcium. Hypocalcemia rarely causes dysrhythmias in the absence of hypokalemia. In contrast, abnormalities in serum potassium concentration can be diagnosed by ECG.

DIGITALIS EFFECT

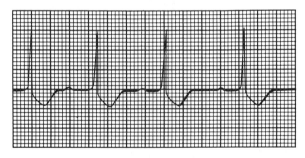

Rate: <100 bpm.
Rhythm: Regular.
PR interval: Normal or prolonged.
QT interval: ST segment sloping ("digitalis effect").

Notes: Digitalis toxicity can be the cause of many common dysrhythmias (e.g., premature ventricular contractions, second-degree heart block). Verapamil, quinidine, and amiodarone cause an increase in serum digitalis concentration.

CORONARY ARTERY DISEASE—Ischemia

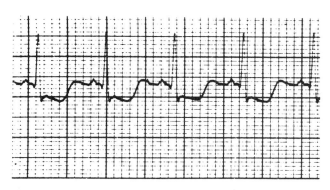

Rate: Variable.

Rhythm: Usually regular, but may show atrial and/or ventricular dysrhythmias.

PR interval: Normal.

QT interval: ST segment depressed; J point depression; T-wave inversion; conduction disturbances. Coronary vasospasm (Prinzmetal) ST segment elevation.

Note: Intraoperative ischemia is usually seen in the presence of "normal" vital signs (e.g., ±20% of preinduction values).

CORONARY ARTERY DISEASE—Myocardial Infarction

Anatomic Site	Leads	ECG Changes	Coronary Artery
Inferior	II, III, aVF	Q, ST, T	Right
Lateral	I, aVL, V_5–V_6	Q, ST, T	Left circumflex
Anterior	I, aVL, V_1–V_4	Q, ST, T	Left
Anteroseptal	V_1–V_4	Q, ST, T	Left anterior descending

SUBENDOCARDIAL MYOCARDIAL INFARCTION (SEMI)

Persistent ST segment depression and/or T-wave inversion in the absence of Q wave. Usually requires additional laboratory data (e.g., isoenzymes) to confirm diagnosis.

TRANSMURAL MYOCARDIAL INFARCTION (TMI)

Q waves seen on ECG useful in confirming diagnosis. Associated with poorer prognosis and more significant hemodynamic impairment; dysrhythmias frequently complicate course.

PAROXYSMAL ATRIAL TACHYCARDIA (PAT)

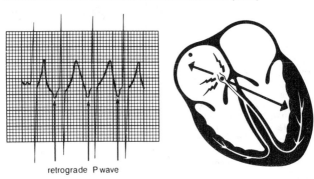

retrograde P wave

Rate: 150–250 bpm.

Rhythm: Regular.

PR interval: Difficult to distinguish because of tachycardia obscuring P wave. P wave may precede, be included in, or follow QRS complex.

QT interval: Normal, but ST segment and T wave may be difficult to distinguish.

Note: Therapy depends on degree of hemodynamic compromise. In contrast to management of PAT in awake patients, synchronized cardioversion rather than pharmacologic treatment is preferred in hemodynamically unstable anesthetized patients.

PREMATURE ATRIAL CONTRACTION (PAC)

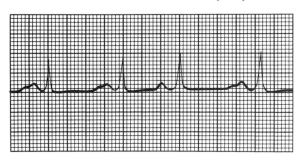

Rate: <100 bpm.
Rhythm: Irregular.
PR interval: P waves may be lost in preceding T waves. PR interval is variable.
QT interval: QRS normal configuration; ST segment and T wave normal.

Note: Nonconducted PAC appearance similar to that of sinus arrest; T waves with PAC may be distorted by inclusion of P wave in the T wave.

PREMATURE VENTRICULAR CONTRACTION (PVC)

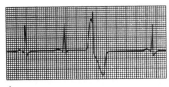

A

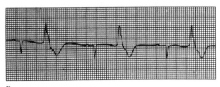

B

Rate: Usually <100 bpm.

Rhythm: Irregular.

PR interval: P wave and PR interval absent; retrograde conduction of P wave can be seen.

QT interval: Wide QRS (> 0.12 second); ST segment cannot be evaluated (e.g., ischemia); T wave opposite direction of QRS with compensatory pause (A). Bigeminy: every other beat a PVC (B); trigeminy: every third beat a PVC. R-on-T occurs when PVC falls in the T wave and can lead to ventricular tachycardia or fibrillation.

Note: If compensatory pause is not seen following an ectopic beat, the complex is most likely supraventricular in origin.

SINUS TACHYCARDIA

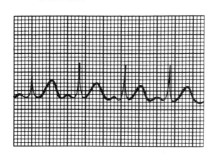

Rate: 100–160 bpm.
Rhythm: Regular.
PR interval: Normal; P wave may be difficult to see.
QT interval: Normal.

Note: Should be differentiated from paroxysmal atrial tachycardia (PAT). With PAT, carotid massage terminates dysrhythmia. Sinus tachycardia may respond to vagal maneuvers but reappears as soon as vagal stimulus removed.

VENTRICULAR FIBRILLATION

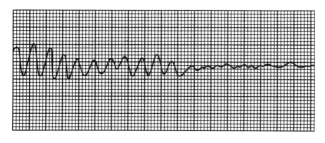

Rate: Absent.
Rhythm: None.
PR interval: Absent.
QT interval: Absent.

Note: "Pseudoventricular fibrillation" may be the result of a monitor malfunction (e.g., ECG lead disconnect). Always check for carotid pulse before instituting therapy.

VENTRICULAR TACHYCARDIA

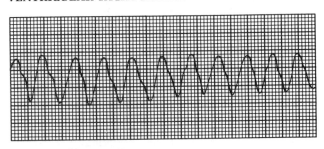

Rate: 100–250 bpm.
Rhythm: No atrial component seen; ventricular rhythm irregular or regular.
PR interval: Absent; retrograde P wave may be seen in QRS complex.
QT interval: Wide, bizarre QRS complex. ST segment and T wave difficult to determine.

Note: In the presence of hemodynamic compromise, immediate DC nonsynchronized cardioversion is required. If the patient is stable, with short bursts of ventricular tachycardia, pharmacologic management is preferred. Should be differentiated from supraventricular tachycardia with aberrancy (SVT-A). Compensatory pause and atrioventricular dissociation suggest a PVC. P waves and SR' (V_1) and slowing to vagal stimulus suggest SVT-A.

WOLFF-PARKINSON-WHITE SYNDROME (WPW)

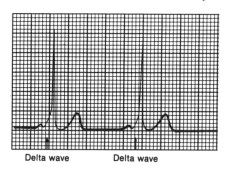

Delta wave   Delta wave

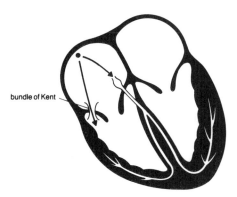

bundle of Kent

Rate: <100 bpm.
Rhythm: Regular.
PR interval: P wave normal; PR interval short (<0.12 second).
QT interval: Duration (> 0.10 second) with slurred QRS complex. Type A has delta wave, RBBB, with upright QRS complex V_1. Type B has delta wave and downward QRS-V_1. ST segment and T wave usually normal.

Note: Digoxin should be avoided in the presence of WPW because it increases conduction through the accessory bypass tract (bundle of Kent) and decreases atrioventricular node conduction; consequently, ventricular fibrillation can occur.

C

Drug List

Adenosine (Adenocard)
    Use(s): antidysrhythmic (paroxysmal supraventricular tachycardia)
    Dose: (iv) 6 mg
    Site of clearance: enzymatic
    Interaction/toxicity: Transient dysrhythmias seen prior to conversion to sinus rhythm. Excessive doses may cause significant hypotension, shortness of breath, and flushing. Adenosine does not convert atrial flutter/atrial fibrillation/ventricular tachycardia to a sinus rhythm but may be used to distinguish diagnostically between paroxysmal supraventricular tachycardia and other tachycardias.

Alfentanil (Alfenta)
    Uses: analgesia
    Dose: (iv) 8–50 $\mu g \cdot kg^{-1}$; induction, 130–245 $\mu g \cdot kg^{-1}$; maintenance 1 $\mu g \cdot kg^{-1} \cdot min^{-1}$
    Site of clearance: hepatic
    Interaction/toxicity: Diazepam potentiates hypotensive action; truncal muscle rigidity may be seen during induction and emergence. Erythromycin delays clearance.

Alprostadil (Prostin)
  Uses: maintains patency of patent ductus arteriosus
  Dose: (iv) 0.1 $\mu g \cdot kg^{-1} \cdot min^{-1}$
  Site of clearance: pulmonary
  Interaction/toxicity: In premature newborns produces apnea
    at higher doses.

Aminocaproic acid (Amicar)
  Uses: inhibits fibrinolysis
  Dose: (iv) infusion 5 g in 250 ml normal saline (NS) first
    hour; then 1.0–1.25 $g \cdot h^{-1}$
  Site of clearance: renal
  Interaction/toxicity: Contraindicated for disseminated
    intravascular coagulation, increased serum potassium
    (impaired renal function).

Aminophylline (various)
  Uses: bronchodilator
  Dose: loading: (iv) 6 $mg \cdot kg^{-1}$ (dilute in 100 ml D5W or NS);
    do not exceed 25 $mg \cdot min^{-1}$ (each 0.6 $mg \cdot kg^{-1}$ increases
    serum theophylline level 1 $\mu g \cdot ml^{-1}$). Maintenance 0.5–1.0
    $mg \cdot kg^{-1} \cdot h^{-1}$ (adjust dose based on serum level)
  Site of clearance: hepatic
  Interaction/toxicity: Increases effects of sympathomimetics,
    digitalis, oral anticoagulants; decreases effects of
    phenytoin, lithium, nondepolarizing muscle relaxants;
    Phenobarbital increases aminophylline metabolism.
    Antagonizes beta blockers; toxicity with halothane
    (dysrhythmias) and ketamine (seizures).

Amiodarone (Cordarone)
  Uses: antidysrhythmic
  Dose: (po) loading dose, 800–1600 mg; maintenance, 400 mg
  Site of clearance: hepatic
  Interaction/toxicity: Increases serum levels of digoxin,
    quinidine, procainamide, phenytoin; potentiates warfarin
    compounds; potentiates bradycardia seen with beta and
    calcium channel blockers. Causes pulmonary alveolitis/
    interstitial pneumonitis; mild liver injury manifested by
    abnormal liver enzyme levels.

Amrinone (Inocor)
  Uses: inotropic support
  Dose: (iv) loading dose, 0.75 $mg \cdot kg^{-1}$; maintenance, 5–10
    $\mu g \cdot kg^{-1} \cdot min^{-1}$
  Site of clearance: renal
  Interaction/toxicity: Marked vasodilator action seen in
    hypovolemic patients. Thrombocytopenia following long-
    term therapy.

Atracurium (Tracrium)
   Uses: nondepolarizing neuromuscular blocker
   Dose: (iv) 0.2–0.5 mg·kg^{-1}
   Site of clearance: plasma (Hofmann elimination) and ester hydrolysis; hepatic
   Interaction/toxicity: Potentiated by volatile anesthetics, hypokalemia, antibiotics (aminoglycosides), lithium, verapamil, trimethaphan, and procainamide. Antagonized by theophylline and phenytoin (decrease action). Releases histamine at high doses.

Atropine (various)
   Uses: antisialagogue; vagolysis
   Dose: (iv) 0.2–1.0 mg
   Site of clearance: renal
   Interaction/toxicity: Potentiated by antihistamines, procainamide, tricyclic antidepressants, and monoamine oxidase inhibitors. Antagonizes effects of cholinesterase inhibitors and metoclopramide.

Benzocaine (Americaine, Hurricaine)
   Uses: topical anesthesia
   Dose: (topical) 200 mg
   Site of clearance: plasma cholinesterase
   Interaction/toxicity: None known.

Bretylium (Bretylol)
   Uses: prophylaxis; treatment of ventricular fibrillation
   Dose: (iv) Loading dose, 5–10 mg·kg^{-1}; maintenance dose, 1–2 mg·min^{-1} (dilute 500 mg in 100 ml D5W or NS)
   Site of clearance: renal
   Interaction/toxicity: Digitalis toxicity may follow initial release of norepinephrine; transient hypertension and increased frequency of dysrhythmias follow initial release of norepinephrine from postganglionic nerve terminals.

Bupivacaine (Marcaine, Sensorcaine)
   Uses: local/regional anesthesia
   Dose: neural/epidural blockade 175 mg (maximum); with epinephrine (1:200,000) 225 mg; spinal 20 mg
   Site of clearance: hepatic
   Interaction/toxicity: Bupivacaine 0.75% not recommended for obstetrics or iv regional anesthesia. Diazepam increases bioavailability. Acute cardiovascular collapse following accidental intravenous injection; cardiac toxicity greater than central nervous system toxicity.

Buprenorphine (Buprenex)
   Uses: analgesia; opioid agonist-antagonist

Dose: (iv/im) 0.3 mg
Site of clearance: hepatic
Interaction/toxicity: Potentiates barbiturates and central nervous system depressants. Potentiated in patients with hepatic disease. May precipitate withdrawal in opioid dependent patient. Increases intracholedochal pressure.

Butorphanol (Stadol)
  Uses: analgesia; opioid agonist-antagonist
  Dose: (iv) 0.2–2 mg
  Site of clearance: hepatic/renal
  Interaction/toxicity: May precipitate withdrawal in opioid-dependent patients.

Calcium chloride (various)
  Uses: electrolyte replacement; inotrope
  Dose: (iv) 500–1000 mg (1 g $= 13.6$ mEq Ca^{2+})
  Site of clearance: gastrointestinal, renal
  Interaction/toxicity: Increases risk of dysrhythmias in digitalized patients; antagonizes verapamil; skin slough (necrosis) seen with extravasation.

Calcium gluconate (various)
  Uses: electrolyte replacement; inotrope
  Dose: (iv) 500–2000 mg (1 g $= 4.5$ mEq Ca^{2+})
  Site of clearance: gastrointestinal, urine
  Interaction/toxicity: Increases risk of dysrhythmias in digitalized patients; antagonizes verapamil; risk of skin slough (necrosis) seen with extravasation.

Captopril (Capoten)
  Uses: antihypertensive; congestive heart failure
  Dose: (po) 25 mg three times a day
  Site of clearance: renal
  Interaction/toxicity: Potentiates the hypotensive effects of anesthetics; elevates serum digoxin level; enhances the hemodynamic effects of vasodilators, calcium channel blockers, and beta blockers.

Chlordiazepoxide (Librium)
  Uses: antianxiety
  Dose: (iv) 50–100 mg
  Site of clearance: hepatic
  Interaction/toxicity: Cimetidine, metoprolol, propranolol decrease elimination. Increases effect of digoxin.

Chloroprocaine (Nesacaine)
  Uses: regional anesthesia
  Dose: neural blockade 800 mg (maximum); with epinephrine (1:200,000) 1000 mg (maximum)

Site of clearance: plasma cholinesterase
Interaction/toxicity: Rapid inadvertent intrathecal injection of low pH and bisulfite-containing solution may be associated with residual motor/sensory deficit.

Chlorpromazine (Thorazine)
  Uses: psychiatric disorders; premedication; vasodilator
  Dose: premedication (im) 0.02 mg·kg^{-1}; (iv) 1 mg
  Site of clearance: hepatic
  Interaction/toxicity: Potentiates sedative hypnotics. Lithium reduces bioavailability. Mephentermine and epinephrine potentiate chlorpromazine-induced hypotension.

Cimetidine (Tagamet)
  Uses: histamine antagonist (H$_2$)
  Dose: premedication (iv) 300 mg (dilute in 20–100 ml NS); (po) 300 mg
  Site of clearance: renal
  Interaction/toxicity: Rapid iv administration may cause hypotension and dysrhythmias. Potentiates respiratory depressant effects of morphine. High serum level associated with confusional states in the elderly. Reduces hepatic metabolism of drugs requiring cytochrome P-450 (beta blockers, calcium channel blockers, theophylline, tranquilizers).

Clonidine (Catapres)
  Uses: antihypertensive
  Dose: (po) 0.1–0.2 mg·day^{-1}
  Site of clearance: renal, hepatic
  Interaction/toxicity: Rebound hypertension follows abrupt withdrawal. Enhances effects of anesthetics, tranquilizers, sedatives, and hypnotics. Tolazoline and tricyclic antidepressants can block antihypertensive effects.

Cocaine (various)
  Uses: topical anesthesia
  Dose: (topical) 1–3 mg·kg^{-1}
  Site of clearance: plasma cholinesterase
  Interaction/toxicity: Potentiates vasopressors; cardiac dysrhythmias and seizures at high doses.

Dantrolene (Dantrium)
  Uses: malignant hyperpyrexia
  Dose: (iv) 1–2.5 mg·kg^{-1} (dilute 20 g in 60 ml sterile distilled H$_2$O)
  Site of clearance: hepatic
  Interaction/toxicity: Skeletal muscle weakness. (See inside back cover for Malignant Hypothermia Protocol.)

Desmopressin acetate (DDAVP, Stimate)
    Uses: antidiuretic hormone, coagulation (von Willebrand's Type I syndrome)
    Dose: (iv) 0.3 $\mu g \cdot kg^{-1}$ (dilute in 50–100 ml NS)
    Site of clearance: renal
    Interaction/toxicity: Chlorpropamide, clofibrate, and carbamazepine potentiate antidiuretic effects.

Dexamethasone (Hexadrol, Decadron)
    Uses: cerebral edema; allergic reactions; replacement therapy
    Dose: (iv) cerebral edema 10 mg, then 4 mg every 6 hours; replacement 2–4 mg twice a day
    Site of clearance: hepatic
    Interaction/toxicity: Increases insulin requirements; phenytoin, phenobarbital, and ephedrine may increase metabolic clearance of steroid.

Dezocine (Dalgan)
    Uses: analgesia; opioid agonist-antagonist
    Dose: (iv) 5 mg every 4 hours; (im) 10 mg every 4 hours
    Site of clearance: hepatic; renal
    Interaction/toxicity: Potentiates barbiturates and central nervous system depressants. Potentiated in patients with hepatic and/or renal disease. May precipitate withdrawal in opioid dependent patient.

Diazepam (Valium)
    Uses: antianxiety
    Dose: sedation (iv) 2.5–5.0 mg; induction (iv) 0.3–0.5 $mg \cdot kg^{-1}$; (po) 5–10 mg
    Site of clearance: hepatic, renal
    Interaction/toxicity: Elimination reduced by cimetidine, metoprolol, propranolol. Increases effect of digoxin.

Digoxin (Lanoxin)
    Uses: heart failure; antidysrhythmic
    Dose: (iv) loading dose 8–12 $\mu g \cdot kg^{-1}$; maintenance dose is one third loading dose
    Site of clearance: renal, hepatic
    Interaction/toxicity: Potentiated by hypokalemia; synergistic with catecholamines, calcium.

Diltiazem (Cardizem)
    Uses: antiarrhythmic (atrial fibrillation/flutter paroxymal supraventricular tachycardia)
    Dose: (iv) 0.25 mg.kg-1 (bolus over 2 min), wait 15 min, if inadequate response 0.35 $mg \cdot kg \cdot^{-1}$ (bolus over 2 min) infusion 2 $\mu g \cdot kg^{-1} \cdot min^{-1}$ or 10 $mg \cdot hr^{-1}$.
    Site of clearance: hepatic, renal

Interaction/toxicity: Potentiated by hepatic and renal disease. Potentiates theophylline and cardiovascular depressant effects of volatile anesthetics. Cimetidine and ranitidine may increase bioavailability. Intensifies sick sinus syndrome, 2nd and 3rd degree AV block, hypotension and cardiogenic shock. Should not be used in patients with Wolf-Parkinson-White Syndrome or short PR interval.

Diphenhydramine (Benadryl)
  Uses: histamine blocker (H_1); allergic reaction
  Dose: (iv) 25–50 mg; (po) 25–50 mg
  Site of clearance: hepatic
  Interaction/toxicity: monoamine oxidase inhibitors intensify effects; may antagonize effect of heparin.

Dobutamine (Dobutrex)
  Uses: inotropic support
  Dose: (iv) 2.5–30 $\mu g \cdot kg^{-1} \cdot min^{-1}$ (dilute 250 mg in 250 ml D5W or NS)
  Site of clearance: hepatic
  Interaction/toxicity: Halogenated anesthetics (especially halothane) sensitize myocardium to sympathomimetic effects (dysrhythmias).

Dopamine (Intropin)
  Uses: inotropic support
  Dose: (iv) 2–20 $\mu g \cdot kg^{-1} \cdot min^{-1}$ (dilute 200 mg in 250 ml D5W or NS)
  Site of clearance: hepatic enzymatic transformation
  Interaction/toxicity: Reduce dose in patients receiving monoamine oxidase inhibitors; combined with phenytoin, causes seizures, hypotension, and bradycardia; halogenated anesthetics (especially halothane) sensitize myocardium to sympathomimetic effects (dysrhythmias).

Doxacurium (Nuromax)
  Uses: Nondepolarizing neuromuscular blocker
  Dose: (iv) 0.05 $mg \cdot kg^{-1}$
  Site of clearance: renal
  Interaction/toxicity: Potentiated by volatile anesthetics, hypokalemia, antibiotics (aminoglycosides), lithium, magnesium, local anesthetics, procainamide, quinidine. Anticonvulsants (phenytoin and carbamazepine) lengthen onset and shorten duration of neuromuscular blockade. Contains benzyl alcohol which may be associated with increased incidence of neurologic complications in neonates. Due to long duration of action not recommended for patients undergoing cesarian section.

Droperidol (Inapsine)
   Uses: antianxiety; antiemetic
   Dose: (iv) 0.625–2.5 mg
   Site of clearance: hepatic
   Interaction/toxicity: Intensifies hypotension of vasodilators; produces extrapyramidal signs.

Edrophonium (Tensilon)
   Uses: anticholinesterase; antidysrhythmic
   Dose: (iv) 0.5–1.0 mg·kg^{-1}
   Site of clearance: hepatic, renal
   Interaction/toxicity: Bradycardia, salivation.

Ephedrine (various)
   Uses: sympathomimetic
   Dose: (iv) 5–10 mg
   Site of clearance: hepatic
   Interaction/toxicity: Potentiated by tricyclic antidepressants and monoamine oxidase inhibitors; halogenated anesthetics sensitize myocardium to sympathomimetic effects (dysrhythmias).

Epinephrine (various)
   Uses: sympathomimetic; allergic reaction
   Dose: (iv) 2–8 μg; infusion, 0.01–0.02 μg·kg^{-1}·min^{-1}
   Site of clearance: enzymatic transformation
   Interaction/toxicity: halogenated anesthetics (especially halothane) sensitize myocardium to sympathomimetic effects (dysrhythmias); potentiated by tricyclic antidepressants, monoamine oxidase inhibitors, and antihistamines.

Epinephrine—racemic (Vaponefrin, microNefrin)
   Uses: bronchodilator, croup (laryngotracheobronchitis)
   Dose: (inhalation) every 4 hours dilute 1:6 with NS
   Site of clearance: enzymatic transformation
   Interaction/toxicity: Halogenated anesthetics (especially halothane) sensitize myocardium to sympathomimetic effects (dysrhythmias).

Ergonovine (Ergotrate)
   Uses: increases uterine contractions
   Dose: (iv) 0.2 mg
   Site of clearance: hepatic
   Interaction/toxicity: Can induce coronary artery spasm.

Esmolol (Brevibloc)
   Uses: supraventricular tachycardia, hypertension
   Dose: (iv) bolus, 0.25–0.5 mg·kg^{-1}; loading dose, 500

$\mu g \cdot kg^{-1} \cdot min^{-1} \times$ 1–2 min; maintenance, 50–200 $\mu g \cdot kg^{-1} \cdot min^{-1}$ (dilute 5 g in 500 ml D5W or NS)
Site of clearance: red blood cell esterase
Interaction/toxicity: Increases digoxin and serum morphine levels.

Ethacrynic acid (Edecrin)
  Uses: diuretic
  Dose: (iv) 50 mg
  Site of clearance: renal
  Interaction/toxicity: Administration with aminoglycoside antibiotics can cause ototoxicity. Reduces renal clearance of lithium. Warfarin dose should be reduced.

Etidocaine (Duranest)
  Uses: regional anesthesia
  Dose: neural blockade 300 mg (with epinephrine 1:200,000)
  Site of clearance: hepatic
  Interaction/toxicity: Not recommended for obstetric anesthesia because of profound motor blockade.

Etomidate (Amidate)
  Uses: induction agent
  Dose: (iv) 0.2–0.3 $mg \cdot kg^{-1}$
  Site of clearance: hepatic
  Interaction/toxicity: Interferes with adrenal function (reduced release of cortisol). Myoclonus and pain with rapid iv injection.

Famotidine (Pepcid)
  Uses: histamine blocker (H_2)
  Dose: (iv) 20 mg every 12 hours (dilute in 10 mg D5W or NS)
  Site of clearance: renal
  Interaction/toxicity: Antacids decrease oral absorption.

Fentanyl (Sublimaze)
  Uses: analgesia
  Dose: (iv) 50–100 μg; induction (iv) 50–100 $\mu g \cdot kg^{-1}$; pediatric 25–50 $\mu g \cdot kg^{-1}$
  Site of clearance: hepatic
  Interaction/toxicity: Diazepam potentiates hypotensive action; truncal muscle rigidity may be seen during induction and emergence.

Fentanyl (Duragesic)
  Uses: Analgesia
  Dose: (transdermal) 2.5 mg transdermal patch (therapeutically equivalent to (im) 15 mg morphine or (po) 90 mg morphine

Site of clearance: hepatic
Interaction/toxicity: Potentiates opioid analgesics, tranquilizers and sedatives.

Flumazenil (Mazicon)
  Uses: benzodiazepine receptor antagonist
  Dose: (iv) 0.1–0.2 mg
  Site of clearance: hepatic
  Interaction/toxicity: Benzodiazepine reversal may be associated with seizures in high risk populations: major hypnotic drug withdrawal, previous seizure activity, and cyclic antidepressant poisoning. May precipitate withdrawal syndrome in benzodiazepine dependent patients.

Flurazepam (Dalmane)
  Uses: antianxiety
  Dose: (po) 15–30 mg
  Site of clearance: hepatic
  Interaction/toxicity: Significantly longer elimination half-time in the elderly.

Furosemide (Lasix)
  Uses: diuretic
  Dose: (iv) 10–20 mg; children, 0.5–1.0 mg·kg^{-1}
  Site of clearance: renal
  Interaction/toxicity: Stimulates release of renal prostaglandin E$_2$ (increases incidence of patent ductus arteriosus in premature infants). Administration with aminoglycoside antibiotics can cause ototoxicity.

Gallamine (Flaxedil)
  Uses: nondepolarizing neuromuscular blocker
  Dose: (iv) 1 mg·kg^{-1}
  Site of clearance: renal
  Interaction/toxicity: Tachycardia. Do not administer to patients with iodide allergy.

Glucagon (Glucagon)
  Uses: treatment of hypoglycemia; relaxes sphincter of Oddi
  Dose: (iv) 0.25–0.50 mg
  Site of clearance: renal
  Interaction/toxicity: Intensifies action of anticoagulants; causes significant increase in blood pressure.

Glycopyrrolate (Robinul)
  Uses: anticholinergic
  Dose: (iv) 0.1–0.4 mg; premedication (iv) 0.004 mg·kg^{-1}

Site of clearance: renal
Interaction/toxicity: None known.

Haloperidol (Haldol)
  Uses: tranquilizer
  Dose: (im) 2–5 mg (not approved for intravenous use)
  Site of clearance: hepatic
  Interaction/toxicity: Co-administration with lithium may
    produce neurotoxicity.

Heparin (various)
  Uses: anticoagulant
  Dose: (iv) 350–450 units·kg^{-1} using activated coagulation
    time (ACT) as therapeutic guide
  Site of clearance: hepatic
  Interaction/toxicity: Increases diazepam plasma levels;
    digitalis and antihistamines interfere with anticoagulant
    properties; nitroglycerin may antagonize heparin.

Hetastarch (Hespan)
  Uses: volume expander
  Dose: (iv) 500–1000 ml
  Site of clearance: enzymatic
  Interaction/toxicity: Anaphylactoid reaction. Large volumes
    may cause coagulopathy.

Hydralazine (Apresoline)
  Uses: antihypertensive
  Dose: (iv) 5–10 mg
  Site of clearance: hepatic
  Interaction/toxicity: Increases bioavailability of beta
    blockers; may require co-administration of beta blockers
    to blunt cardiac stimulation.

Hydrocortisone (Solu-Cortef)
  Uses: anti-inflammatory; steroid replacement; allergic
    reaction
  Dose: (iv) 100–200 mg
  Site of clearance: hepatic
  Interaction/toxicity: Increases insulin requirements;
    phenytoin; phenobarbital, and ephedrine may increase
    metabolic clearance.

Isoproterenol (Isuprel)
  Uses: inotrope/chronotrope; bronchodilator
  Dose: (iv) 0.05–0.1 μg·kg^{-1}·min^{-1} (dilute 1 mg in 250 ml
    D5W or NS)
  Site of clearance: hepatic
  Interaction/toxicity: Halogenated anesthetics (especially

halothane) sensitize myocardium to sympathomimetic
effects (dysrhythmias); effects of monoamine oxidase
inhibitors and tricyclic antidepressants are potentiated.

Ketamine (Ketalar)
  Uses: induction agent; anesthesia
  Dose: (iv) 1–2 mg·kg^{-1}; (im) 5–10 mg·kg^{-1}
  Site of clearance: hepatic
  Interaction/toxicity: Potentiates action of sedatives,
    hypnotics, and opioids; dysphoric reactions; increases
    cerebral blood flow and intraocular pressure. Increases
    upper airway secretions and heightens laryngeal reflexes.

Ketorolac (Toradol)
  Uses: Analgesic
  Dose: (im) 30–60 mg every 4 hours
  Site of clearance: renal
  Interaction/toxicity: Potentiates nonsteroidal anti-
    inflammatory drugs. Reversibly inhibits platelet
    aggregation. May cause renal toxicity and is potentiated by
    renal impairment.

Labetalol (Normodyne, Trandate)
  Uses: Beta blockade and alpha$_1$-adrenergic blockade;
    antihypertensive
  Dose: (iv) 0.25 mg·kg^{-1}
  Site of clearance: hepatic
  Interaction/toxicity: Cimetidine increases bioavailability;
    halothane or diazepam prolongs effects.

Lidocaine (Xylocaine)
  Uses: local anesthetic; antidysrhythmic
  Dose: antidysrhythmic (iv) 1 mg·kg^{-1}, then infusion 2–4
    mg·min^{-1} (20–50 μg·kg^{-1}·min^{-1}); anesthetic (topical) < 4
    mg·kg^{-1}; infiltration, 4 mg·kg^{-1}; (with epinephrine
    1:200,000) 7 mg·kg^{-1}
  Site of clearance: hepatic
  Interaction/toxicity: Beta blockers decrease hepatic
    clearance; cimetidine increases serum level. Plasma
    concentration > 8 μg·ml^{-1} may cause seizures,
    respiratory/cardiac depression.

Lorazepam (Ativan)
  Uses: antianxiety agent
  Dose: (iv) 1–2 mg; premedicant (po) 50 μg·kg^{-1} (maximum
    4 mg)
  Site of clearance: hepatic; urine
  Interaction/toxicity: Cimetidine, metoprolol, propranolol
    decrease elimination. Increases effect of digoxin.

Magnesium (various)
 Uses: toxemia; pre-eclampsia; hypomagnesemia
 Dose: (iv) 1–4 g; infusion $<$ 3 ml·min^{-1} (4 g in 250 ml)
 Site of clearance: renal
 Interaction/toxicity: Potentiates neuromuscular blockade
  (nondepolarizing/depolarizing), potentiates central
  nervous system effects of anesthetics, hypnotics, and
  opioids. Toxicity seen with serum levels $>$ 7–10 mEq·l^{-1}.

Mannitol (Osmitrol)
 Uses: osmotic diuretic
 Dose: (iv) 12.5–25.0 g; neurosurgery, 0.5–2 g·kg^{-1} (10–20%
  solution over 30–60 minutes)
 Site of clearance: renal
 Interaction/toxicity: Abrupt increases in intravascular
  volume.

Meperidine (Demerol)
 Uses: analgesia; antishivering
 Dose: (iv) 25 mg; pediatric, 1–2 mg·kg^{-1}; (im) 1.5 mg·kg^{-1}
 Site of clearance: hepatic
 Interaction/toxicity: Combined with monoamine oxidase
  inhibitors can cause hyperthermia and death. High doses
  may cause seizures.

Mephentermine (Wyamine)
 Uses: sympathomimetic
 Dose: (iv) 15–30 mg
 Site of clearance: hepatic
 Interaction/toxicity: Pressor effect exaggerated in patients
  treated with monoamine oxidase inhibitors; halogenated
  anesthetics (especially halothane) sensitize myocardium
  to sympathomimetic effects (dysrhythmias).

Mepivacaine (Carbocaine)
 Uses: regional; local anesthesia
 Dose: nerve blockade, 400 mg; epidural, 400 mg; (with
  epinephrine 1:200,000) 500 mg
 Site of clearance: hepatic
 Interaction/toxicity: Beta blockers decrease hepatic
  clearance; cimetidine increases serum level. High plasma
  concentration causes seizures, respiratory/cardiac
  depression.

Methadone (Dolophine)
 Uses: analgesia; opioid addiction
 Dose: (iv) 10 mg (every 8 hours); (po) 2.5–10 mg
 Site of clearance: hepatic
 Interaction/toxicity: Phenytoin reduces bioavailability by
  increasing hepatic clearance.

Methohexital (Brevital)
    Uses: induction agent; cardioversion; electroconvulsive
      shock therapy
    Dose: 1.0–1.5 mg·kg^{-1}
    Site of clearance: hepatic
    Interaction/toxicity: Infrequent allergic reactions;
      myoclonus, hiccups, and seizures

Methyldopa (Aldomet, Methyldopate)
    Uses: antihypertensive
    Dose: (iv) 250–500 mg four times a day; children, 20–40
      mg·kg^{-1}·day^{-1} (maximum 65 mg·kg^{-1})
    Site of clearance: hepatic, renal
    Interaction/toxicity: Reduces anesthetic requirements,
      potentiates sympathomimetics and levodopa.
      Concommitant treatment with propranolol may cause
      paradoxical hypertension.

Methylergonovine (Methergine)
    Uses: increases uterine contractions
    Dose: (im) 0.2 mg
    Site of clearance: hepatic
    Interaction/toxicity: Acute hypertension; additive effects
      with sympathomimetics.

Methylprednisolone (Solu-Medrol)
    Uses: anti-inflammatory, allergic reaction, steroid
      replacement
    Dose: (iv) 10–40 mg
    Site of clearance: hepatic
    Interaction/toxicity: Increases insulin requirements;
      phenytoin, phenobarbital, and ephedrine may increase
      metabolic clearance of steroid.

Metoclopramide (Reglan)
    Uses: stimulates gastric emptying; antiemetic
    Dose: (iv) 10 mg; (po) 10–15 mg
    Site of clearance: renal
    Interaction/toxicity: Antagonized by anticholinergics and
      opioids; potentiated by sedatives, hypnotics, opioids, and
      tranquilizers. Potentiates extrapyramidal effects of
      phenothiazines.

Metocurine (Metubine)
    Uses: nondepolarizing neuromuscular blocker
    Dose: (iv) 0.2–0.4 mg·kg^{-1}
    Site of clearance: renal
    Interaction/toxicity: Histamine release. Cross-sensitivity in
      patients allergic to other muscle relaxants. Do not
      administer to patients with iodide allergy.

Metoprolol (Lopressor)
   Uses: cardioselective beta blocker; antidysrhythmic
   Dose: (iv) 2–5 mg
   Site of clearance: hepatic
   Interaction/toxicity: Increases digoxin and morphine serum
      levels.

Midazolam (Versed)
   Uses: premedicant; induction agent
   Dose: (iv) 1–4 mg sedation; induction 0.10–0.20 mg·kg^{-1};
      (im) 0.05–0.1 mg·kg^{-1}
   Site of clearance: renal
   Interaction/toxicity: Intensifies effects of sedatives,
      hypnotics, opioids, and tranquilizers.

Mivacurium (Mivacron)
   Uses: nondepolarizing neuromuscular blocker
   Dose: (iv) 0.08–0.15 mg·kg^{-1}; (infusion) 4–8 µg·kg^{-1}·min^{-1}
   Site of clearance: plasma cholinesterase
   Interaction/toxicity: Potentiated by volatile anesthetics,
      hypokalemia, antibiotics (aminoglycosides), lithium,
      magnesium local anesthetics, procainamide, quinidine.
      Chronic administration of oral contraceptives,
      glucocorticoids, monoamine oxidase inhibitors, or
      echothiophate enhances neuromuscular block by
      decreasing plasma cholinesterase activity. Releases
      histamine at high doses.

Morphine (various)
   Uses: analgesia
   Dose: (iv) 2–10 mg; pediatric, 0.05–0.1 mg·kg^{-1}; epidural,
      2–5 mg; intrathecal, 0.2–0.6 mg; (im) 0.1–0.2 mg·kg^{-1}
   Site of clearance: hepatic
   Interaction/toxicity: Hypotension and respiratory
      depression. Potentiates cimetidine; increases
      anticoagulation with warfarin. Releases histamine in high
      doses.

Nalbuphine (Nubain)
   Uses: analgesia; opioid agonist-antagonist
   Dose: (iv) 10 mg
   Site of clearance: hepatic
   Interaction/toxicity: Does not antagonize effects of opioids
      in nondependent patients (kappa receptor).

Naloxone (Narcan)
   Uses: opioid antagonist
   Dose: (iv) 50–100 µg as needed; pediatric (iv), 10 µg·kg^{-1}
   Site of clearance: hepatic
   Interaction/toxicity: Can cause abrupt cardiovascular

stimulation and pulmonary edema; causes withdrawal in opioid-dependent patients.

Neostigmine (Prostigmine)
  Uses: anticholinesterase
  Dose: (iv) 1.25–5.0 mg
  Site of clearance: hepatic
  Interaction/toxicity: Bradycardia, salivation.

Nicardipine (Cardene IV)
  Uses: antihypertensive, antidysrhythymic and antianginal
  Dose: (iv) 1–2 $\mu g \cdot kg^{-1} \cdot min^{-1}$ or 10 $mg \cdot h^{-1}$ (dilute in 250 ml; incompatible with Ringers' lactate)
  Site of clearance: hepatic
  Interaction/toxicity: Cimetidine and ranitidine may increase bioavailability. Potentiated in patient with liver disease may increase hepatic portal pressure in cirrhotic patients.

Nifedipine (Procardia, Adalat)
  Uses: coronary vasospasm; angina; antihypertensive
  Dose: (po) 10–20 mg three times a day.
  Site of clearance: hepatic, renal
  Interaction/toxicity: Decreases platelet aggregation. Cimetidine and ranitidine may increase bioavailability. Potentiates theophylline.

Nimodipine (Nimotop)
  Uses: prevent cerebral arterial spasm (subarachnoid hemorrhage)
  Dose: (po) 60 mg every 4 hours × 21 days
  Site of clearance: hepatic
  Interaction/toxicity: Potentiated in patients with hepatic disease. Potentiates effects of antihypertensive drugs.

Nitroglycerin (Tridil, Nitrol IV, Nitrostat IV)
  Uses: vasodilator; antianginal; controlled hypotension
  Dose: (iv) 1–3 $\mu g \cdot kg^{-1} \cdot min^{-1}$ (dilute 50 mg in 250 ml D5W or NS)
  Site of clearance: hepatic, renal
  Interaction/toxicity: Increases bioavailability of dihydroergotamine. Methemoglobinemia seen with high doses, especially in individuals with methemoglobin reductase deficiency. Treat with oxygen and methylene blue (0.2 $ml \cdot kg^{-1}$ iv). Dose may be increased to 1–2 $mg \cdot kg^{-1}$.

Nitroprusside (Nipride, Nitropress)
  Uses: antihypertensive; vasodilator; controlled hypotension

Dose: (iv) 0.5–8.0 µg·kg^{-1}·min^{-1} (dilute 50 mg in 250 ml D5W)

Site of clearance: hepatic

Interaction/toxicity: Cyanide toxicity may occur at doses >10 µg·kg^{-1}·min^{-1}. Tachyphylaxis, elevated mixed venous oxygen tension (saturation), and acidosis suggest diagnosis of cyanide toxicity. Hydroxocobalamin may reduce risk of cyanide toxicity. Treatment of cyanide toxicity is intravenous administration of sodium thiosulfate, 150 mg·kg^{-1} over 15 minutes. Thiocyanate ion can be removed by hemodialysis.

Norepinephrine (Levophed)

Uses: vasoconstrictor

Dose: (iv) 0.1–0.5 µg·kg^{-1}·min^{-1} (dilute 4 mg in 250 ml D5W)

Site of clearance: enzymatic

Interaction/toxicity: Monoamine oxidase inhibitors and tricyclic antidepressants may cause severe hypertension. Halogenated anesthetics (especially halothane) may sensitize myocardium to sympathomimetic effects (dysrhythmias). Furosemide may decrease arterial vasoconstrictor properties. Extravasation may cause skin slough.

Ondansetron (Zofran)

Uses: Antiemetic

Dose: (iv) 0.15 mg·kg^{-1} (dilute in 50 ml D5W)

Site of clearance: hepatic

Interaction/toxicity: Potentiated by hepatic disease.

Oxytocin (Pitocin)

Uses: increases uterine contraction

Dose: (iv) 10 units; infusion, 0.002 units·min^{-1}

Site of clearance: hepatic

Interaction/toxicity: Potentiates sympathomimetics.

Pancuronium (Pavulon)

Uses: nondepolarizing neuromuscular blocker

Dose: (iv) 0.05–0.10 mg·kg^{-1}

Site of clearance: renal, hepatic

Interaction/toxicity: Potentiated by volatile anesthetics, hypokalemia, antibiotics (aminoglycosides), magnesium local anesthetics, procainamide, quinidine. Conditions associated with increased volume of distribution (e.g., slower circulation time, edematous states and old age) may be associated with delay in onset. Prolongation of neuromuscular blockade may occur in patients with renal and/or hepatic disease. Patients receiving tricyclic antidepressants who are anesthetized with halothane and receive pancuronium may develop cardiac dysrhythmias.

Pentobarbital (Nembutal)
 Uses: hypnotic; premedication
 Dose: (iv) 50–100 mg; (im) 1–2 mg·kg^{-1}
 Site of clearance: hepatic/renal
 Interaction/toxicity: Barbiturates decrease the effects of theophylline, beta-adrenergic blockers, corticosteroids, and tricyclic antidepressants. Monoamine oxidase inhibitors increase action.

Pentazocine (Talwin)
 Uses: analgesia; opioid agonist-antagonist
 Dose: (im) 30 mg every 4 hours; (po) 50 mg every 4 hours
 Site of clearance: hepatic; renal
 Interaction/toxicity: Potentiates barbiturates and central nervous system depressants. Potentiated in patients with hepatic and/or renal disease. May precipitate withdrawal in opioid dependent patient.

Phentolamine (Regitine)
 Uses: arterial dilator
 Dose: (iv) 2.5–5.0 mg
 Site of clearance: Not known.
 Interaction/toxicity: Vasoconstrictor effects of epinephrine and ephedrine are blocked by phentolamine.

Phenylephrine (Neo-Synephrine)
 Uses: vasoconstrictor
 Dose: (iv) 50–100 μg; infusion, 0.5–1 μg·kg^{-1}·min^{-1} (dilute 4 mg in 250 ml D5W or NS)
 Site of clearance: hepatic
 Interaction/toxicity: Effects potentiated by oxytocic drugs, monoamine oxidase inhibitors, and tricyclic antidepressants.

Phenytoin (Dilantin)
 Uses: anticonvulsant; antidysrhythmic
 Dose: (iv) 100–200 mg; children, 10–15 mg·kg^{-1}
 Site of clearance: hepatic
 Interaction/toxicity: Increased effects seen with cimetidine and diazepam; decreased effects seen with barbiturates, theophylline, and antacids. Decreases effectiveness of corticosteroids, dicumarol, haloperidol, quinidine, furosemide, dopamine, and nondepolarizing muscle relaxants. Increases toxicity of lithium.

Physostigmine (Antilirium)
 Uses: anticholinesterase; nonspecific reversal of central

nervous system side-effects of benzodiazepines, scopolamine, and ketamine.
Dose: (iv) 0.5–1.0 mg; pediatric, 0.02 mg·kg^{-1}·min^{-1}
Site of clearance: cholinesterase enzyme
Interaction/toxicity: Rapid administration can cause bradycardia, salivation, and seizures.

Phytonadione (AquaMEPHYTON, Konakion)
  Uses: hepatic synthesis of prothrombin (II); proconvertin (VII); plasma thromboplastin (IX); and Stuart factor (X).
  Dose: (iv slow) 2.5–10.0 mg; pediatric, 0.5–2.0 mg
  Site of clearance: hepatic
  Interaction/toxicity: Severe reaction resembling anaphylaxis has been seen even with administration of dilute phytonadione.

Pipercuronium (Arduan)
  Uses: nondepolarizing neuromuscular blocker
  Dose: (iv) 0.07 mg·kg^{-1}
  Site of clearance: renal
  Interaction/toxicity: Potentiated by volatile anesthetics, hypokalemia, antibiotics (aminoglycosides), lithium, magnesium, local anesthetics, procainamide, quinidine. Conditions associated with increased volume of distribution (e.g., slower circulation time, edematous states and old age) may be associated with delay in onset. Contains benzyl alcohol, which may be associated with increased incidence of neurologic complications in neonates. Due to long duration of action not recommended for patient undergoing cesarian section.

Prilocaine (Citanest)
  Uses: regional anesthesia
  Dose: nerve block, 600 mg
  Site of clearance: hepatic
  Interaction/toxicity: Methemoglobinemia may be associated with doses > 500 mg; treat with methylene blue (iv), 1–2 mg·kg^{-1} over 5 minutes.

Procainamide (Pronestyl)
  Uses: antidysrhythmic
  Dose: (iv) 100 mg; loading dose (infusion), 500 mg over 30 minutes; then 2–6 mg·min^{-1} (dilute 1000 mg in 500 ml D5W)
  Site of clearance: hepatic
  Interaction/toxicity: Enhances anticholinergic drugs, potentiates neuromuscular blockers.

Procaine (Novocain)
  Uses: regional anesthesia

Dose: nerve block 1000 mg; epidural 1000 mg; spinal 50–200 mg
Site of clearance: plasma cholinesterase
Interaction/toxicity: Potential for allergic reaction with repeated use.

Prochlorperazine (Compazine)
  Uses: antiemetic; antipsychotic
  Dose: (iv) 5–10 mg: pediatric, 0.1 mg·kg^{-1}
  Site of clearance: hepatic
  Interaction/toxicity: Hypersensitivity reaction may manifest as jaundice; extrapyramidal symptoms.

Promethazine (Phenergan)
  Uses: antiemetic
  Dose: (im) 12.5–25.0 mg; pediatric, 1 mg·kg^{-1}
  Site of clearance: hepatic
  Interaction/toxicity: Hypersensitivity reaction may manifest as jaundice.

Propofol (Diprivan)
  Uses: induction agent
  Dose: (iv) induction, 1.5–2.5 mg·kg^{-1}; infusion, 0.1–0.2 mg·kg^{-1}·min^{-1}; bolus, 25–50 mg
  Site of clearance: hepatic
  Interaction/toxicity: Hypotension, respiratory depression, and pain with injection. Prepared in lipid emulsion; infection potential, allergic reaction.

Propranolol (Inderal)
  Uses: beta blockade; antidysrhythmic, antihypertensive
  Dose: (iv) 0.5–1.0 mg
  Site of clearance: hepatic
  Interaction/toxicity: Increases digoxin, local anesthesia, and morphine serum levels. Bradycardia, hypotension, and bronchospasm can be seen.

Protamine (various)
  Uses: heparin antagonist
  Dose: titrated on the basis of coagulation test, e.g., activated coagulation time (ACT); protamine, 1 mg, neutralizes 90 units heparin (lung) or 115 units heparin (intestinal mucosa).
  Site of clearance: Not known.
  Interaction/toxicity: Potentiates vasodilators; anaphylactic reactions especially in patients with fish allergy or diabetics treated with protamine-containing insulin solutions; complement-mediated pulmonary vasoconstriction.

Pyridostigmine (Regonol, Mestinon)
  Uses: anticholinesterase; myasthenia gravis
  Dose: (iv) 0.2 mg·kg^{-1}
  Site of clearance: renal, hepatic
  Interaction/toxicity: Bradycardia, salivation.

Ranitidine (Zantac)
  Uses: histamine antagonist (H$_2$)
  Dose: (po) 150 mg; (iv) 50 mg (diluted in 100 ml NS or D5W)
  Site of clearance: hepatic
  Interaction/toxicity: Bradycardia with intravenous
    administration.

Ritodrine (Yutopar)
  Uses: uterine relaxation
  Dose: (iv) 0.1–0.3 mg·min^{-1}
  Site of clearance: renal
  Interaction/toxicity: Cardiovascular effects (dysrhythmias
    and hypotension) seen with meperidine and general
    anesthetics. Concomitant use of corticosteroids may lead
    to pulmonary edema.

Scopolamine (various)
  Uses: anticholinergic; amnesia
  Dose: (im) 0.2–0.4 mg
  Site of clearance: renal
  Interaction/toxicity: Central nervous system excitation or
    sedation (central anticholinergic syndrome).
    Antihistamines, procainamide, sedatives, hypnotics, and
    opioids intensify effect. Amnesia, vertigo, and dry mouth.

Secobarbital (Seconal)
  Uses: hypnotic; premedication
  Dose: (iv) 50–100 mg; (im) 1–2 mg·kg^{-1}
  Site of clearance: hepatic
  Interaction/toxicity: Barbiturates decrease the effects of
    theophylline. Beta-adrenergic blockers, corticosteroids,
    tricyclic antidepressants, and monoamine oxidase
    inhibitors increase action.

Succinylcholine (Anectine, Sucostrin, Quelicin)
  Uses: depolarizing neuromuscular blocker
  Dose: (iv) 1–1.5 mg·kg^{-1}
  Site of clearance: plasma cholinesterase enzyme
  Interaction/toxicity: Elevates serum potassium, especially in
    burn patients and patients with spinal cord injury or
    progressive neuromuscular disease; trigger for malignant
    hyperthermia, causes increased intraocular pressure. Can
    cause bradycardia, especially with repeated

administration at short intervals (<5 minutes). Cross-sensitivity in patients allergic to other muscle relaxants.

Sufentanil (Sufenta)
  Uses: analgesia
  Dose: (iv) 5–10 μg; (iv anesthesia) 5–10 μg·kg^{-1}; pediatric, 1.0–2.5 μg·kg^{-1}
  Site of clearance: hepatic
  Interaction/toxicity: Benzodiazepines potentiate hypotensive action; truncal muscle rigidity may be seen during induction and emergence. Bradycardia.

Terbutaline (Brethaire, Bricanyl)
  Uses: bronchodilator; premature labor
  Dose: (iv) 0.25 mg or 10 mg·kg^{-1}·min^{-1}; (inhalation, 2 breaths)
  Site of clearance: hepatic
  Interaction/toxicity: Potentiates monoamine oxidase inhibitors; halogenated anesthetics sensitize (especially halothane) myocardium to sympathomimetic effects (dysrhythmias).

Tetracaine (Pontocaine)
  Uses: regional/topical anesthesia
  Dose: spinal, 8–15 mg; topical, 80 mg
  Site of clearance: plasma cholinesterase, hepatic
  Interaction/toxicity: Beta blockers decrease hepatic clearance; cimetidine increases serum level. Plasma concentration > 8 μg·ml^{-1} may cause seizures, respiratory/cardiac depression.

Thiopental (Pentothal)
  Uses: induction agent
  Dose: (iv) 3–5 mg·kg^{-1}; (rectal) 25 mg·kg^{-1}
  Site of clearance: hepatic
  Interaction/toxicity: Releases histamine; may cause hypotension or respiratory depression; may trigger porphyria, allergic reactions.

Trimethaphan (Arfonad)
  Uses: vasodilator (ganglionic blocker)
  Dose: 2–4 mg·min^{-1} (dilute 500 mg in 500 ml D5W); pediatric, 50–150 μg·kg^{-1}·min^{-1}
  Site of clearance: plasma cholinesterase
  Interaction/toxicity: Histamine release. Produces mydriasis, ileus, dilation, and respiratory depression.

***d*-Tubocurarine** (various)
  Uses: nondepolarizing neuromuscular blocker

Dose: (iv) 0.3–0.5 mg·kg^{-1}
Site of clearance: renal
Interaction/toxicity: Potentiated by volatile anesthetics, hypokalemia, antibiotics (aminoglycosides), lithium, magnesium, local anesthetics, procainamide, quinidine, monoamine oxidase inhibitors, trimethephan and propranolol. Prolongation of neuromuscular blockade may occur in patients with renal and/or hepatic disease. Releases histamine.

Vasopressin (Pitressin)
Uses: neurogenic diabetes insipidus
Dose: (im) 5–10 units
Site of clearance: renal, hepatic
Interaction/toxicity: Coronary artery vasoconstriction, allergic reactions, hypertension.

Vecuronium (Norcuron)
Uses: nondepolarizing neuromuscular blocker
Dose: (iv) 0.05–0.1 mg·kg^{-1}
Site of clearance: hepatic, renal
Interaction/toxicity: Potentiated by volatile anesthetics, hypokalemia, antibiotics (aminoglycosides), magnesium, local anesthetics, procainamide, quinidine. Conditions associated with increased volume of distribution (e.g., slower circulation time, edematous states and old age) may be associated with delay in onset. Prolongation of neuromuscular blockade may occur in patients with renal and/or hepatic disease. Theophylline and phenytoin decrease effects. Bradycardia may occur with rapid administration in patients receiving opioids.

Verapamil (Calan, Isoptin)
Uses: antidysrhythmic, antihypertensive
Dose: (iv) 1.25–2.5 mg
Site of clearance: renal
Interaction/toxicity: Potentiates beta blockers, theophylline; increases digoxin levels. Barbiturates may decrease bioavailability. Cimetidine increases bioavailability.

Warfarin (Coumadin)
Uses: anticoagulant
Dose: (po) 10–15 mg (adjust dose for prothrombin time 1.5–2.0 times control)
Site of clearance: hepatic
Interaction/toxicity: Platelet aggregation inhibitors (e.g., salicylates, dipyridamole, indomethacin), procoagulant inhibition factors (e.g., quinidine) increase risk of hemorrhage. Decreased effect with enzyme inducers (e.g., barbiturates, phenytoin).

Anesthesia Apparatus Checkout Recommendations, 1992

This checkout, or a reasonable equivalent, should be conducted before administration of anesthesia. These recommendations are only valid if the anesthesia system includes an ascending bellows ventilator and the following monitors: capnograph, pulse oximeter, oxygen analyzer, respiratory volume monitor (spirometer), and breathing system pressure monitor with high and low pressure alarms. This is a guideline which users are encouraged to modify to accommodate differences in equipment design and variations in local clinical practice. Such local modifications should have appropriate peer review. Users should refer to the operator's manual for specific procedures and precautions.

EMERGENCY VENTILATION EQUIPMENT
  1. Emergency Equipment is Available and Functioning

HIGH-PRESSURE SYSTEM
  2. Check Oxygen Cylinder Supply
     a. Open O_2 cylinder and verify at least half full (about 1000 psi).
     b. Close cylinder.
  3. Check Central Pipeline Supplies
     a. Hoses are properly connected and pipeline gauges read 45-55 psi.

LOW-PRESSURE SYSTEM
  4. Check Initial Status of Low-Pressure System
     a. Flow control valves and vaporizers are off.
     b. Check fill level and tighten vaporizer filler caps.
     c. Remove O_2 monitor sensor from circuit.

FDA Draft ver. 2.4, 1/1/92.

5. Perform Machine Low-Pressure Leak Check
   a. Verify that the machine master switch and flow control valves are OFF.
   b. Attach "Suction Bulb" to common (fresh) gas outlet.
   c. Repeatedly pump until fully collapsed.
   d. Verify bulb stays *fully* collapsed for at least 5 seconds.
   e. Open one vaporizer at a time and repeat 'b' and 'c' as above.
   f. Remove suction bulb, and reconnect fresh gas hose.
6. Turn On Machine Master Switch
   and all other necessary electrical equipment.
7. Test Flow Meters
   a. Adjust flow of all gases through their full range, checking for smooth operation of floats and undamaged flow tubes.
   b. Attempt to create a hypoxic O_2/N_2O mixture and verify correct changes in flow and/or alarm.

BREATHING SYSTEM

8. Check Initial Status of Breathing System
   a. Selector switch is in "Bag" mode.
   b. Breathing circuit is complete, undamaged, and unobstructed.
   c. CO_2 absorbent is adequate.
9. Install Accessory Equipment
   to be used during the case.
10. Calibrate O_2 Monitor
   a. Calibrate to read 21% in room air.
   b. Reinstall sensor in circuit and flush breathing system with O_2.
   c. Monitor should now read greater than 90%.
11. Perform Breathing System Leak Check
   a. Set all gas flows to zero (or minimum).
   b. Close APL valve and occlude Y-piece.
   c. Pressurize breathing system to 30 cm H_2O with O_2 flush.
   d. Gauge value shouldn't noticeably drop in 10 seconds.

SCAVENGER SYSTEM

12. Check APL Valve and Scavenger System
   a. Pressurize breathing system to 50 cm H_2O and ensure it remains intact.
   b. Open APL valve and ensure that a pressure decrease occurs as the valve is opened.
   c. Ensure proper scavenging connections and adjust waste gas vacuum.
   d. Fully open APL valve, and occlude Y-piece.
   e. With minimum O_2 flow, ensure negligible negative pressure at the absorber pressure gauge.

f. With O_2 flush activated, ensure negligible positive pressure at the absorber pressure gauge.

VENTILATOR

13. Functional Test of Ventilator and Unidirectional Valves
   a. Place reservoir bag on Y-piece.
   b. Set appropriate ventilator parameters for next patient.
   c. Set O_2 flow to minimum, other gas flows to zero.
   d. Turn ventilator ON and pressurize system with O_2 flush.
   e. Ensure cycling of ventilator and free movement of bellows.
   f. *Check for proper action of unidirectional valves.*
   g. Exercise breathing circuit accessories to assure appropriate function.
   h. Turn ventilator OFF, and return bag to bag mount.

MONITORS

14. Check, Calibrate, and Set Alarm Limits of All Monitors
   Capnograph   Pulse Oximeter
   Oxygen Analyzer   Respiratory Volume Monitor (Spirometer)
   Pressure Monitor with High and Low Airway Pressure Alarms

FINAL POSITION

15. Check Final Status of Machine
   a. All flow meters to zero (or minimum).
   b. Vaporizers off.
   c. Selector switch to "Bag" mode.
   d. APL valve open.
   e. Patient suction level appropriate.
   f. Patient breathing system ready to use.

E

American Heart Association Resuscitation Protocols

Basic and Advanced Cardiac Life Support for Adults, Children, and Infants

Foreign Body Airway Obstruction in Adults, Children, and Infants

Adult
    Universal Algorithm For Adult Emergency Cardiac Care (ECC)
    Ventricular Fibrillation/Pulseless Ventricular Tachycardia
    Electromechanical Dissociation/Pulseless Electrical Activity
    Asystole
    Tachycardia
    Bradycardia
    Electrical Cardioversion
    Hypotension, Shock, and Acute Pulmonary Edema
    Acute Myocardial Infarction
    Hypothermia

Pediatric
    Bradycardia Decision Tree
    Asystole and Pulseless Arrest Decision Tree
    Drugs
    Infusion Medications

Neonatal (Delivery Room/Newborn)
    Drug Sequence
    Delivery Room Overview
    Therapeutic Guidelines

Conveying News of a Sudden Death to Family Members

Recommendations for Critical Incident Debriefing

For more detailed information the reader is referred to the Emergency Cardiac Care Committee and Subcommittees, American Heart Association. Guidelines for Cardiopulmonary Resuscitation and Emergency Cardiac Care. JAMA 1992;268(16):2171–2183.

AMERICAN HEART ASSOCIATION TREATMENT SEQUENCES FOR FOREIGN BODY AIRWAY OBSTRUCTION IN ADULTS, CHILDREN, AND INFANTS

	Objectives	Actions		
		Adult (over 8 yr)	Child (1 to 8 yr)	Infant (under 1 yr)
Conscious Victim	1. Assessment: Determine airway obstruction.	Ask, "Are you choking?" Determine if victim can cough or speak.		Observe breathing difficulty.
	2. Act to relieve obstruction.	Perform subdiaphragmatic abdominal thrusts (Heimlich maneuver).		Give 4 back blows.
				Give 4 chest thrusts.
	Be persistent.	Repeat Step 2 until obstruction is relieved or victim becomes unconscious.		
Victim Who Becomes Unconscious	3. Position the victim; call for help.	Turn on back as a unit, supporting head and neck, face up, arms by sides. Call out, "Help!" If others come, activate EMS.		
	4. Check for foreign body.	Perform tongue-jaw lift and finger sweep.	Perform tongue-jaw lift. Remove foreign object only if you actually see it.	
	5. Give rescue breaths.	Open the airway with head-tilt/chin-lift. Try to give rescue breaths.		
	6. Act to relieve obstruction.	Perform subdiaphragmatic abdominal thrusts (Heimlich maneuver).		Give 4 back blows.
				Give 4 chest thrusts.
	7. Check for foreign body.	Perform tongue-jaw lift and finger sweep.	Perform tongue-jaw lift. Remove foreign object only if you actually see it.	
	8. Try again to give rescue breaths.	Open the airway with head-tilt/chin-lift. Try to give rescue breaths.		
	9. Be persistent.	Repeat Steps 6–8 until obstruction is relieved.		

(continued)

AMERICAN HEART ASSOCIATION TREATMENT SEQUENCES FOR FOREIGN BODY AIRWAY OBSTRUCTION IN ADULTS, CHILDREN, AND INFANTS (continued)

	Objectives	Actions		
		Adult (over 8 yr)	Child (1 to 8 yr)	Infant (under 1 yr)
Unconscious Victim	1. Assessment: Determine unresponsiveness.	Tap or gently shake shoulder. Shout. "Are you okay?"		Tap or gently shake shoulder.
	2. Call for help; position the victim.	Turn on back as a unit, supporting head and neck, face up, arms by sides. Call out, "Help!" If others come, activate EMS.		
	3. Open the airway.	Head-tilt/chin-lift		Head-tilt/chin-lift, but do not tilt too far.
	4. Assessment: Determine breathlessness.	Maintain an open airway. Ear over mouth: observe chest. Look, listen, feel for breathing (3–5 seconds)		
	5. Give rescue breaths.	Make mouth-to-mouth seal.		Make mouth-to-nose-and-mouth seal.
	6. Try again to give rescue breaths.	Try to give rescue breaths. Reposition head. Try rescue breaths again.		
	7. Activate the EMS system.	If someone responded to the call for help, that person should activate the EMS system.		
	8. Act to relieve obstruction.	Perform subdiaphragmatic abdominal thrusts (Heimlich maneuver).		Give 4 back blows. Give 4 chest thrusts.
	9. Check for foreign body.	Perform tongue-jaw lift and finger sweep.	Perform tongue-jaw lift. Remove foreign object only if you actually see it.	

| | 10. Rescue breaths. | Open the airway with head-tilt/chin-lift. Try again to give rescue breaths. |
| | 11. Be persistent. | Repeat Steps 8–10 until obstruction is relieved. |

Reproduced with permission from Albarran-Sotelo R, Flint LS (eds): Instructor's Manual for Basic Life Support. Dallas, American Heart Association, 1987.

AMERICAN HEART ASSOCIATION BASIC LIFE SUPPORT SEQUENCES FOR ADULTS, CHILDREN, AND INFANTS

	Objectives	Actions		
		Adult (over 8 yr)	Child (1 to 8 yr)	Infant (under 1 yr)
A. Airway	1. Assessment: Determine unresponsiveness	Tap or gently shake shoulder.		
		Say, "Are you okay?"		Observe
	2. Get help.	Call out "Help!"		
	3. Position the victim.	Turn on back as a unit, supporting head and neck if necessary. (4–10 seconds)		
	4. Open the airway.	Head-tilt/chin-lift		
B. Breathing	5. Assessment: Determine breathlessness.	Maintain open airway. Place ear over mouth, observing chest. Look, listen, feel for breathing. (3–5 seconds)		
	6. Give 2 rescue breaths.	Maintain open airway		
		Seal mouth to mouth		mouth to nose/mouth
		Give 2 rescue breaths, 1½ to 2 seconds (adult), 1 to 1½ seconds (children) each. Observe chest rise. Allow lung deflation between breaths.		

(continued)

585

AMERICAN HEART ASSOCIATION BASIC LIFE SUPPORT SEQUENCES FOR ADULTS, CHILDREN, AND INFANTS (continued)

		Actions		
	Objectives	Adult (over 8 yr)	Child (1 to 8 yr)	Infant (under 1 yr)
	7. Option for obstructed airway	a. Reposition victim's head. Try again to give rescue breaths.		
		b. Activate the EMS system.		
		c. Give 6–10 subdiaphragmatic abdominal thrusts (the Heimlich maneuver).		Give 4 back blows.
				Give 4 chest thrusts.
		d. Tongue-jaw lift and finger sweep	Tongue-jaw lift, but finger sweep only if you see a foreign object.	
		If unsuccessful, repeat a, c, and d until successful.		
C. Circulation	8. Assessment: Determine pulselessness.	Feel for carotid pulse with one hand; maintain head-tilt with the other. (5–10 seconds)		Feel for brachial pulse; keep head-tilt.
	9. Activate EMS system.	If someone responded to call for help, send them to activate the EMS system.		
	Begin chest compressions: 10. Landmark check	Run middle finger along bottom edge of rib cage to notch at center (tip of sternum).		Imagine a line drawn between the nipples.
	11. Hand position	Place index finger next to finger on notch:		Place 2–3 fingers on sternum, 1 finger's width below line. Depress ½–1 in.
		Two hands next to index finger. Depress 1½–2 in.	Heel of one hand next to index finger. Depress 1–1½ in.	

586

		Adult	Child	Infant
CPR Cycles	12. Compression rate.	80–100 per minute		At least 100 per minute
	13. Compressions to breaths.	2 breaths to every 15 compressions.		1 breath to every 5 compressions.
	14. Number of cycles.	4 (52–73 seconds)	10 (60–87 seconds)	10 (45 seconds or less)
	15. Reassessment.	Feel for carotid pulse. (5 seconds)		Feel for brachial pulse.
		If no pulse, resume CPR, starting with 2 breaths.		If no pulse, resume CPR, starting with 1 breath.
Option for entrance of 2nd rescuer: "I know CPR. Can I help?"	1st rescuer ends CPR.	End cycle with 2 rescue breaths.		End cycle with 1 rescue breath.
	2nd rescuer checks pulse (5 seconds).	Feel for carotid pulse		Feel for brachial pulse.
	If no pulse, 2nd rescuer begins CPR.	Begin one-rescuer CPR, starting with 2 breaths.		Begin one-rescuer CPR, starting with 1 breath.
	1st rescuer monitors 2nd rescuer.	Watch for chest rise and fall during rescue breathing; check pulse during chest compressions.		
Option for pulse return	If no breathing, give rescue breaths.	1 breath every 5 seconds	1 breath every 4 seconds	1 breath every 3 seconds

Modified from Albarran-Sotelo R, Flint LS (eds): Instructor's Manual for Basic Life Support. Dallas, American Heart Association, 1987.

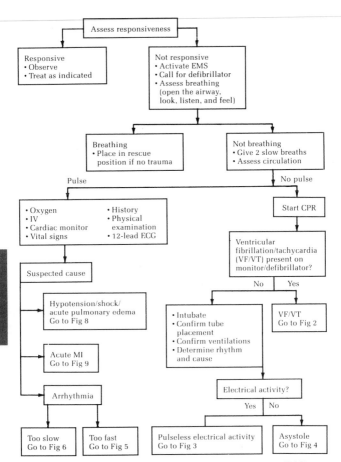

Figure 1. Universal algorithm for adult emergency cardiac care (ECC).

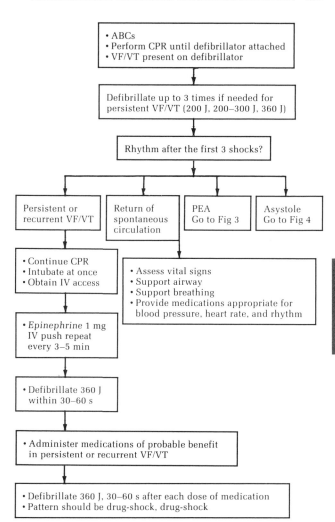

Figure 2. Algorithm for ventricular fibrillation and pulseless ventricular tachycardia (VF/VT).

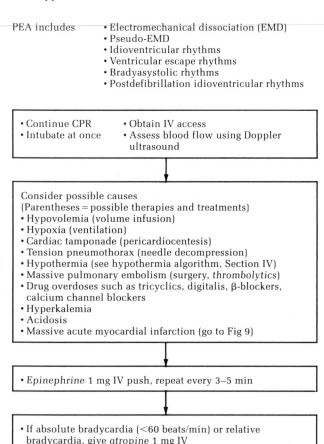

PEA includes —— • Electromechanical dissociation (EMD)
                 • Pseudo-EMD
                 • Idioventricular rhythms
                 • Ventricular escape rhythms
                 • Bradyasystolic rhythms
                 • Postdefibrillation idioventricular rhythms

---

| • Continue CPR | • Obtain IV access |
| • Intubate at once | • Assess blood flow using Doppler ultrasound |

↓

Consider possible causes
(Parentheses = possible therapies and treatments)
• Hypovolemia (volume infusion)
• Hypoxia (ventilation)
• Cardiac tamponade (pericardiocentesis)
• Tension pneumothorax (needle decompression)
• Hypothermia (see hypothermia algorithm, Section IV)
• Massive pulmonary embolism (surgery, *thrombolytics*)
• Drug overdoses such as tricyclics, digitalis, β-blockers, calcium channel blockers
• Hyperkalemia
• Acidosis
• Massive acute myocardial infarction (go to Fig 9)

↓

• *Epinephrine* 1 mg IV push, repeat every 3–5 min

↓

• If absolute bradycardia (<60 beats/min) or relative bradycardia, give *atropine* 1 mg IV
• Repeat every 3–5 min up to a total of 0.04 mg/kg

Figure 3. Algorithm for pulseless electrical activity (PEA) (electromechanical dissociation [EMD]).

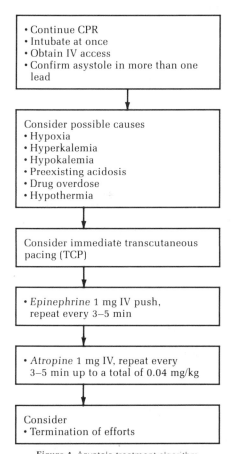

Figure 4. Asystole treatment algorithm.

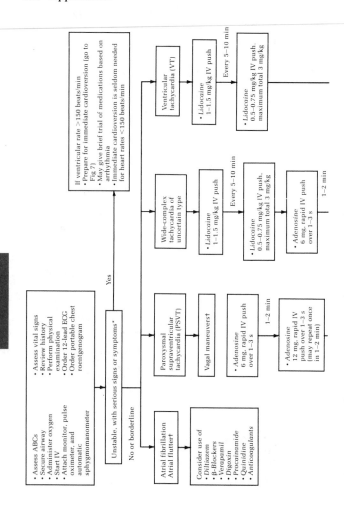

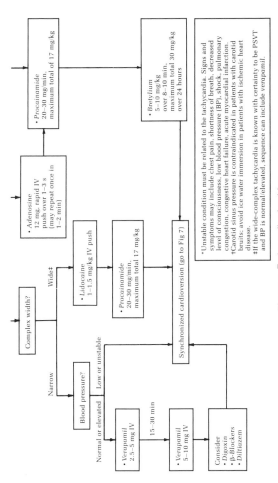

Figure 5. Tachycardia algorithm.

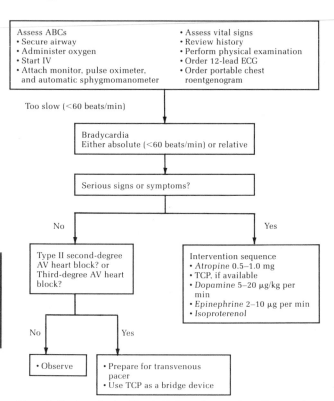

Figure 6. Bradycardia algorithm (with the patient not in cardiac arrest).

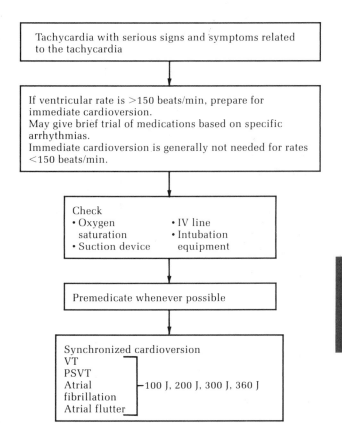

Figure 7. Electrical cardioversion algorithm (with the patient not in cardiac arrest).

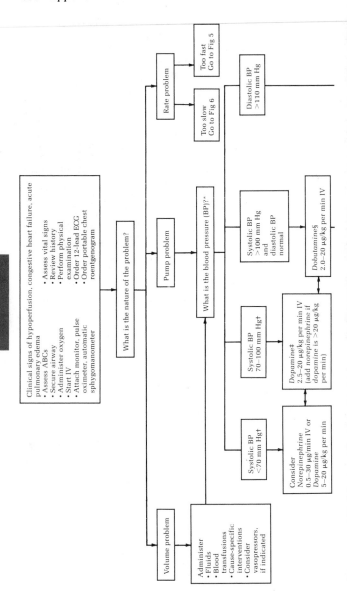

Clinical signs of hypoperfusion, congestive heart failure, acute
pulmonary edema
• Assess ABCs
• Secure airway
• Administer oxygen
• Start IV
• Attach monitor, pulse
oximeter, automatic
sphygomanometer
• Assess vital signs
• Review history
• Perform physical
examination
• Order 12-lead ECG
• Order portable chest
roentgenogram

What is the nature of the problem?

Volume problem

Pump problem

Rate problem

Administer
• Fluids
• Blood
transfusions
• Cause-specific
interventions
• Consider
vasopressors,
if indicated

What is the blood pressure (BP)?*

Systolic BP
<70 mm Hg†

Systolic BP
70–100 mm Hg†

Systolic BP
70–100 mm Hg†

Systolic BP
>100 mm Hg
and
diastolic BP
normal

Consider
Norepinephrine
0.5–30 µg/min IV or
Dopamine
5–20 µg/kg per min

Dopamine‡
2.5–20 µg/kg per min IV
(add norepinephrine if
dopamine is >20 µg/kg
per min)

Dobutamine§
2.0–20 µg/kg per min IV

Too slow
Go to Fig 6

Too fast
Go to Fig 5

Diastolic BP
>110 mm Hg

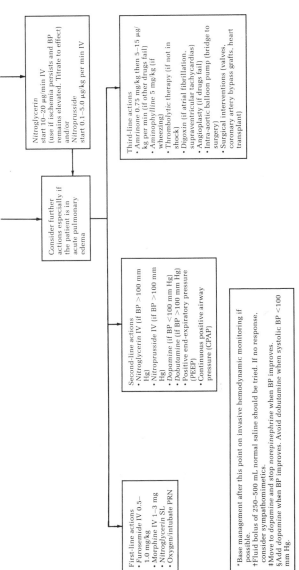

First-line actions
• Furosemide IV 0.5–1.0 mg/kg
• Morphine IV 1–3 mg
• Nitroglycerin SL
• Oxygen/intubate PRN

Second-line actions
• Nitroglycerin IV (if BP >100 mm Hg)
• Nitroprusside IV (if BP >100 mm Hg)
• Dopamine (if BP <100 mm Hg)
• Dobutamine (if BP >100 mm Hg)
• Positive end-expiratory pressure (PEEP)
• Continuous positive airway pressure (CPAP)

Consider further actions especially if the patient is in acute pulmonary edema

Nitroglycerin
start 10–20 µg/min IV
(use if ischemia persists and BP remains elevated. Titrate to effect)
and/or
Nitroprusside
start 0.1–5.0 µg/kg per min IV

Third-line actions
• Amrinone 0.75 mg/kg then 5–15 µg/kg per min (if other drugs fail)
• Aminophylline 5 mg/kg (if wheezing)
• Thrombolytic therapy (if not in shock)
• Digoxin (if atrial fibrillation, supraventricular tachycardias)
• Angioplasty (if drugs fail)
• Intra-aortic balloon pump (bridge to surgery)
• Surgical interventions (valves, coronary artery bypass grafts, heart transplant)

* Base management after this point on invasive hemodynamic monitoring if possible.
† Fluid bolus of 250–500 mL normal saline should be tried. If no response, consider sympathomimetics.
‡ Move to dopamine and stop norepinephrine when BP improves.
§ Add dopamine when BP improves. Avoid dobutamine when systolic BP <100 mm Hg.

Figure 8. Algorithm for hypotension, and acute pulmonary edema.

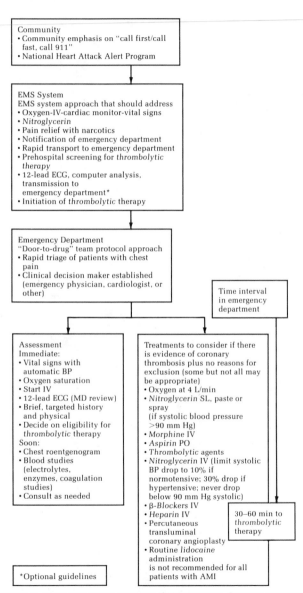

Figure 9. Acute myocardial infarction (AMI) algorithm. Recommendations for early treatment of patients with chest pain and possible AMI.

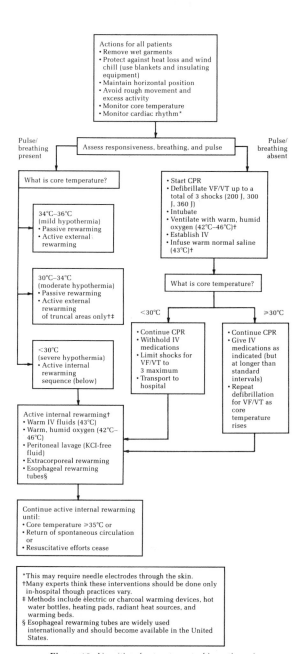

Actions for all patients
• Remove wet garments
• Protect against heat loss and wind chill (use blankets and insulating equipment)
• Maintain horizontal position
• Avoid rough movement and excess activity
• Monitor core temperature
• Monitor cardiac rhythm*

Assess responsiveness, breathing, and pulse

Pulse/breathing present

Pulse/breathing absent

What is core temperature?

34°C–36°C (mild hypothermia)
• Passive rewarming
• Active external rewarming

30°C–34°C (moderate hypothermia)
• Passive rewarming
• Active external rewarming of truncal areas only†‡

<30°C (severe hypothermia)
• Active internal rewarming sequence (below)

• Start CPR
• Defibrillate VF/VT up to a total of 3 shocks (200 J, 300 J, 360 J)
• Intubate
• Ventilate with warm, humid oxygen (42°C–46°C)†
• Establish IV
• Infuse warm normal saline (43°C)†

What is core temperature?

<30°C
• Continue CPR
• Withhold IV medications
• Limit shocks for VF/VT to 3 maximum
• Transport to hospital

≥30°C
• Continue CPR
• Give IV medications as indicated (but at longer than standard intervals)
• Repeat defibrillation for VF/VT as core temperature rises

Active internal rewarming†
• Warm IV fluids (43°C)
• Warm, humid oxygen (42°C–46°C)
• Peritoneal lavage (KCl-free fluid)
• Extracorporeal rewarming
• Esophageal rewarming tubes§

Continue active internal rewarming until:
• Core temperature ≥35°C or
• Return of spontaneous circulation or
• Resuscitative efforts cease

*This may require needle electrodes through the skin.
†Many experts think these interventions should be done only in-hospital though practices vary.
‡ Methods include electric or charcoal warming devices, hot water bottles, heating pads, radiant heat sources, and warming beds.
§ Esophageal rewarming tubes are widely used internationally and should become available in the United States.

Figure 10. Algorithm for treatment of hypothermia.

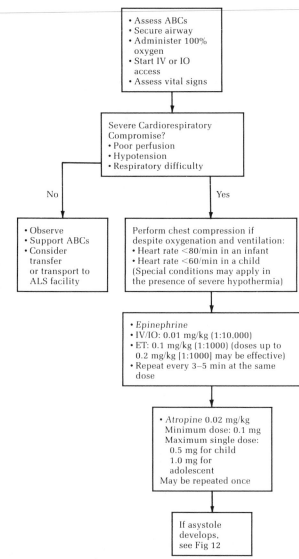

Figure 11. Pediatric Bradycardia decision tree. ABCs indicates airway, breathing, and circulation; ALS, advanced life support; ET, endotracheal; IO, intraosseous; and IV, intravenous.

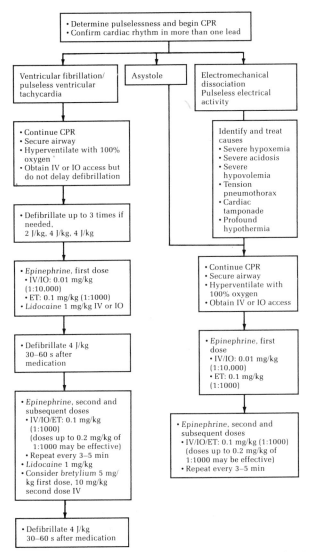

Figure 12. Pediatric asystole and pulseless arrest decision tree. CPR indicates cardiopulmonary resuscitation; ET, endotracheal; IO, intraosseous; and IV, intravenous.

Drugs Used in Pediatric Advanced Life Support*

Drug	Dose	Remarks
Adenosine	0.1 to 0.2 mg/kg Maximum single dose: 12 mg	Rapid IV bolus
Atropine sulfate	0.02 mg/kg per dose	Minimum dose: 0.1 mg Maximum single dose: 0.5 mg in child, 1.0 mg in adolescent
Bretylium	5 mg/kg; may be increased to 10 mg/kg	Rapid IV
Calcium chloride 10%	20 mg/kg per dose	Give slowly
Dopamine hydrochloride	2–20 μg/kg per minute	α-Adrenergic action dominates at ≥15–20 μg/kg per minute
Dobutamine hydrochloride	2–20 μg/kg per minute	Titrate to desired effect
Epinephrine For bradycardia	IV/IO: 0.01 mg/kg (1:10,000) ET: 0.1 mg/kg (1:1000)	Be aware of effective dose of preservatives administered (if preservatives are present in epinephrine preparation) when high doses are used

For asystolic or pulseless arrest	First dose: IV/IO: 0.01 mg/kg (1:10,000) ET: 0.1 mg/kg (1:1000) Doses as high as 0.2 mg/kg may be effective Subsequent doses: IV/IO/ET: 0.1 mg/kg (1:1000) Doses as high as 0.2 mg/kg may be effective	Be aware of effective dose of preservative administered (if preservatives present in epinephrine preparation) when high doses are used
Epinephrine infusion	Initial at 0.1 µg/kg per minute Higher infusion dose used if asystole present	Titrate to desired effect (0.1–1.0 µg/kg per minute)
Lidocaine	1 mg/kg per dose	
Lidocaine infusion	20–50 µg/kg per minute	
Sodium bicarbonate	1 mEq/kg per dose or $0.3 \times kg \times$ base deficit	Infuse slowly and only if ventilation is adequate

*IV indicates intravenous route; IO, intraosseous route; and ET, endotracheal route.

INFUSION MEDICATIONS FOR PEDIATRIC CARDIOPULMONARY RESUSCITATION

Infusion Medications, by Weight and Age, for Infants and Children 0–10 Years

Add 0.6 mg (3 ml)* of isoproterenol
0.6 mg (0.6 ml)* of epinephrine
60.0 mg (1.5 ml)* of dopamine   *To* 100 ml of diluent
60.0 mg (2.4 ml)* of dobutamine

Infuse at 1 ml·kg^{-1}·h^{-1} or according to following table in order

To give 0.1 µg·kg^{-1}·min^{-1} isoproterenol
0.1 µg·kg^{-1}·min^{-1} epinephrine
10 µg·kg^{-1}·min^{-1} dopamine
10 µg·kg^{-1}·min^{-1} dobutamine

Age	50th Percentile Weight (kg)	Infusion Rate (ml·h)
Newborn	3	3.0
1 Month	4	4.0
3 Months	5.5	5.5
6 Months	7.0	7.0
1 Year	10.0	10.0
2 Years	12.0	12.0
3 Years	14.0	14.0
4 Years	16.0	16.0
5 Years	18.0	18.0
6 Years	20.0	20.0
7 Years	22.0	22.0
8 Years	25.0	25.0
9 Years	28.0	28.0
10 Years	34.0	34.0

These are starting doses. Adjust concentration to dose and fluid tolerance.

*Based on the following concentrations:
isoproterenol = 0.2 mg·ml^{-1}
epinephrine = 1:1000 (1 mg·ml^{-1})
dopamine = 40 mg·ml^{-1}
dobutamine = 25 mg·ml^{-1}

Chamedies L. (ed): Textbook of Pediatric Advanced Life Support. Reproduced with permission of the American Heart Association, Dallas, 1988.

DRUG SEQUENCE

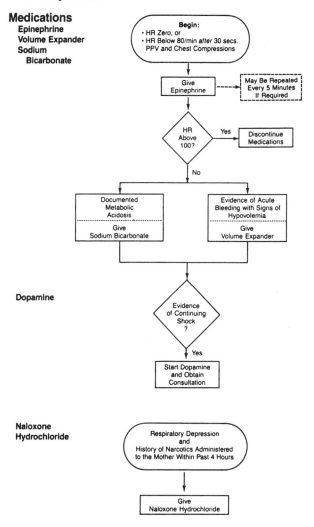

Medications
Epinephrine
Volume Expander
Sodium
  Bicarbonate

Dopamine

Naloxone
Hydrochloride

Begin:
• HR Zero, or
• HR Below 80/min *after* 30 secs. PPV and Chest Compressions

Give Epinephrine → May Be Repeated Every 5 Minutes If Required

HR Above 100? — Yes → Discontinue Medications

No

Documented Metabolic Acidosis
Give Sodium Bicarbonate

Evidence of Acute Bleeding with Signs of Hypovolemia
Give Volume Expander

Evidence of Continuing Shock?

Yes

Start Dopamine and Obtain Consultation

Respiratory Depression and History of Narcotics Administered to the Mother Within Past 4 Hours

Give Naloxone Hydrochloride

Bloom RS, Cropley C, Drew CR: Textbook of Neonatal Resuscitation. Reproduced with permission of the American Heart Association, American Academy of Pediatrics, Dallas, 1987.

DELIVERY ROOM OVERVIEW

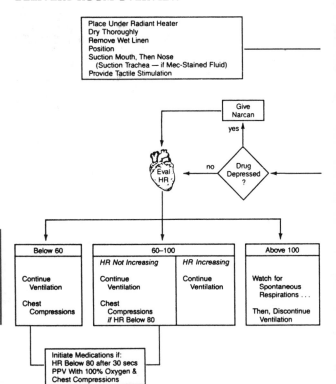

Bloom RS, Cropley C, Drew CR: Textbook of Neonatal Resuscitation. Reproduced with permission of the American Heart Association, American Academy of Pediatrics, Dallas, 1987.

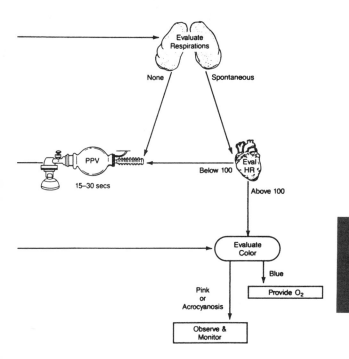

THERAPEUTIC GUIDELINES

Drug or Volume Expander	Concentration to Administer	Preparation (Based on Recommended Concentration)	Dosage	Route/Rate
Epinephrine	1:10,000	1 ml in a syringe Can dilute 1:1 with normal saline if giving IT	$0.1–0.3 \text{ ml·kg}^{-1}$	iv or IT Give rapidly
Volume Expanders	Whole blood 5% albumin/ saline solution Normal saline Ringer's lactate	40 ml to be given by syringe or iv drip	10 ml·kg^{-1}	Give over 5–10 minutes
Sodium Bicarbonate	0.5 mEq·ml^{-1} (4.2% solution)	20 ml in a syringe or two 10-ml prefilled syringes	2 mEq·kg^{-1}	iv Give slowly over at least 2 minutes (1 mEq·kg^{-1}·min^{-1})
Naloxone Hydrochloride	Narcan Neonatal 0.02 mg·ml^{-1}	2 ml in a syringe	0.5 ml·kg^{-1}	iv, im, sc, or IT Give rapidly

im = intramuscular; iv = intravenous; IT = intratracheal; sc = subcutaneous.

Adapted from Bloom RS, Cropley C, Drew CR: Textbook of Neonatal Resuscitation. Reproduced with permission of the American Heart Association, American Academy of Pediatrics, Dallas, 1987.

Conveying News of a Sudden Death to Family Members

Call the family if they have not been notified. Explain that their loved one has been admitted to the emergency department and that the situation is serious. Survivors should not be told of the death over the telephone.

Obtain as much information as possible about the patient and the circumstances surrounding the death. Carefully go over the events as they happened in the emergency department.

Ask someone to take family members to a private area. Walk in, introduce yourself, and sit down. Address the closest relative.

Briefly describe the circumstances leading to the death. Go over the sequence of events in the emergency department. Avoid euphemisms such as "he's passed on," "she's no longer with us," or "he's left us." Instead, use the words "death," "dying," or "dead."

Allow time for the shock to be absorbed. Make eye contact, touch, and share. Convey your feelings with a phrase such as "You have my (our) sincere sympathy" rather than "I (we) am sorry."

Allow as much time as necessary for questions and discussion. Go over the events several times to make sure everything is understood and to facilitate further questions.

Allow the family the opportunity to see their relative. If equipment is still connected, let the family know.

Know in advance what happens next and who will sign the death certificate. Physicians may impose burdens on staff and family if they fail to understand policies about death certification and disposition of the body. Know the answers to these questions before meeting the family.

Enlist the aid of a social worker or the clergy if not already present.

Offer to contact the patient's attending or family physician and to be available if there are further questions. Arrange for follow-up and continued support during the grieving period.

Recommendations for Critical Incident Debriefing

The debriefing should occur as soon as possible after the event, with all team members present.

Call the group together, preferably in the resuscitation room. State that you want to have a "code debriefing."

Review the events and conduct of the code. Include the contributory pathophysiology leading to the code, the decision tree followed, and any variations.

Analyze the things that were done wrong and especially the things that were done right. Allow free discussion.

Ask for recommendations/suggestions for future resuscitative attempts.

All team members should share their feelings, anxieties, anger, and possible guilt.

Team members unable to attend the debriefing should be informed of the process followed, the discussion generated, and the recommendations made.

The team leader should encourage team members to contact him or her if questions arise later.

F

ASA Standards

Standards for Basic Intra-Operative Monitoring
Guidelines for Regional Anesthesia in Obstetrics
Standards for Postanesthesia Care

Reprinted with permission of the American Society of Anesthesiologists.

STANDARDS FOR BASIC
INTRA-OPERATIVE MONITORING

(Approved by House of Delegates on October 21, 1986 and last amended on October 23, 1990, to become effective by January 1, 1991)

These standards apply to all anesthesia care although, in emergency circumstances, appropriate life support measures take precedence. These standards may be exceeded at any time based on the judgment of the responsible anesthesiologist. They are intended to encourage high quality patient care, but observing them cannot guarantee any specific patient outcome. They are subject to revision from time to time, as warranted by the evolution of technology and practice. This set of standards addresses only the issue of basic intra-operative monitoring, which is one component of anesthesia care. In certain rare or unusual circumstances, 1) some of these methods of monitoring may be clinically impractical, and 2) appropriate use of the described monitoring methods may fail to detect untoward clinical developments. Brief interruptions of continual[†] monitoring may be unavoidable. *Under extenuating circumstances, the responsible anesthesiologist may waive the requirements marked with an asterisk (*); it is recommended that when this is done, it should be so stated (including the reasons) in a note in the patient's medical record.* These standards are not intended for application to the care of the obstetrical patient in labor or in the conduct of pain management.

> [†]Note that "continual" is defined as "repeated regularly and frequently in steady rapid succession," whereas "continuous" means "prolonged without any interruption at any time."

STANDARD I
QUALIFIED ANESTHESIA PERSONNEL SHALL BE PRESENT IN THE ROOM THROUGHOUT THE CONDUCT OF ALL GENERAL ANESTHETICS, REGIONAL ANESTHETICS AND MONITORED ANESTHESIA CARE.

OBJECTIVE

Because of the rapid changes in patient status during anesthesia, qualified anesthesia personnel shall be continuously present to monitor the patient and provide anesthesia care. In the event there is a direct known hazard, e.g., radiation, to the anesthesia personnel which might require intermittent remote observation of the patient, some provision for monitoring the patient must be made. In the event that an emergency requires the temporary absence of the person primarily responsible for the anesthetic, the best judgment of the anesthesiologist will be exercised in comparing the emergency with the anesthetized patient's condition and in the selection of the person left responsible for the anesthetic during the temporary absence.

STANDARD II

DURING ALL ANESTHETICS, THE PATIENT'S OXYGENATION, VENTILATION, CIRCULATION AND TEMPERATURE SHALL BE CONTINUALLY EVALUATED.

OXYGENATION

OBJECTIVE

To ensure adequate oxygen concentration in the inspired gas and the blood during all anesthetics.

METHODS

1. Inspired gas: During every administration of general anesthesia using an anesthesia machine, the concentration of oxygen in the patient breathing system shall be measured by an oxygen analyzer with a low oxygen concentration limit alarm in use.*

2. Blood oxygenation: During all anesthetics, a quantitative method of assessing oxygenation such as pulse oximetry shall be employed.* Adequate illumination and exposure of the patient are necessary to assess color.*

VENTILATION

OBJECTIVE

To ensure adequate ventilation of the patient during all anesthetics.

METHODS

1. Every patient receiving general anesthesia shall have the adequacy of ventilation continually evaluated. While qualitative clinical signs such as chest excursion, observation of the reservoir breathing bag and auscultation of breath sounds may be adequate, quantitative monitoring of the CO_2 content and/or volume of expired gas is encouraged.

2. When an endotracheal tube is inserted, its correct positioning in the trachea must be verified by clinical assessment and by identification of carbon dioxide in the expired gas.* End-tidal CO_2 analysis, in use from the time of endotracheal tube placement, is encouraged.

3. When ventilation is controlled by a mechanical ventilator, there shall be in continuous use a device that is capable of detecting disconnection of components of the breathing system. The device must give an audible signal when its alarm threshold is exceeded.

4. During regional anesthesia and monitored anesthesia care, the adequacy of ventilation shall be evaluated, at least, by continual observation of qualitative clinical signs.

CIRCULATION

OBJECTIVE

To ensure the adequacy of the patient's circulatory function during all anesthetics.

METHODS

1. Every patient receiving anesthesia shall have the electro-cardiogram continuously displayed from the beginning of anesthesia until preparing to leave the anesthetizing location.*

2. Every patient receiving anesthesia shall have arterial blood pressure and heart rate determined and evaluated at least every five minutes.*

3. Every patient receiving general anesthesia shall have, in addition to the above, circulatory function continually evaluated by at least one of the following: palpation of a pulse, auscultation of heart sounds, monitoring of a tracing of intra-arterial pressure, ultrasound peripheral pulse monitoring, or pulse plethysmography or oximetry.

BODY TEMPERATURE

OBJECTIVE

To aid in the maintenance of appropriate body temperature during all anesthetics.

METHODS

There shall be readily available a means to continuously measure the patient's temperature. When changes in body temperature are intended, anticipated or suspected, the temperature shall be measured.

GUIDELINES FOR REGIONAL
ANESTHESIA IN OBSTETRICS

(Approved by House of Delegates on October 12, 1988 and last amended on October 30, 1991

These guidelines apply to the use of regional anesthesia or analgesia in which local anesthetics are administered to the parturient during labor and delivery. They are intended to encourage quality patient care but cannot guarantee any specific patient outcome. Because the availability of anesthesia resources may vary, members are responsible for interpreting and establishing the guidelines for their own institutions and practices. These guidelines are subject to revision from time to time as warranted by the evolution of technology and practice.

GUIDELINE I

REGIONAL ANESTHESIA SHOULD BE INITIATED AND MAINTAINED ONLY IN LOCATIONS IN WHICH APPROPRIATE RESUSCITATION EQUIPMENT AND DRUGS ARE IMMEDIATELY AVAILABLE TO MANAGE PROCEDURALLY RELATED PROBLEMS.

Resuscitation equipment should include, but is not limited to sources of oxygen and suction, equipment to maintain an airway and perform endotrachael intubation, a means to provide positive pressure ventilation, and drugs and equipment for cardiopulmonary resuscitation.

GUIDELINE II

REGIONAL ANESTHESIA SHOULD BE INITIATED BY A PHYSICIAN WITH APPROPRIATE PRIVILEGES AND MAINTAINED BY OR UNDER THE MEDICAL DIRECTIONS[1] OF SUCH AN INDIVIDUAL.

Physicians should be approved through the institutional credentialing process to initiate and direct the maintenance of obstetric anesthesia and to manage procedurally related complications.

GUIDELINE III

REGIONAL ANESTHESIA SHOULD NOT BE ADMINISTERED UNTIL (1) THE PATIENT HAS BEEN EXAMINED BY A QUALIFIED INDIVIDUAL[2]; and (2) THE MATERNAL AND FETAL STATUS AND PROGRESS OF LABOR HAVE BEEN EVALUATED BY A PHYSICIAN WITH PRIVILEGES IN OBSTETRICS WHO IS READILY AVAILABLE TO SUPERVISE THE LABOR AND MANAGE ANY OBSTETRIC COMPLICATIONS THAT MAY ARISE.

Under circumstances defined by department protocol, qualified personnel may perform the initial pelvic examination. The physician responsible for the patient's obstetric care should be informed of her status so that a decision can be made regarding present risk and further management.[2]

GUIDELINE IV

AN INTRAVENOUS INFUSION SHOULD BE ESTABLISHED BEFORE THE INITIATION OF REGIONAL ANESTHESIA AND MAINTAINED THROUGHOUT THE DURATION OF THE REGIONAL ANESTHETIC.

GUIDELINE V

REGIONAL ANESTHESIA FOR LABOR AND/OR VAGINAL DELIVERY REQUIRES THAT THE PARTURIENT'S VITAL SIGNS AND THE FETAL HEART RATE BE MONITORED AND DOCUMENTED BY A QUALIFIED INDIVIDUAL. ADDITIONAL MONITORING APPROPRIATE TO THE CLINICAL CONDITION OF THE PARTURIENT AND THE FETUS SHOULD BE EMPLOYED WHEN INDICATED. WHEN EXTENSIVE REGIONAL BLOCKADE IS ADMINISTERED FOR COMPLICATED VAGINAL DELIVERY, THE STANDARDS FOR BASIC INTRAOPERATIVE MONITORING[3] SHOULD BE APPLIED.

GUIDELINE VI

REGIONAL ANESTHESIA FOR CESAREAN DELIVERY REQUIRES THAT THE STANDARDS FOR BASIC INTRAOPERATIVE MONITORING[3] BE APPLIED AND THAT A PHYSICIAN WITH PRIVILEGES IN OBSTETRICS BE IMMEDIATELY AVAILABLE.

GUIDELINE VII

QUALIFIED PERSONNEL, OTHER THAN THE ANESTHESIOLOGIST ATTENDING THE MOTHER, SHOULD BE IMMEDIATELY AVAILABLE TO ASSUME RESPONSIBILITY FOR RESUSCITATION OF THE NEWBORN.[2]

The primary responsibility of the anesthesiologist is to provide care to the mother. If the anesthesiologist is also requested to provide brief assistance in the care of the newborn, the benefit to the child must be compared to the risk to the mother.

GUIDELINE VIII

A PHYSICIAN WITH APPROPRIATE PRIVILEGES SHOULD REMAIN READILY AVAILABLE DURING THE REGIONAL ANESTHETIC TO MANAGE ANESTHETIC COMPLICATIONS UN-

TIL THE PATIENT'S POSTANESTHESIA CONDITION IS SATISFACTORY AND STABLE.

GUIDELINE IX

ALL PATIENTS RECOVERING FROM REGIONAL ANESTHESIA SHOULD RECEIVE APPROPRIATE POSTANESTHESIA CARE. FOLLOWING CESAREAN DELIVERY AND/OR EXTENSIVE REGIONAL BLOCKADE, THE STANDARDS FOR POSTANESTHESIA CARE[4] SHOULD BE APPLIED.

1. A Postanesthesia Care Unit (PACU) should be available to receive patients. The design, equipment and staffing should meet requirements of the facility's accrediting and licensing bodies.
2. When a site other than the PACU is used, equivalent postanesthesia care should be provided.

GUIDELINE X

THERE SHOULD BE A POLICY TO ASSURE THE AVAILABILITY IN THE FACILITY OF A PHYSICIAN TO MANAGE COMPLICATIONS AND TO PROVIDE CARDIOPULMONARY RESUSCITATION FOR PATIENTS RECEIVING POSTANESTHESIA CARE.

[1]Anesthesia Care Team (approved by ASA House of Delegates 10/14/87).
[2]Guidelines for Perinatal Care (American Academy of Pediatrics and American College of Obstetricians and Gynecologists, 1988).
[3]Standards for Basic Intra-Operative Monitoring (approved by ASA House of Delegates 10/21/86 and last amended 10/23/90).
[4]Standards for Postanesthesia Care (approved by ASA House of Delegates 10/12/88 and last amended 10/23/90).

STANDARDS FOR
POSTANESTHESIA CARE

Approved by House of Delegates on October 12, 1988 and last amended on October 23, 1990)

These Standards apply to postanesthesia care in all locations. These Standards may be exceeded based on the judgment of the responsible anesthesiologist. They are intended to encourage high quality patient care, but cannot guarantee any specific patient outcome. They are subject to revision from time to time as warranted by the evolution of technology and practice. *Under extenuating circumstances, the responsible anesthesiologist may waive the requirements marked with an asterisk (*); it is recommended that when this is done, it should be so stated (including the reasons) in a note in the patient's medical record.*

STANDARD I

ALL PATIENTS WHO HAVE RECEIVED GENERAL ANESTHESIA, REGIONAL ANESTHESIA, OR MONITORED ANESTHESIA CARE SHALL RECEIVE APPROPRIATE POSTANESTHESIA MANAGEMENT.

1. A Postanesthesia Care Unit (PACU) or an area which provides equivalent postanesthesia care shall be available to receive patients after surgery and anesthesia. All patients who receive anesthesia shall be admitted to the PACU except by specific order of the anesthesiologist responsible for the patient's care.

2. The medical aspects of care in the PACU shall be governed by policies and procedures which have been reviewed and approved by the Department of Anesthesiology.

3. The design, equipment and staffing of the PACU shall meet requirements of the facility's accrediting and licensing bodies.

4. The nursing standards of practice shall be consistent with those approved in 1986 by the American Society of Post Anesthesia Nurses (ASPAN).

STANDARD II

A PATIENT TRANSPORTED TO THE PACU SHALL BE ACCOMPANIED BY A MEMBER OF THE ANESTHESIA CARE TEAM WHO IS KNOWLEDGEABLE ABOUT THE PATIENT'S CONDITION. THE PATIENT SHALL BE CONTINUALLY EVALUATED AND TREATED DURING TRANSPORT WITH MONITORING AND SUPPORT APPROPRIATE TO THE PATIENT'S CONDITION.

STANDARD III

UPON ARRIVAL IN THE PACU, THE PATIENT SHALL BE RE-EVALUATED AND A VERBAL REPORT PROVIDED TO THE RESPONSIBLE PACU NURSE BY THE MEMBER OF THE ANESTHESIA CARE TEAM WHO ACCOMPANIES THE PATIENT.

1. The patient's status on arrival in the PACU shall be documented.

2. Information concerning the preoperative condition and the surgical/anesthetic course shall be transmitted to the PACU nurse.

3. The member of the Anesthesia Care Team shall remain in the PACU until the PACU nurse accepts responsibility for the nursing care of the patient.

STANDARD IV

THE PATIENT'S CONDITION SHALL BE EVALUATED CONTINUALLY IN THE PACU.

1. The patient shall be observed and monitored by methods appropriate to the patient's medical condition. Particular attention should be given to monitoring oxygenation, ventilation and circulation. During recovery from all anesthetics, a quantitative method of assessing oxygenation such as pulse oximetry shall be employed in the initial phase of recovery.*[†] This is not intended for application during the recovery of the obstetric patient in whom regional anesthesia was used for labor and vaginal delivery.

2. An accurate written report of the PACU period shall be maintained. Use of an appropriate PACU scoring system is encouraged for each patient on admission, at appropriate intervals prior to discharge, and at the time of discharge.

3. General medical supervision and coordination of patient care in the PACU should be the responsibility of an anesthesiologist.

4. There shall be a policy to assure the availability in the facility of a physician capable of managing complications and providing cardiopulmonary resuscitation for patients in the PACU.

[†]To become effective as soon as feasible, but no later than January 1, 1992.

STANDARD V

A PHYSICIAN IS RESPONSIBLE FOR THE DISCHARGE OF
THE PATIENT FROM THE POSTANESTHESIA CARE UNIT.

1. When discharge criteria are used, they must be approved
   by the Department of Anesthesiology and the medical
   staff. They may vary depending upon whether the patient
   is discharged to a hospital room, to the ICU, to a short stay
   unit, or home.

2. In the absence of the physician responsible for the discharge, the PACU nurse shall determine that the patient
   meets the discharge criteria. The name of the physician ac-
   cepting responsibility for discharge shall be noted on the
   record.

G

Difficult Airway Algorithm

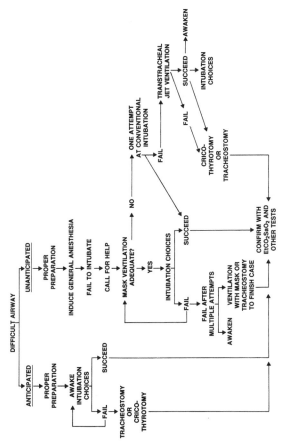

Anesthetic Considerations Introduced By Rare and Coexisting Diseases

ALZHEIMER'S DISEASE

Avoid drugs likely to accentuate dementia (anticholinergics, sedatives)

Inhaled anesthetics with short-term effects are logical

EPILEPSY

Continue anticonvulsant therapy in perioperative period but consider possible drug interactions (accelerated metabolism, resistance to muscle relaxants)

Consider avoidance of drugs with known ability to evoke seizure-like activity.

Enflurane

Methohexital

Opioids (high doses)

Ketamine (?)

GLUCOSE-6-PHOSPHATE DEHYDROGENASE DEFICIENCY

Premature erythrocyte destruction

Avoid drugs that may trigger a hemolytic crisis

Nonopioid analgesics

Antibiotics

Sulfonamides

Avoid drugs associated with methemoglobin

Prilocaine

Nitroprusside

GUILLAIN-BARRÉ SYNDROME

Absence of compensatory reflex responses (hypotension with position changes, blood loss, positive airway pressure)

Stimulus-induced activation of the sympathetic nervous system (may necessitate alpha and beta blockade)

Succinylcholine-induced hyperkalemia

MULTIPLE SCLEROSIS

Exacerbation may follow anesthesia

Body temperature increases may exacerbate symptoms

Possible need for corticosteroid supplementation

Succinylcholine-induced hyperkalemia (?)

MUSCULAR DYSTROPHY

Myocardial dysfunction (cardiac arrest with induction)

Succinylcholine-induced hyperkalemia

Delayed gastric emptying

Retention of pulmonary secretions

Unpredictable susceptibility to malignant hyperthermia

MYASTHENIC SYNDROME

Increased sensitivity to succinylcholine and nondepolarizing muscle relaxants

MYOTONIC DYSTROPHY

Succinylcholine-induced skeletal muscle contracture

Increased sensitivity to ventilatory depressant effects of anesthetics

Cardiac dysrhythmias

Delayed gastric emptying

PARKINSON'S DISEASE

Continue drug therapy in perioperative period but consider side effects (hypovolemia, cardiac dysrhythmias)

Avoid dopamine antagonists (droperidol, metoclopramide)

Succinylcholine-induced hyperkalemia (?)

RHEUMATOID ARTHRITIS

Cervical spine involvement (atlantoaxial subluxation, odontoid compression)

Synovitis of the temporomandibular joint

Crycoarytenoid arthritis (hoarseness)
Pericarditis
Aortic regurgitation
Pulmonary fibrosis
Peripheral nerve compression
Hepatitis
Anemia
Drug-induced side effects (aspirin, corticosteroids)

SICKLE CELL DISEASE

Maintain oxygenation (sickling begins at PaO_2 <50 mm Hg)
Maintain intravascular fluid volume (venous stasis allows PO_2
   to decline)
Avoid hypothermia and associated vasoconstriction
Consider impact of pre-existing abnormalities
   Anemia $(7–8 \text{ g} \cdot \text{dl}^{-1})$
   Pulmonary infarction
   Renal infarction
   Cholelithiasis
   Infection (asplenia)

The authors thank the authors and publishers listed below for permission to reprint the following material:

Figure 4-2: From Willis BA, Pender JW, Mapleson W: Rebreathing in a T-piece: Volunteer and theoretical studies of the Jackson-Rees modification of Ayre's T-piece during spontaneous respiration. Br J Anaesth 47:1239, 1975.

Figure 4-3: Redrawn from Bain JA, Spoerel WE: A streamlined anaesthetic system. Can Anesth Soc J 19:426, 1972.

Figure 5-4: From Cormack RS, Lehane J: Difficult tracheal intubation in obstetrics. Anaesthesia 39:1105, 1984.

Figure 6-1: Modified from Wadsworth TG: The cubital tunnel and the external compression syndrome. Anesth Analg 53:303, 1974.

Figure 7-2: From Brown M, Vender JS: Noninvasive oxygen monitoring. Crit Care Clin 4:493, 1988.

Figure 7-3: From Brown BR, Blitt CD, Vaughn RW: Clinical Anesthesiology, p. 139. St. Louis, CV Mosby, 1985.

Figure 7-7: From Mark JB: Central venous pressure monitoring: Clinical insights beyond the numbers. J. Cardiothorac Vasc Anesth 5:163, 1991.

Figure 7-8: From Dizon CT, Barash PG: The value of monitoring pulmonary artery pressure in clinical practice.

Figure 10-1: From Herker LA: Hemostasis Manual, P. 4. Seattle, University of Washington Press, 1970.

Figures 14-2, 14-3, 14-4, and 14-5: From Eger EI: Isoflurane: A review. Anesthesiology 55:559, 1981.

Figure 14-6: With permission from the International Anesthesia Research Society and from Johnston RR, Eger EI, Wilson C: A comparative interaction of epinephrine with enflurane, isoflurane and halothane in man. Anesth Analg 55:709, 1976.

Figure 15-2: From Taylor P: Are neuromusclar blocking agents more efficacious in pairs? Anesthesiology 63:1, 1985.

Figure 17-1: From Covino BG, Scott DB: Handbook of Epidural Anaesthesia and Analgesia, p. 25. Orlando, Grune & Stratton, 1985.

Figure 17-4: Reproduced with permission: Lee JA, Atkinson RS: Sir Robert MacIntosh's Lumbar Puncture and Spinal Analgesia: Intradural and Extradural, p. 138. Edinburgh, Churchill-Livingstone, 1978.

Figures 18-1, 18-2, 18-5 through 18-12: From Mulroy M: Handbook of Regional Anesthesia. Boston, Little, Brown, 1988.

Figure 19-1: From Michenfelder JD: Anesthesia and the Brain, pp 6, 94–130. New York, Churchill Livingstone, 1988.

Figure 19-2: Modified from Miller JD, Garibi J, Pickard JD: The effects of induced changes of cerebrospinal fluid volume during continuous monitoring of ventricular pressure. Arch Neurol 128:265, 1973.

Figure 20-1: From Wilson RS: Endobronchial intubation. In Kaplan JA (ed): Thoracic Anesthesia. New York, Churchill-Livingstone, 1983.

Figures 20-2 and 20-3: From Benumof JL: Intraoperative considerations for all thoracic surgery. In Benumof JL: Anesthesia for Thoracic Surgery. Philadelphia, WB Saunders, 1987.

Figure 21-1: From Tinker JH: Cardiopulmonary bypass: Technical aspects. In Thomas SJ (ed): Manual of Cardiac Anesthesia, p. 375. New York, Churchill-Livingstone, 1984.

Figure 27-1: From Vaughan RW: Pulmonary and cardiovascular derangements. In Brown BR (ed): Anesthesia and the Obese Patient. Contemporary Anesthesia Practice Series, p. 19. Philadelphia, FA Davis, 1982.

Figure 32-1: Modified from Smith RM: Anesthesia for Infants and Children, 4th ed. St. Louis, CV Mosby, 1980.

Figure 34-1: From Hilgenberg JC: Inhalation and intravenous drugs in the elderly patient. Seminars in Anesthesia 5:44, 1986.

Figure 41-1: From Lubenow TR, Ivankovich AD: Organization of an acute pain management service. In Stoelting RK, Barash PG, Gallagher TJ (eds): Advances in Anesthesia, pp. 1–28, 57–137. Chicago, Mosby Year Book, 1991.

Table 41-9: Modified from El-Baz NM, Faber LP, Jensik RJ: Continuous epidural infusion of morphine for treatment of pain after thoracic surgery. A new technique. Anesth Analg 63:757, 1984.

INDEX

Page numbers followed by t and f indicate tables and figures, respectively.

ISBN 0-397-51297-X